S0-BAM-818

VETERINARY MEDICAL TERMINOLOGY

Title identified in:
Doody's Review Service
http://www.doody.com/dej/
Core or Essential Title

Title identified in:
RCL: Resources for College Libraries
ISBN: 9780835248556, 2006

no newer ed.
as of 6/2015

SEP 30 2000

WITHDRAWN

VETERINARY MEDICAL TERMINOLOGY

Second Edition

Authored and Illustrated by

Dawn E. Christenson, L.V.T.
Instructor
College of Veterinary Medicine
Michigan State University
East Lansing, Michigan

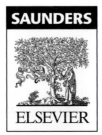

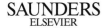

SAUNDERS
ELSEVIER

11830 Westline Industrial Drive
St. Louis, Missouri 63146

VETERINARY MEDICAL TERMINOLOGY

ISBN: 978-0-7216-9726-0

Copyright © 2009 by Saunders, an imprint of Elsevier Inc.

All rights reserved. No part of this publication may be reproduced or transmitted in any form
or by any means, electronic or mechanical, including photocopying, recording, or any information
storage and retrieval system, without permission in writing from the publisher. Permissions may
be sought directly from Elsevier's Rights Department: phone: (+1) 215 239 3804 (US) or (+44) 1865
843830 (UK); fax: (+44) 1865 853333; e-mail: healthpermissions@elsevier.com. You may also
complete your request on-line via the Elsevier website at http://www.elsevier.com/permissions.

Notice

Neither the Publisher nor the Author assumes any responsibility for any loss or injury and/or
damage to persons or property arising out of or related to any use of the material contained in
this book. It is the responsibility of the treating practitioner, relying on independent expertise
and knowledge of the patient, to determine the best treatment and method of application for
the patient.

The Publisher

Previous edition copyrighted 1997

Library of Congress Control Number: 2007943081

Vice President and Publisher: Linda Duncan
Publisher: Penny Rudolph
Managing Editor: Teri Merchant
Developmental Editor: Shelly Stringer
Publishing Services Manager: Julie Eddy
Project Manager: Laura Loveall
Designer: Paula Catalano

Working together to grow
libraries in developing countries

www.elsevier.com | www.bookaid.org | www.sabre.org

ELSEVIER   BOOK AID
            International   Sabre Foundation

Printed in Canada

Last digit is the print number: 9 8 7 6 5 4 3 2 1

This text is designed to be used in self-study or to augment other veterinary related courses. It has been created to assist veterinary technology, preveterinary, and veterinary students alike. It should be used with a comprehensive, unabridged medical dictionary. The text is intended to provide students with a basic foundation in the language of veterinary medicine—veterinary medical terminology. Through the years as a veterinary technician educator, I have learned that if students are to be successful, they must immediately apply what they have learned. That is why anatomy, physiology, and disease concepts are included at an introductory level. The scientific information provides immediate application of the terminology that is found at the beginning of each chapter. It is my hope that the scientific information brings to life the language and gives students an insatiable desire to learn even more. When learning any "foreign" language, simply memorizing words does not make one fluent in the language. The words must be read, spoken, and used in context. Repetition and practice with the language makes one fluent. Facts memorized without reinforcement or application will soon be forgotten. To forget medical terminology is to do your future patients a disservice. A commitment to life-long learning is essential to the success of every veterinary professional and the patients they serve.

NEW LEARNING RESOURCES ON EVOLVE

Your professional success is important—so important that we have gone to great lengths to create multiple tools to help you in your quest to become fluent with medical terminology. Many students find pronouncing medical terms very difficult. No student wants to sound foolish by mispronouncing terms when talking with classmates or instructors. The cavalry just arrived! We have created an Evolve website to accompany this new edition. The website features outstanding student learning resources: An audio glossary and four interactive games to reinforce the concepts introduced in this text.

Audio Glossary

On the accompanying Evolve site for this text, you'll find over 4500 veterinary medical terms that are pronounced, spelled out, and defined. You'll be able to see the term spelled correctly, hear the term pronounced accurately, and see correct usage of each term in a sample sentence. This will add a whole new sensory dimension to the learning process to help you achieve competency with both the spoken and written language.

Interactive Games

To further help you immerse yourself in the language (without drowning), we have created four interactive games for the Evolve site: Hangman, Part Puzzler, Listen and Spell, and Word Shop. Hangman is a fun way to interact with the terms. Believe it or not, the more fun you have with a subject, the better you'll remember it. Part Puzzler will give you practice dividing terms appropriately. Listen and Spell provides the audio pronunciation for a word. You listen to the word, and then type the word as you think it should appear. That is a fabulous way to hone your spelling skill. Finally, Word Shop provides a definition and then permits you to drag and drop word parts in the order necessary to create the correct term that matches the definition.

Answers to Exercises in the Book

The Evolve site also contains the answers to review questions and crossword puzzles found in the book. We decided that you would find your study of terminology to be more meaningful if you studied the book, answered the questions, worked the crossword puzzles, and then checked the Evolve site to see how close you came to acing the questions. We think that making it a little harder for you to find the correct answers will pay off for you in the long run.

All of these electronic features should make learning medical terminology fun and easy. These features also provide convenient and effective means for you to assess your progress in the learning process.

FLASH CARDS NOW AVAILABLE FOR PURCHASE

For years, I have watched students labor over creating "flash cards" of word parts that they could use to study medical terminology anytime and anywhere. That time spent creating the flash cards could have been devoted to actually studying and learning various word parts. To help you manage your study time wisely, we have also created Saunders Veterinary Terminology Flash Cards. That's right—printed, illustrated, well-organized, color flash cards have been created with you in mind. Now, you have a convenient, effective tool that you can use anywhere to help you master prefixes, suffixes, combining forms, and abbreviations. Make a stop at your school book store to check out these new flash cards.

TEACHING RECOMMENDATIONS

Between the book and all of the ancillary resources, learning medical terminology has never been easier. It is strongly recommended that students complete Chapters 1 through 4, in succession, before moving on to any subsequent chapters. The remaining chapters are organized by body system. While they may be completed in any order, recommendations for "prerequisite" chapters may be noted in the beginning of some. The prerequisites may not be essential, but will serve to maximize student learning and understanding.

Dear Student:

I remember when I was a student, the way that I struggled with learning medical terminology. The intensity and complexity of my professional education were overwhelming at times. This "foreign language" just complicated matters. Medical terminology has at times confused me, frightened me, and put me to sleep.

Through my experiences as a student, as a practicing veterinary technician, and as a teacher, I have found that medical terminology does not have to be an ominous "monster" or a millstone. Learning medical terminology can actually be an adventure and FUN! Look at medical terms the way a forensic scientist pursues Crime Scene Investigation. Each word part holds a clue to unraveling the mystery of the term's meaning. All you need is a little curiosity (and a dictionary). I still have that curiosity. Yes, even today, after over 25 years as a veterinary technician educator, I have an insatiable curiosity for learning new terms and increasing the depth of my vocabulary. Whenever I run across a term or a word part that I'm unfamiliar with, I look it up! I want to know its origins. Sometimes looking at those Greek and Latin origins can be quite amusing.

I know that medical terminology "feels" awkward at first. What language doesn't? You're probably wondering how you will ever remember all of the terms, what they mean, and (good grief!) how to spell them. Once you begin to use them on a regular basis, they will become a part of you. You'll take them for granted. You might even feel adventurous and begin making up pseudomedical terms just for fun. Then you can talk in "code" with some of your professional friends and colleagues. Terms like stomatomegaly, ornithencephaly, aerocephalon, or condylocephalus could enter conversations. (Pull out a dictionary to figure those out, and have a good laugh.) Someday you'll be in casual conversation with family or friends and someone will stop you. "What did you say? Why do you always have to use such big words?" You'll feel like you've really arrived when you're having a conversation with practitioners, who are experts in the field, and you understand everything that they're talking about. That is SO gratifying. You'll get there. Trust me. Just give it time. When will you "arrive"? No one knows. It sneaks up on you. Someday you'll simply recognize, "I'm there!" Being persistent and consistent with anything is the key to success. Someone once said that success is a journey, not a destination. Enjoy the journey. I hope that this book will help you on that journey, and I hope that you'll have some fun along the way. And never forget, you're not simply learning this for yourself . . . you're ultimately learning it for your patients. You need to talk the medical lingo, but you also need to serve as an interpreter for the human counterparts of your patients. You are the future of veterinary medicine. Whatever you do, follow what Winston Churchill once said, "Never, never, never give up!"

Grace and peace,

How is it possible? I have completed 17 chapters of text and illustrations. Yet, this is the most difficult piece of this book to write. I am at a loss for words that will adequately express my most sincere gratitude. This wouldn't be so hard if I didn't have so much to be grateful for. So much has happened since the first edition of this text was published. The storms of life have tossed me to and fro and definitely delayed the completion of this edition. (Thank you, Teri, for your patience. I couldn't have asked for a more understanding editor.)

Through all of the challenges and hard work I have grown, especially in my faith. I am so thankful for faith, friends, and family – angels here on earth. Bea, mijn beste vriendin, you are such a heaven-sent blessing for me. You've seen me through thick and thin. You and my awesome church family have provided me with the support and encouragement that I have so desperately needed to accomplish this enormous task in my "spare time." You and they have carried me through the difficult times and celebrated each little step along the way. I couldn't have done this without you. To my siblings: Tom, I've always looked up to you, big brother. Unknowingly, you've set the bar for my success. I hope your baby sister is doing you proud. Sharon, you supported me through the first rendition of this book and even endured reading the foreign subject matter. (Sorry, Sis—that version was really boring.) Throughout this edition, you've been an encouragement. I'm grateful, Sis. I hope that you are pleased with the results. Although, I know that my illustrative abilities cannot hold a candle to your abilities as an artist. Jan, you're amazing. You've beaten lymphoma twice now . . . and through all of the "stuff" you've had to endure, you never complained. You just toughed it out and rose above. You go, bro! I pray that you never have to face that demon ever again. To my fellow volunteers with Eaton Community Hospice, thank you for being an inspiration to human kind. I have learned so much from you and from our wonderful patients and their families.

Many thanks to fellow educators everywhere for sharing your ideas and expertise, for using the first edition of this book, and for toiling day after day doing what you do best . . . teaching. To my students, thank you for the innumerable lessons you've taught me, helping me to become a better educator. Mom and dad, I wish you were here to see the completion of this. I hope you're smiling down from the heavens. You instilled in me my core values, work ethic, and showed me what it means to be courageous. I miss you both.

Consultant

Beatrix VanKampen, BS, LVT
Veterinary Teaching Hospital
Michigan State University
East Lansing, Michigan

ATTENTION!
Student, the following information is IMPORTANT to your SUCCESS:

Many of the definitions given in the introductory sections of each chapter are literal translations from the Greek and Latin roots. These literal translations simplify definitions and to reduce the volume of information to be absorbed. This follows the "KISS" principle of "Keep It Simple Silly!" It makes learning to recognize and interpret word parts and terms much, much easier. It is important to read each chapter in its entirety to gain a greater understanding of the meanings and applications of these terms. As stated in the preface, it is strongly recommended that you complete Chapters 1 through 4, in sequence, before moving on to any subsequent chapters. A medical dictionary is an ESSENTIAL companion and resource for this text. Don't study without one!

CONTENTS

CHAPTER 1

Introduction to Veterinary Medical Terminology

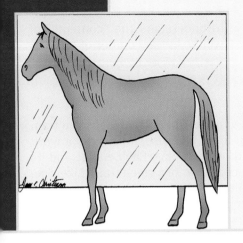

GOALS AND OBJECTIVES

By the conclusion of this chapter, the student will be able to:

1. Recognize common root words, prefixes, suffixes, and combining vowels.
2. Understand the function of root words, prefixes, suffixes, and combining vowels.
3. Divide simple and compound words into their respective parts.
4. Understand the function of combining forms.
5. Recognize, correctly pronounce, and appropriately use common directional terms.
6. Recognize the planes of the body.
7. Demonstrate a basic understanding of directional terminology as it relates to the body and to radiography.

INTRODUCTION TO WORD STRUCTURE

Words, even medical terms, can be likened to trains. They each contain important parts. Without each of the necessary parts, the train cannot run and the word cannot stand alone.

Root Word

The root word is the foundation of a word. It gives substance or meaning to the word, much like each of the boxcars in a train give it mass and value. Just like those train cars, roots come in a variety of sizes, shapes, and "colors," each holding a special cargo (meaning) within. So, it is from the root that the majority of the meaning for a given word is derived. Words may contain one or more roots, as in football (root 1 = foot, root 2 = ball). Some medical terms may have many roots within them. You should not be alarmed by the length of a medical term. Once you begin to recognize various root words (just like brand names and logos on the train cars), you will begin to understand the "contents" of the word. Like railroad barons, your "wealth" will be in the number of boxcars (roots) you possess.

Prefix

The prefix is like the train's engine with its whistle. The engine leads the train and its whistle announces the approaching train. Likewise, a prefix is a word part that precedes the root, modifying the root's meaning. Each engine and its whistle (or horn) is unique and changes the character of a given train. Likewise, each prefix with its own unique meaning alters the impression of the overall meaning of a word. While it is true that the engine with its whistle can run under its own power, without the rest of the boxcars, it is not a complete train. Prefixes are really no different. Alone they do possess some meaning, but they are not complete words without the rest of the word parts. When written alone, prefixes are followed by a hyphen (e.g., pre-, a prefix meaning "before").

Suffix

In earlier days of the railroad, trains always had a caboose. Today, the caboose has become the very last car of the train, with a special red light at the rear of that car. Regardless, the caboose, like a suffix, is always last. A suffix is a word part that follows the root word, modifying the root's meaning. In a word containing a suffix, it is the suffix that determines whether the word is classified as a noun, adjective, or another type of word. Alone, a caboose is not a complete train. Likewise, suffixes may not stand alone as words. When written alone, suffixes are preceded by a hyphen (e.g., -ad, a suffix meaning "toward"). When reading the meaning of a word containing a suffix, begin by reading the meaning of the suffix first. For example, in the word craniad (crani/ad), the root crani(o)- [head], when combined with the suffix -ad [toward], is interpreted as meaning "toward the head."

Compound Word

A word constructed of two or more roots is a compound word (like a typical long train). The roots may or may not be joined by a combining vowel. *Mediolateral* is a compound word. Given the following information, medi(o)- [middle]/o/later(o)- [side]/al [pertaining to], the basic interpretation of the word mediolateral would be "pertaining to the middle and the side." Application of directional terms like this will be discussed later in this chapter.

Combining Form

A combining form is an incomplete word constructed of a root word, prefix, or suffix with a combining vowel. The combining vowel is nothing more than the coupler or connector between the cars (i.e., word parts). In combining forms, the standard combining vowel (shown in parentheses) is "o." Medi(o)- is a combining form meaning "middle." Later(o)- is a combining form meaning "side." When joined in the compound word mediolateral, note that the combining vowel "o" is used between the two roots. However, the second combining vowel "o" is dropped before the suffix -al. In most cases, the combining vowel should be dropped when it precedes a suffix beginning with a vowel. (Think of it as a caboose built with its own strongest coupler. The existing coupler on the car may create a weak connection to the caboose. Therefore, the boxcar's coupler may need to be removed temporarily.) The combining vowel "o," shown in most combining forms, may not be appropriate for use in the creation of some words. For example, with the adjective posterior (poster/i/or; "pertaining to the rear"), the combining form poster(o)- is joined to the suffix -or by the combining vowel "i." Consult an unabridged medical dictionary to ensure correct spelling of any medical term. (Try to think of the dictionary as a "railroad operator's manual." For any new railroad owner to ensure the smooth operation and appropriate maintenance of the trains and rails, one should consult the operator's manual from time to time. Avoiding this could lead to costly mistakes.)

General Rules

1. Read the meaning of medical terms beginning with the suffix, then proceed to the first part of the word and follow through.
2. Drop the combining vowel before a suffix beginning with a vowel.
3. Retain the combining vowel between two roots.
   These rules hold true for most medical terms.

INTRODUCTION TO RELATED TERMS[1]

Divide each of the following terms into its respective parts ("R," root; "P," prefix; "S," suffix; "CV," combining vowel).

1. **Example: Anterior** (adj.)   (R) _anter_   (CV) _____i_____ (S) _____or_____
   anterior (an-te're-or; pertaining to the front)

2. **Caudad** (adj.)   (R) _____ (S) _____
   caudad (kaw'dad; toward the tail)

3. **Cranial** (adj.)   (R) _____ (S) _____
   cranial (kra'ne-al; pertaining to the head)

4. **Caudocranial** (adj.)   (R) _____ (CV) _____ (R) _____ (S) _____
   caudocranial (kaw'do-kra'ne-al; pertaining to the tail and head; directionally pertaining to coursing from the tail to the head)

---

[1]Note that directional terminology used in this text adheres to the standardized nomenclature accepted by veterinary anatomists and the American College of Veterinary Radiologists (ACVR).

5. **Craniocaudal** (adj.)   (R) _____ (CV) _____ (R) _____ (S) _____
    craniocaudal (kra′ne-o-kaw″-dal; pertaining to the head and tail; directionally pertaining to coursing from the head to the tail)

6. **Dorsal** (adj.)   (R) _____ (S) _____
    dorsal (dor′sal; pertaining to the back; clinically refers to the dorsum of the head, neck, trunk, and tail oriented the same as the surface of the back)

7. **Palmar** (adj.)   (R) _____ (S) _____
    palmar (pal′mar; pertaining to the "palm"; in veterinary medicine refers to the sole of the forefeet of domestic animals)

8. **Dorsopalmar** (adj.)   (R) _____ (CV) _____ (R) _____ (S) _____
    dorsopalmar (dor″so-pal′mar; pertaining to the dorsum and "palm"; directionally pertaining to coursing from the dorsum to the sole of the forefoot)

9. **Plantar** (adj.)   (R) _____ (S) _____
    plantar (plan′tar; pertaining to the sole; in veterinary medicine refers to the sole of the hindfeet of domestic animals)

10. **Dorsoplantar** (adj.)   (R) _____ (CV) _____ (R) _____ (S) _____
    dorsoplantar (dor″so-plan′tar; pertaining to the dorsum and sole; directionally pertaining to coursing from the dorsum to the sole of the hindfoot)

11. **Ventral** (adj.)   (R) _____ (S) _____
    ventral (ven′tral; pertaining to the belly; clinically refers to those surfaces of the head, neck, trunk, and tail oriented the same as the belly surface)

12. **Dorsoventral** (adj.)   (R) _____ (CV) _____ (R) _____ (S) _____
    dorsoventral (dor″so-ven′tral; pertaining to the back and the belly; directionally pertaining to coursing from the dorsum to the belly)

13. **Lateral** (adj.)   (R) _____ (S) _____
    lateral (lat′er-al; pertaining to the side)

14. **Medial** (adj.)   (R) _____ (S) _____
    medial (me′de-al; pertaining to the middle)

15. **Mediolateral** (adj.)   (R) _____ (CV) _____ (R) _____ (S) _____
    mediolateral (me″de-o-lat′er-al; pertaining to the middle and the side; directionally pertaining to coursing from the middle to the side)

16. **Palmarodorsal** (adj.)   (R) _____ (CV) _____ (R) _____ (S) _____
    palmarodorsal (pal′mar-o-dor″sal; pertaining to the "palm" and dorsum; directionally pertaining to coursing from the sole to the dorsum of the forefoot)

17. **Plantarodorsal** (adj.)   (R) _____ (CV) _____ (R) _____ (S) _____
    plantarodorsal (plan′tar-o-dor″sal; pertaining to the sole and dorsum; directionally pertaining to coursing from the sole to the dorsum of the hindfoot)

18. **Posterior** (adj.)   (R) _____ (CV) _____ (S) _____
    posterior (pos-ter′e-or; pertaining to the rear)

19. **Rostral** (adj.)   (R) _____ (S) _____
    rostral (ros′tral; pertaining to the nose)

20. **Contralateral** (adj.)   (P) _____ (R)_____ (S) _____
    contralateral (kon″trah-lat′er-al; pertaining to the opposite side; antonym = ipsilateral)

21. **Ipsilateral** (adj.)   (P) _____ (R) _____ (S)_____
    ipsilateral (ip″sĭ-lat′er-al; pertaining to the same side; antonym = contralateral)

INTRODUCTION TO BODY PLANES

The body is divided by three principal planes. The 3-dimensional configuration of these planes is much like the plywood structure shown in Figure 1-1. Each sheet of plywood is perpendicular to the other two, just as each of the principal body planes are perpendicular to one another. Let's attempt to transpose the plywood structure to the body. But first, let's change each of the sheets of plywood into magic Plexiglas sheets that are able to penetrate the body unnoticed and without harm. Why discuss these seemingly invisible, nonexistent planes in such detail? All of our directional terminology is built on the relationship of the body to these planes. Let's look at each plane individually.

The **median plane** (me′de-an) divides the body into equal right and left halves (Fig. 1-2). It can also be referred to as the midsagittal plane (mid-, because it extends through the middle of the body, and sagittal, because it is straight like an arrow). **Sagittal planes** (saj′ĭ-tal) can be thought of as accessory planes and are any planes, to the right or to the left, that lie parallel to the median plane (Fig. 1-3). Sagittal planes permit us to divide extremities longitudinally into *medial* and *lateral* aspects. The next principal plane is the dorsal plane that divides the animal into *dorsal* and *ventral* portions (Fig. 1-4). If the horse in Figure 1-4 was wading in a pond, the surface of the water would represent the **dorsal plane.** The submerged portions of the horse's trunk would lie ventral to that plane, and the exposed portions would be considered dorsal to it. If the horse

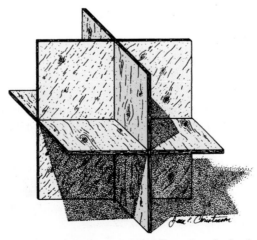

FIGURE 1-1   Plywood structure representing the body planes.

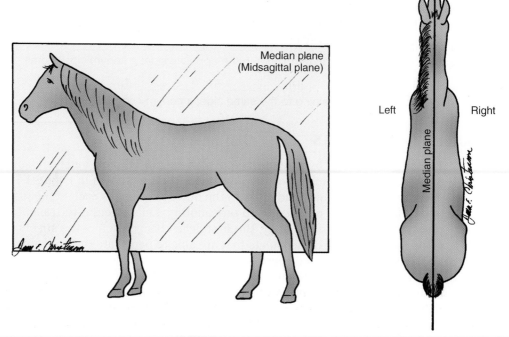

FIGURE 1-2   Median plane.

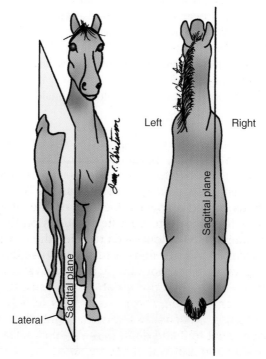

FIGURE 1-3   Sagittal plane.

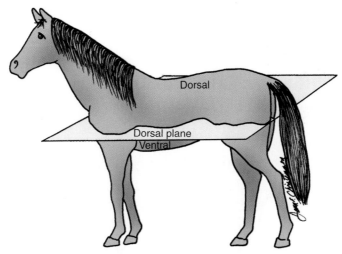

FIGURE 1-4   Dorsal plane.

was swimming, the ventral surfaces of its head and neck would be submerged and the dorsal portions would be dry. Finally, the **transverse plane** (trans-vers′) divides the trunk of the animal into *cranial* and *caudal* regions (Fig. 1-5), much like a magician "saws the lady in half." The transverse plane of the body is perpendicular to both the dorsal and median planes. Extremities each have their own transverse planes. Imagine a line drawn from the shoulder straight down the center of the front leg to the foot. This line would be the limb's axis. The transverse plane of that limb would be perpendicular to the axis and would divide the limb into *distal* (dis′tal; [distant]) and *proximal* (prok′sĭ-mal; [close]) portions (Fig. 1-6). Again, think of the horse wading through a knee-deep stream. The surface of the water becomes the transverse plane of each leg.

APPLICATION OF DIRECTIONAL TERMS

Whether describing the location of a wound on an animal or producing radiographs (x-rays) of its body parts, directional terminology is critical. Imagine navigating around the world without points of latitude and longitude or the references of east, west, north, or south. Just as GPS (Global Positioning System) permits us to find a specific location on the globe, directional terminology permits us to navigate to specific locations on the body. Military leaders use GPS and similar navigational aids to guide their troops to enemy targets. A veterinary professional who finds a tumor will use directional terminology to guide the surgeon to the tumor for efficient removal of the mass. The key to using directional terminology appropriately is to use a suitable point of reference on the animal. For example, if you were to try to describe the location of the right elbow of a dog, you could say that the right elbow lies at a midpoint *proximal* to the right front foot and *distal* to the right shoulder. Without the reference points of the shoulder and foot, the terms *"proximal"* and *"distal"* would have no value in locating the right elbow. It is also important to remember that domestic

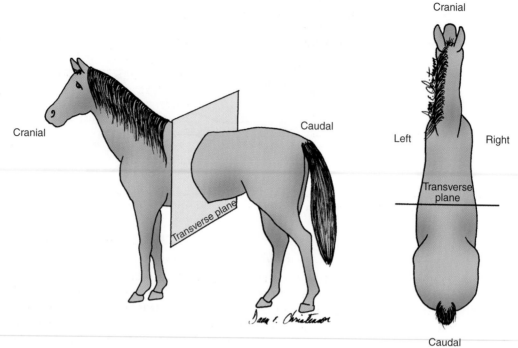

FIGURE 1-5   Transverse plane.

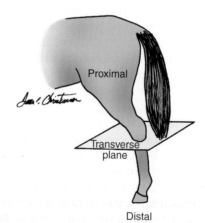

FIGURE 1-6   Transverse plane of an extremity.

animals walk on four limbs (usually with *contralateral* front and rear limbs moving simultaneously; horses who "pace" tend to walk with *ipsilateral* limbs moving together). For quadripeds (i.e., with four feet) the basic structure and orientation of their bodies make reference to various aspects appropriate in some circumstances and inappropriate in others (Table 1-1). Along the head, neck, trunk, and tail, references are made to physical attributes, such as the back and belly, to describe dorsal ("upper") and ventral ("lower") surfaces

TABLE 1-1	Directional terms applicable to radiographic views of body parts	
Head	**Neck, trunk, and tail**	**Limbs***
Left	Left	Cranial (proximal limb only)
Right	Right	Caudal (proximal limb only)
Rostral	Cranial	Dorsal (distal limb only)
Caudal	Caudal	Palmar (distal forelimb only)
Dorsal	Dorsal	Plantar (distal hindlimb only)
Ventral	Ventral	Proximal
		Distal
		Medial
		Lateral

*Radiographs of extremities must always be marked with regard to right versus left limbs.

(see Fig. 1-4). Because the neck, trunk, and proximal limbs (i.e., proximal to the carpus and tarsus[2]) are physically connected between the head and the tail, it is appropriate to use the terms *cranial* and *caudal* to describe anterior and posterior locations, respectively, on those body parts. "Distal" and "proximal" are inappropriate for use directionally along the trunk, because the trunk serves as the reference point for those terms. The trunk could be likened to the center of the universe. Points along the extremities are like the near and distant planets and stars, but are all referenced to the central, originating point (i.e., the trunk). Not only do limbs have proximal and distal points, each limb has a *lateral* surface and a *medial* surface (i.e., nearest the median plane). Anterior and posterior aspects of the limbs are subdivided into proximal and distal parts. (It should be noted that many veterinary professionals simplify directional limb terminology by merely using anterior and posterior. While this is acceptable, to be most accurate, the limbs should be subdivided and referenced appropriately.) As stated earlier, on the proximal portions of the limbs, *"cranial"* is used to refer to the anterior surfaces and *"caudal"* is used to refer to the posterior surfaces. Distal to the carpus and tarsus, *"dorsal"* is used to refer to the anterior aspects of the limbs and feet. The posterior aspect of the distal forelimb and the sole of the forefoot are referred to as the *palmar* surfaces. (Hint: Think of the pads of a cat's front paw being like the palm of your own hand.) The posterior aspect of the distal hindlimb and the sole of the hindfoot are referred to as the *plantar* surfaces. (This is why plantar warts in people are so named, because of the location of the warts on the sole of the foot.) Finally, because the most anterior structure on the head of any animal is the nose, it is used as a common point of reference on the head. Therefore, rather than referring to anterior locations on the head, *rostral* is used. (Note: Cranial cannot be used to describe a location on the head because we are already at the head; that would be like telling someone to go to the city when he or she is already in the city. The question becomes, "Where in the city should they go?") For visualization of appropriate directional terms as they relate to the body, refer to Figure 1-7 and Figure 1-8 (on pp. 10 and 11).

---

[2]If necessary, see Figures 6-11, 6-13, and 6-15 in Chapter 6 of this text for clarification of these joint locations.

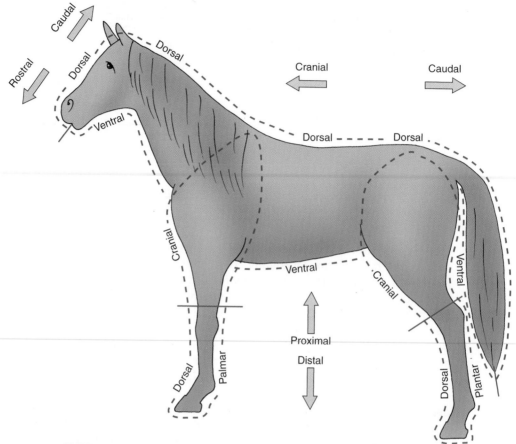

FIGURE 1-7 Directional terms related to body surfaces of large animals.

We begin to combine many of the directional terms for the production of radiographs. The combination of terms is based on the direction of passage of the beam of radiation through the body part. If it is difficult to visualize a beam of radiation penetrating the body, the analogy of the penetration of a bullet may help. The directional terms are combined in the order of passage of the "bullet" (beam) sequentially through each body surface (i.e., entry and exit points). For example, if a bullet was fired straight through the left thigh of an animal with the entry wound on the lateral aspect of the thigh and the exit wound on the medial thigh, the directional term used to describe the path of the bullet would be *lateromedial* (LM). A radiograph taken of an animal's chest, such that the beam of radiation penetrates from his back to the underside of his chest, before reaching the x-ray film, describes a *dorsoventral* (DV) radiographic view of the chest. A radiograph taken of the *proximal* limb of an animal, such that the beam of radiation passes through the limb from front to rear, describes a *craniocaudal* (CrCd) view. A similar view of the *distal* forelimb is called a *dorsopalmar* (DPa) view (see Figs. 1-9 through 1-11), whereas a similar view of the

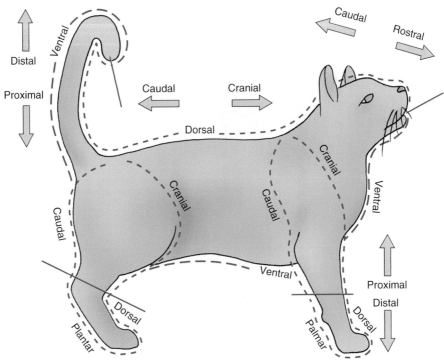

FIGURE 1-8   Directional terms related to body surfaces of companion animals.

distal hindlimb is called a *dorsoplantar* (DPl) view. For those who simplify radiographic terminology, each of these three views (CrCd, DPa, and DPl) could be referred to as AP *(anteroposterior)* views. Note that the radiographic views discussed to this point orient the beam of radiation parallel or perpendicular to the various planes of the body. In special circumstances, to help visualize particular aspects of a body part, the beam may be angled so that it is neither parallel nor perpendicular to any body plane (i.e., tangent). Any radiographic view that is neither parallel nor perpendicular to any body plane is said to be oblique (o-blĭk, o-blēk). In such a view, the term "oblique" usually follows the directional terms used to describe the overall beam penetration. For instance, if the overall penetration of the beam through a limb was in a dorsopalmer direction (i.e., with the beam angled such that it was tangent to the limb [~45° angle], entering on the dorsal aspect and exiting on the palmar aspect), the radiographic view would be labeled as a dorsopalmer oblique (DPaO) view of that body part. Because the directional terminology in radiography can become lengthy at times, Table 1-2 provides standardized abbreviations for the terms. Standardized terminology is still being adopted by some veterinary professionals; therefore, Table 1-3 provides comparisons between some standardized and obsolete terminology.

Of course, the directional terms and their abbreviations mean nothing radiographically, unless each film is marked appropriately. Note that in Figure 1-9 radiographic markers have been placed on the cassette, lateral to the dog's foot/limb. The "Lt" indicates that it is the left limb. The "DPa" indicates the

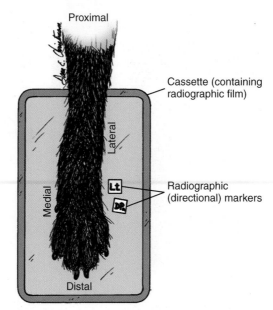

FIGURE 1-9   Dorsal view, distal left front limb (canine).

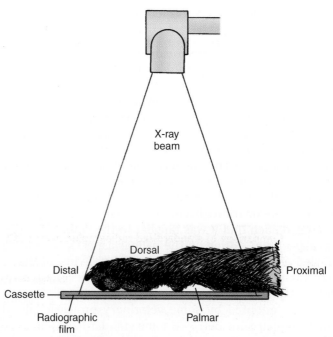

FIGURE 1-10   Lateral view (schematic) x-ray penetration of distal left front limb (canine).

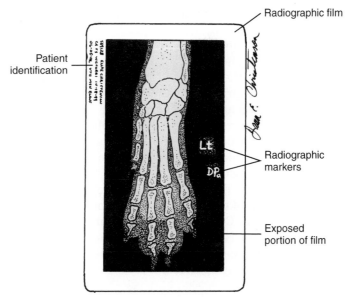

Radiographic film

Patient identification

Radiographic markers

Exposed portion of film

FIGURE 1-11 Dorsopalmar radiograph (schematic), distal left front limb (canine).

TABLE 1-2	Directional terms and abbreviations		
Directional term	**Abbreviation**	**Directional term**	**Abbreviation**
Left	Lt	Medial	M
Right	Rt	Lateral	L
Dorsal	D	Proximal	Pr
Ventral	V	Distal	Di
Cranial	Cr	Palmar	Pa
Caudal	Cd	Plantar	Pl
Rostral	R	Oblique	O

TABLE 1-3	Comparison of standardized radiographic nomenclature and obsolete terminology	
	Official/standardized terminology	**Obsolete terminology**
	Craniocaudal (CrCd)	Anteroposterior (AP)
	Caudocranial (CdCr)	Posteroanterior (PA)
	Dorsopalmar (DPa)	Anteroposterior (AP)
	Dorsoplantar (DPl)	Anteroposterior (AP)
	Palmarodorsal (PaD)	Posteroanterior (PA)
	Plantarodorsal (PlD)	Posteroanterior (PA)

radiographic view (dorsopalmar). Figure 1-10 demonstrates the x-ray beam penetration. The final radiograph produced (Fig. 1-11) results from variations in exposure of the film to the x-ray beam. Greater exposure to the radiation creates darker images. The shades of black, gray, and "white" (transparent on an actual film) appear on the developed radiograph because of differences in tissue densities. The black surrounding the limb (see Fig. 1-11) has resulted because the film in those regions has been fully exposed to the x-ray beam. This is typical of air density (i.e., the radiation can pass freely through air and contact the film). The densest material on this particular film is contained in the lead markers. The lead letters of those markers completely block the beam. Because the film in those areas is not exposed, the letters appear "white" (transparent). Bones are denser than air but less dense than lead. Bones block a large part of the x-ray beam. Because much of the beam is blocked by the bony structures, very little of the film is exposed. Consequently, those areas of the film appear very light gray to white (clear). Notice that the remainder of the extremity is radiographically gray. This is typical of tissue and fluid density. The more tissue or fluid present, the lighter the gray on the film.

SELF-TEST

Using the previous information in this chapter, complete the following crossword puzzle using the most appropriate term. Do not use abbreviations.

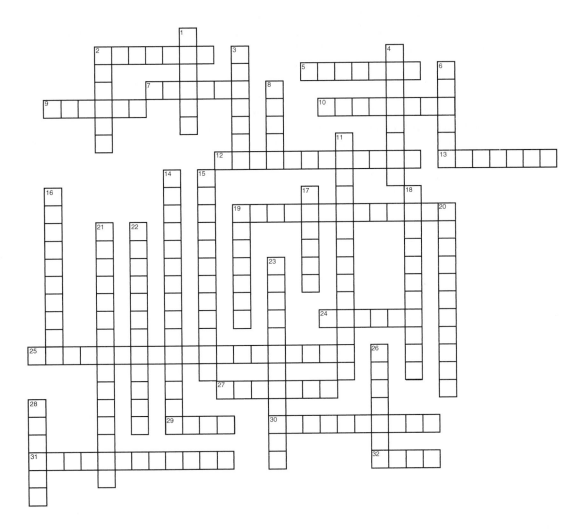

ACROSS

2   The surface of a horse's rear foot where the sole is found
5   Pertaining to the side
7   The surface of a limb that lies nearest the midsagittal plane
9   A word part that follows a root and modifies its meaning
10   In relation to the trunk of the body, the hip is the most _____ point on the rear limb

12	A radiographic view in which the beam passes through the surface of the belly and then the back, before reaching the film
13	Toward the nose
19	An incomplete word that is formed by joining a root word with a vowel (usually in parentheses)(2 words)
24	The horizontal body plane that divides an animal into ventral and dorsal portions
25	A radiographic view created by passage of the beam through the medial surface of the elbow to the side of the elbow, at a tangent angle that is neither parallel nor perpendicular to any body plane
27	Pertaining to the belly
29	Word part considered the foundation of a word
30	A permanent film image created by exposure of special film to x-rays that have passed through the body
31	In the rear foot, pertaining to the dorsum and sole
32	The opposite of right

DOWN

1	Toward the tail
2	Word part before a root that modifies its meaning
3	Neither parallel nor perpendicular; cf. tangent
4	A plane that lies parallel to the median plane
6	The surface of a forepaw where the pads are found
8	Not left
11	A single-letter word part that is used to join other word parts (2 words)
14	Pertaining to the rear and the front
15	A perpendicular radiographic view of the skull in which the beam penetrates the top of the skull before penetrating the lower jaw
16	A plane that divides the trunk of the body into cranial and caudal portions
17	In relation to the trunk of the body, the foot is at a _____ point on the limb
18	A radiographic view of the front foot such that the beam passes through the top of the toes and then through the pads
19	When describing the relationship between the chest and the abdomen, the chest lies _____ to the abdomen
20	Another name for median plane
21	Pertaining to the front and the rear
22	Pertaining to the head and tail
23	A radiographic view of a limb in which the beam penetrates from the inner surface of the leg to the side
26	Pertaining to the nose
28	Pertaining to the tail

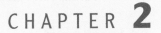

CHAPTER 2

The Cell

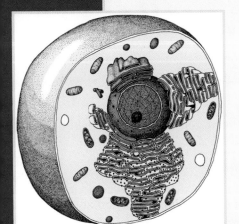

GOALS AND OBJECTIVES

By the conclusion of this chapter, the student will be able to:

1. Recognize common root words, prefixes, and suffixes related to cells.
2. Divide simple and compound words into their respective parts.
3. Recognize, correctly pronounce, and appropriately use common medical terms related to cells.
4. Recognize anatomic components of animal cells.
5. Demonstrate a basic understanding of animal cell physiology.

INTRODUCTION TO RELATED TERMS

Divide each of the following terms into its respective parts ("R," root; "P," prefix; "S," suffix; "CV," combining vowel).

1. **Microscopic** (adj.)   (P) _____ (CV) _____ (R) _____ (S) _____
   microscopic (mi″kro-skop′ik; pertaining to a small view; clinically refers to something that requires visualization by use of a microscope)

2. **Cytology**[1] (n.)   (R) _____ (CV) _____ (S) _____
   cytology (si-tol′o-je; the study of cells)

3. **Lysosomal** (adj.)   (R) _____ (CV) _____ (R) _____ (S) _____
   lysosomal (li″so-so′mal; pertaining to a dissolving/destructive body)

---

[1]Cytology: Note that the true suffix for the word is technically the letter "y." The interpretive meaning of "y" as a suffix is "the process of." It implies action. Therefore any word ending in the letter "y" will have action implicated in it and should be used accordingly. For the purpose of simplifying medical terms in this text, the letter "y" will be shown collectively with the adjacent word part as a suffix. In the case of cytology, the adjacent word part is -log-. The collective meaning of the "suffix" -logy is "the study of." Hence, the meaning of cytology is interpreted as "the study of cells."

4. **Intracellular** (adj.)   (P) _____ (R) _____ (S) _____
intracellular (in"trah-sel'u-lar; pertaining to within cells)

5. **Extracellular** (adj.)   (P) _____ (R) _____ (S) _____
extracellular (eks"trah-sel'u-lar; pertaining to outside of cells)

6. **Nuclear** (adj.)   (R) _____ (S) _____
nuclear (nu'kle-ar; pertaining to a nucleus)

7. **Chromosome[2]** (n.)   (R) _____ (CV) _____ (S)_____
chromosome (kro'mo-sōm; a colored body)

8. **Nucleolus** (n.)   (R) _____ (S) _____
nucleolus (nu-kle'o-lus; a small nucleus)

9. **Endoplasmic** (adj.)   (P) _____ (R) _____ (S) _____
endoplasmic (en"do-plaz'mik; pertaining to within matter)

10. **Centriole** (n.)   (R) _____ (CV) _____ (S) _____
centriole (sen'trĭ-ōl; a small center)

11. **Cytoplasmic** (adj.)   (R) _____ (CV) _____ (R) _____ (S) _____
cytoplasmic (si"to-plaz'mik; pertaining to cell matter [cytoplasm])

12. **Vacuole** (n.)   (R) _____ (S) _____
vacuole (vak'u-ōl; a small emptiness)

13. **Chromatic** (adj.)   (R) _____ (S) _____
chromatic (kro-mat'ik; pertaining to color)

14. **Phagocytosis[3]** (n.)   (R) _____ (CV) _____ (R) _____
(CV) _____ (S) _____
phagocytosis (fag"o-si-to'sis; process of eating [by] cells)

15. **Pinocytosis** (n.)   (R) _____ (CV) _____ (R) _____
(CV) _____ (S) _____
pinocytosis (pi"no-si-to'sis; process of drinking [by] cells)

16. **Exocytosis** (n.)   (P) _____ (CV) _____ (R) _____
(CV) _____ (S) _____
exocytosis (eks"o-si-to'sis; processing out of a cell)

17. **Mitosis** (n.)   (R) _____ (CV) _____ (S) _____
mitosis (mi-to'sis; a condition of "thread"; clinically refers to cellular reproduction)

---

[2]Chromosome: Note that the true suffix for the word is technically the letter "e." The interpretive meaning of "e" as a suffix is "the presence of." As a suffix, "e" creates nouns (i.e., persons, places, or things). For the purpose of simplifying medical terms in this text, the letter "e" will be shown collectively with the adjacent word part as a root. In the case of chromosome, the adjacent word part is the root -som-. The collective meaning of the "root" -some is "a body." Hence, the meaning of chromosome is interpreted as "a colored body."
[3]Phagocytosis: Note that the suffix -sis may appear alone or with a number of combining vowels (e.g., -osis, -asis, -esis, -iasis). The interpretive meaning of the suffix -sis is usually "the process of" or "a condition of."

18. **Nuclei**[4] (n.)   (R) _____ (S) _____
    nuclei (nu'kle-i; plural of nucleus)

19. **Intercellular** (adj.)   (P) _____ (R) _____ (S) _____
    intercellular (in"ter-sel'u-lar; pertaining to between cells)

20. **Organelle** (n.)   (R) _____ (S) _____
    organelle (or"gan-el'; a tiny organ)

21. **Physiology** (n.)   (R) _____ (CV) _____ (S) _____
    physiology (fiz"e-ol'o-je; the study of function)

22. **Reticular** (adj.)   (R) _____ (S) _____
    reticular (rĕ-tik'u-lar; pertaining to a net)

23. **Ribosomal** (adj.)   (R) _____ (CV) _____ (R) _____ (S) _____
    ribosomal (ri'bo-so-mal; pertaining to an RNA body)

24. **Centromere** (n.)   (P) _____ (CV) _____ (S) _____
    centromere (sen'tro-mĕr; a central part)

CELLULAR ANATOMY AND PHYSIOLOGY

Cells are the smallest functional units of the body. They are so small that they cannot be studied without the aid of a microscope. In fact, many of the intracellular organelles are so small that an electron microscope must be used to visualize them. There are a plethora of cell types within the body of any animal, each uniquely different both anatomically (structurally) and physiologically (functionally). For the purpose of this discussion, an average, basic cell is presented. The reader should recognize that the intracellular organelles and details of cellular physiology will vary among different cells of the body.

Cellular Anatomy

A basic animal cell is shown in Figure 2-1. A portion of the cell has been removed for easy viewing of its anatomic features.

Cellular membrane

The cellular membrane is the outermost structure that forms an envelope or "skin" around all of the intracellular components. It is composed of lipids[5] and proteins.

Cytoplasm

The cytoplasm is a colorless fluid that gives the cell mass and suspends all of the intracellular organelles.

---

[4]Nuclei: As a general rule, many medical terms ending in "i" or "a" indicate the plural form of the word.

[5]Lipid is derived from [Gr. *lipos,* fat]; lip(o)- is a combining form meaning "fat."

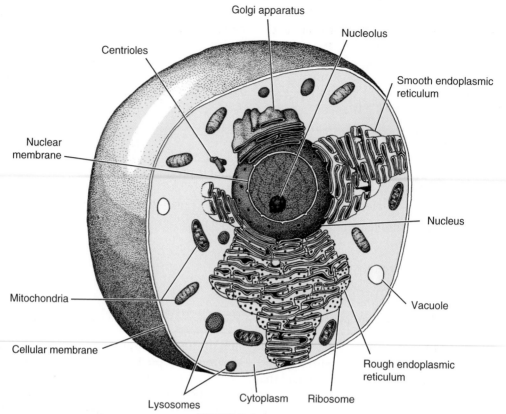

FIGURE 2-1   Animal cell.

Smooth endoplasmic reticulum
> The smooth endoplasmic reticulum is a complex network of canals and flattened sacs throughout the cytoplasm of the cell. It is "smooth" because it has no ribosomes.

Rough endoplasmic reticulum
> The rough endoplasmic reticulum is also a network of canals and flattened sacs throughout the cytoplasm of the cell. It appears rough microscopically because of the many ribosomes attached to it.

Ribosomes
> The ribosomes are tiny, spherical organelles attached to the membrane of the rough endoplasmic reticulum. They are responsible for the production of things like proteins.

Mitochondrion (mi"to-kon'dre-on; mitochondria — plural, mi"to-kon'dre-ah)
> Under the electron microscope, the mitochondria appear as tiny, elongated granules with thread-like ridges over their surfaces. The texture is created by the intricate maze of partitions within the mitochondrial interior. They are like tiny generators.

Lysosome

The lysosomes are small, enzyme-filled sacs. The enzymes within them literally dissolve particles that they come in contact with.

Vacuole

Vacuoles often appear microscopically as small, empty, cytoplasmic spaces, much like the appearance of holes in Swiss cheese. Actually, vacuoles are vesicles[6] that often contain either food for the cell or waste products to be removed from the cell.

Golgi apparatus[7]

The Golgi apparatus is a specialized series of flattened sacs and vesicles near the nucleus. It "packages" cellular products.

Nucleus

The nucleus is a large, intracellular organelle formed of loosely woven chromatin. The chromatin, when the cell is stained in the laboratory, readily accepts the stain, giving it a colorful appearance microscopically. The chromatin is actually made up of loosely woven DNA, which when undergoing mitosis will become organized into the rod-like chromosomes that contain the blueprints of the cell.

Nuclear membrane

The nuclear membrane forms a porous envelope ("skin") around the nucleus.

Nucleolus

Nucleoli are small, dense structures within the nucleus that are composed mainly of RNA and protein. They usually are visible only in very active cells.

Centriole

The centrioles are two cylindrical structures found near the nucleus and the Golgi apparatus. The centrioles lie perpendicular to one another and are important during mitosis.

Cellular Physiology

It was stated previously that cells are separate, functional compartments that make up the tissues of the body. A strong understanding of cellular anatomy and physiology is essential to gaining an understanding of individual body systems and the body as a whole. Unfortunately, many students have found cellular physiology difficult to comprehend. Actually, the structure and function of cells are quite basic, similar to those of a large corporation.

The basic structure of both the cell and the corporation are based on very detailed blueprints. The design of each structure and the materials used to build it may differ in various respects, but the overall organization of the cell and the corporation are much the same. Each has a protective outer structure (i.e., the **cellular membrane** and the corporation's foundation, roof, and outer walls). The cement, mortar, and brick used to fabricate the outer building of the corporation are replaced in the cell by strong, water-impervious lipids and proteins

---

[6]Vesicle is derived from [L. *vesicula*], meaning "tiny bladder." A vesicle is a small sac-like structure.
[7]The Golgi (gol´je) apparatus is named after Camillo Golgi, an Italian scientist who was the co-winner of the Nobel Prize for medicine and physiology in 1906.

in the cellular membrane. Where the corporation uses vents and windows to provide ventilation for the interior, the semipermeable[8] cellular membrane provides for easy passage of lipid-soluble molecules, such as oxygen and carbon dioxide. So, by simple diffusion,[9] cellular respiration is accomplished. In other words, oxygen and carbon dioxide diffuse freely to and fro across the cellular membrane between the intracellular and the extracellular fluids.

Just as the corporation has doors and service doors to allow entry of people, supplies, and products, the cellular membrane provides for passage of liquids and large molecules. Rather than having actual doors that open and close, however, the cellular membrane indents and forms a vesicle around the substance to be taken into the cell. The vesicle, when completely formed, breaks free from the cellular membrane and can then be transported to an area of need intracellularly. Pinocytosis is the name given to the intake ("drinking") of liquids by a cell, via the previously described process. Small, water-soluble molecules, like glucose, are taken into the cell through a mechanism called active transport (facilitated diffusion). For active transport to take place, the extracellular glucose molecule is temporarily attached to a protein molecule on the surface of the cellular membrane (sort of like a tennis ball sticking to a Velcro mitt). This protein molecule actively transports the glucose molecule (much like a revolving door) through the cellular membrane.

Phagocytosis (Fig. 2-2) is a process of a cell taking in large objects, such as large protein particles or organisms like bacteria, and "digesting" them. The process begins much like pinocytosis, with the formation of a vesicle around the object. The object itself is like the raw ore and other crude materials taken into the corporation; it must be refined before it can be used. Therefore, the "food" vesicle of the cell will be joined with a **lysosome.** Just as a foundry would melt down the ore, the lysosomal enzymes digest the object into usable components. Some of the refined by-products may provide fuel for the cell (simple sugars), and others provide building blocks (amino acids) for other production purposes intracellularly. Waste products are expelled from the cell using a reverse process called exocytosis. Similar to corporate dumping of wastes into rivers and streams, cells send waste vesicles to the surface of the cell where the cellular membrane opens, exposing and expelling the contents of the vesicles into the intercellular fluid of the body (see Chapter 5).

All energy for cellular function is provided through the **mitochondria,** just as the internal physical plant and generators provide needed electricity for the corporation. Glucose, rather than coal or petroleum products, provides the fuel for these little powerhouses. Without the energy generated by the mitochondria, other cellular organelles could not carry out their functions.

The smooth and rough **endoplasmic reticula** provide mechanisms for transporting fuel, products, and by-products throughout the cell, much like hallways

---

[8]Semipermeable: [*semi-* partial, *permeable* to pass through] a semipermeable membrane permits passage of some things but not others.

[9]Diffusion is the movement of particles (molecules) across a semipermeable membrane from an area of high concentration to an area of low concentration (cf. osmosis, "Introduction to Related Terms," Chapter 5).

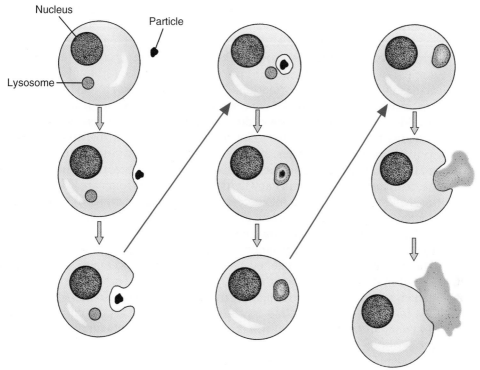

FIGURE 2-2   Phagocytosis.

and elevators provide for transport of products and the like throughout the corporation. The **rough endoplasmic reticulum** is of particular importance because of its close association with the ribosomes. The **ribosomes** are small production units. Where one production unit within the corporation may be responsible for making oblong widgets, another unit may be responsible for producing round gadgets. The principal ribosomal products are proteins of all shapes and sizes. Some of the products may be used for internal needs, such as repairs and general maintenance. Any of the products intended for export and global distribution must be packaged. Only one packaging department exists within the cell—the **Golgi apparatus.** All products and by-products are sent, by way of the endoplasmic reticula, to the Golgi apparatus, where those products are packaged into small vesicles (much like shrink-wrap). Again using the endoplasmic reticula, the packaged proteins, like mucus from a secretory cell, can be transported to the cellular membrane for exocytosis. Other proteins, like lysosomal enzymes, are packaged and distributed (e.g., as lysosomes) throughout the cytoplasm of the cell for later use.

The core of any corporate operation is the executive offices. All detailed information about corporate structure, products, production rates, profits, and losses are stored in the executive offices. The **nucleus** of a cell is much like the executive offices of the corporation. Of course, the nucleus is not enclosed in lavish oak and mahogany woodwork with bright brass fixtures; instead, it is enclosed in a porous nuclear membrane. All of the critical information and original "documents" (DNA [deoxyribonucleic acid]) about the cell and its functions are stored within the nuclear chromatin, as opposed to filing cabinets. The **nucleolus,** like any good executive secretary, is responsible for communicating with the other intracellular organelles. For example, "work orders" and "photocopies" of blueprints are sent to the ribosomes in the form of RNA (ribonucleic acid) messages and information. Each ribosome receives from the nucleolus an RNA "photocopy" of an original DNA template for a protein to be produced, along with the work order for the quantity needed. So, the nucleolus controls protein production. The nucleolus even has the authority and ability to form new ribosomes, if the need exists for additional production units. If the communication needs of a corporation exceed the capabilities of one executive secretary, temporary help may be hired. Temporary support staff, in the case of a cell, comes in the form of additional nucleoli. Whenever multiple nucleoli are visible in a nucleus, the cell is assumed to be very active.

A peak time of activity for a cell is before **mitosis,** or cellular reproduction. During this process every aspect of the cell must be reproduced in fine detail. This situation could be likened to a corporation developing a daughter plant out of state or perhaps out of the country. To be as successful as the original, the plant must be duplicated in every detail. (After all, that's why many fast-food franchises are so successful.) Likewise, the cell must duplicate its every detail. The actual phases of mitosis are explained in the following paragraphs.

During the *prophase*[10] (Fig. 2-3), the nuclear membrane, like the modular wall of an office, is temporarily disassembled. The nuclear chromatin begins to reorganize and becomes tightly coiled into chromosomes. The DNA chains have been duplicated so that each chromosome is actually formed of two chromatids (the original and a duplicate) joined by a temporary attachment called a centromere (like a piece of removable tape holding two documents together). This gives the chromosomes the appearance of an X shape. At this time, too, the centrioles are duplicated. The two pairs of centrioles begin to move to opposite sides of the cell, while forming thin, spindle-like fibers between them.

During the *metaphase*[11] (Fig. 2-4), the chromosomes line up midway between the centrioles. The centromere of each chromosome is attached to a spindle fiber.

During the *anaphase*[12] (Fig. 2-5), the chromatids separate and each (the original and the duplicate) is drawn in opposite directions by the attached spindle fibers, toward the associated centrioles. The centrioles act as powerful magnets, drawing the chromatids toward opposite ends of the cell. Microscopically, the spindle fibers and chromatids have a thread-like appearance that's why this whole process is called *mitosis* (literally meaning: a condition of thread). The other cellular organelles and the cytoplasm are also equally divided between the two sides. The cellular membrane begins to constrict, outlining the two daughter cells.

---

[10]Pro-, a prefix meaning "before."
[11]Meta-, a prefix meaning "after" or "beyond."
[12]Ana-, a prefix meaning "back, up, again."

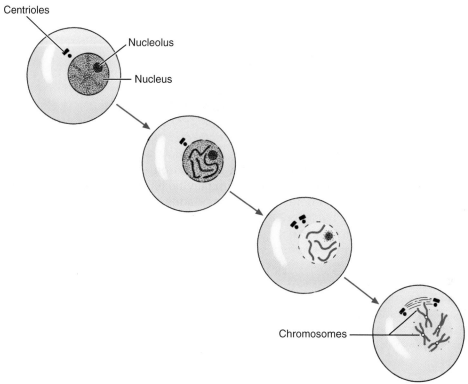

FIGURE 2-3   Mitosis: Prophase.

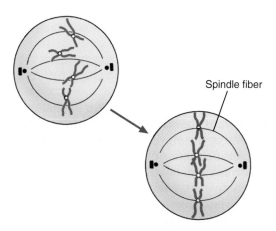

FIGURE 2-4   Mitosis: Metaphase.

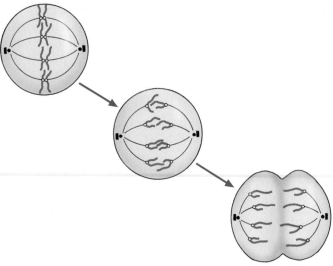

FIGURE 2-5   Mitosis: Anaphase.

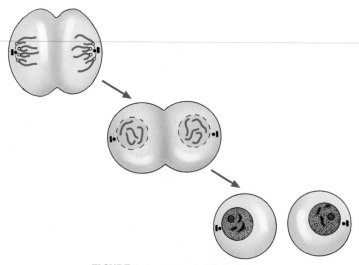

FIGURE 2-6   Mitosis: Telophase.

During the *telophase*[13] (Fig. 2-6), migration of the chromosomes to the centrioles is completed. Soon, the cytoplasmic and cellular membrane divisions will also be completed. Within each new daughter cell, the chromosomes unwind into loosely woven chromatin, while new nuclear membranes envelope the new nuclei. The new daughter cells are identical, yet separate, fully functional entities—just like a new fast-food franchise. Heavy protein production within each new cell is required for further cellular development, such that the reproductive cycle may

---

[13]Telo-, a prefix meaning "end."

be repeated. Do mistakes in construction happen? Unfortunately, yes, they do. If such a mistake is duplicated and perpetuated with the creation of each new franchise, the whole market place may suffer. In the cellular world, this is how cancer develops.

SELF-TEST

Using the previous information in this chapter, complete the following crossword puzzle using the most appropriate medical term(s).

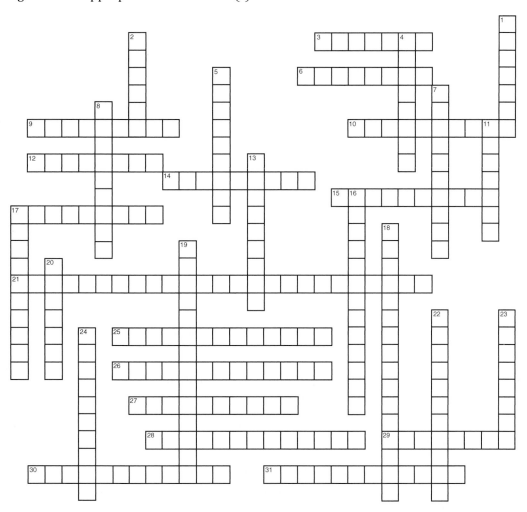

ACROSS

3   Cytoplasmic inclusion that appears as a hole microscopically
6   Initial stage of mitosis
9   Movement across a semipermeable membrane from an area of high concentration to an area of low concentration

10	Tightly coiled, connected strands of original and duplicate DNA, visible only during mitosis (literally meaning: "a colored body")
12	The study of cells
14	Stage of mitosis when chromosomes line up midway between centrioles (its prefix means "after" or "beyond")
15	Paired, cylindrical organelles responsible for chromatid migration during mitosis
17	Colorless fluid that suspends intracellular organelles
21	Organelle composed of highly organized networks of tubes for the transport of proteins produced by its attached ribosomes (3 words)
25	Anything within a cell
26	A type of membrane that permits passage of some things and not others
27	An instrument used to view tiny objects, like cells
28	Pertaining to between cells
29	Intracellular organelle that produces proteins
30	The process of cellular "eating"
31	"Powerhouses" of cells, providing energy for cellular functions

DOWN

1	A small sac
2	Plural of nucleus
4	Cytoplasmic vesicle containing "digestive" enzymes
5	Final stage of mitosis (its prefix means "end")
7	The process of cellular expulsion of waste products
8	Intracellular organelle composed of RNA and protein; responsible for interorganelle communication; literally means "a tiny nut"
11	Cellular reproduction
13	Loosely woven _____ stores DNA in the nucleus when a cell is not reproducing (microscopically gives the nucleus *color*)
16	Anything outside a cell
17	Temporary attachment between original and duplicate chromatids during mitosis
18	The outermost "wall" of a cell (2 words)
19	Intracellular organelle responsible for packaging secretory products (2 words)
20	Control center of cell; containing all DNA information
22	The process of cellular "drinking"
23	Stage of mitosis when chromatids separate and are drawn to centrioles (its prefix means "back," "up," "again")
24	The study of function

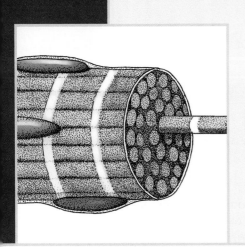

CHAPTER 3

Body Structure and Organization

GOALS AND OBJECTIVES

By the conclusion of this chapter, the student will be able to:

1. Recognize common root words, prefixes, and suffixes related to the body and biology.
2. Divide simple and compound words into their respective parts.
3. Recognize, correctly pronounce, and appropriately use common medical terms related to the body and animal physiology.
4. Demonstrate an understanding of basic chemistry, including atomic structure and molecular bonds.
5. Demonstrate an understanding of general body structure and organization.
6. Demonstrate an understanding of the functional relationships of body tissues and organs.

INTRODUCTION TO RELATED TERMS

Divide each of the following terms into its respective parts ("R," root; "P," prefix; "S," suffix; "CV," combining vowel).

1. **Hematopoietic** (adj.)   (R) _____ (CV) _____ (R) _____ (S) _____
   hematopoietic (hem"ah-to-poi-et'ik; pertaining to blood production)

2. **Lymphatic** (adj.)   (R) _____ (CV) _____ (S) _____
   lymphatic (lim-fat'ik; pertaining to lymph [L. "water"])

3. **Musculoskeletal** (adj.)   (R) _____ (CV) _____ (R) _____ (S) _____
   musculoskeletal (mus"ku-lo-skel'ĕ-tal; pertaining to the muscles and skeleton)

4. **Cardiovascular** (adj.)   (R) _____ (CV) _____ (R) _____ (S) _____
   cardiovascular (kar"de-o-vas'ku-lar; pertaining to the heart and vessels)

5. **Respiratory** (adj.)   (P) _____ (R) _____ (S) _____
respiratory (rĕ-spi′rah-to″re; pertaining to again breathing)

6. **Neurological** (adj.)   (R) _____ (CV) _____ (R) _____
                                         (CV) _____ (S) _____
neurological (nu-ro-loj′ik-al; pertaining to nerve study)

7. **Alimentary** (adj.)   (R) _____ (S) _____
alimentary (al″ĕ-men′tar-e; pertaining to food)

8. **Urinary** (adj.)   (R) _____ (S) _____
urinary (u′rĭ-ner″e; pertaining to urine)

9. **Reproductive** (adj.)   (P) _____ (R) _____ (S) _____
reproductive (re″pro-duk′tiv; pertaining to again producing [i.e., offspring])

10. **Endocrine** (adj.)   (P) _____ (R) _____
endocrine (en′do-krin; to secrete inside)

11. **Integumentary** (adj.)   (R) _____ (S) _____
integumentary (in-teg-u-men′tar-e; pertaining to covering over)

12. **Visceral** (adj.)   (R) _____ (S) _____
visceral (vis′er-al; pertaining to the viscera [organs])

13. **Cranium** (n.)   (R) _____ (S) _____
cranium (kra′ne-um; the head)

14. **Thoracic** (adj.)   (R) _____ (S) _____
thoracic (tho-ras′ik; pertaining to the thorax [chest])

15. **Abdominal** (adj.)   (R) _____ (S) _____
abdominal (ab-dom′ĭ-nal; pertaining to the abdomen [belly])

16. **Epithelial** (adj.)   (R) _____ (S) _____
epithelial (ep″ĭ-the′le-al; pertaining to epithelium[1])

17. **Endothelial** (adj.)   (R) _____ (S) _____
endothelial (en″do-the′le-al; pertaining to endothelium[2])

18. **Cuboidal** (adj.)   (R) _____ (S) _____
cuboidal (ku-boi′dal; pertaining to resembling a cube)

19. **Squamous** (adj.)   (R) _____ (S) _____
squamous (skwa′mus; pertaining to scales)

20. **Columnar** (adj.)   (R) _____ (S) _____
columnar (ko-lum′nar; pertaining to columns [pillars])

---

[1]Epithelium: derived from the prefix epi- [upon] and [L. *thele*, nipple], epithelium is a superficial tissue found on any exposed surface of the body.
[2]Endothelium: derived from the prefix endo- [within, inside] and [L. *thele*], endothelium is a type of epithelium found lining the interior surfaces of vessels and the like.

21. **Myocyte** (n.)   (R) _____ (CV) _____ (R) _____
    myocyte (mi′o-sīt; a muscle cell)

22. **Homeostasis** (n.)   (R) _____ (CV) _____ (S) _____
    homeostasis (ho″me-o-sta′sis; standing unchanged; clinically refers to that state
    of balance or equilibrium, albeit normal function within the body)

23. **Pathology** (n.)   (R) _____ (CV) _____ (S) _____
    pathology (pah-thol′o-je; the study of disease)

24. **Synergism** (n.)   (P) _____ (R) _____ (S) _____
    synergism (sin′er-jizm; the state of working together; *syn-* [together], *erg(o)-* [work])

25. **Symbiosis** (n.)   (P) _____ (R) _____ (S) _____
    symbiosis (sim″bi-o′sis; the state of living together; *sym-* [together], *bio-* [life])

26. **Biology** (n.)   (R) _____ (S) _____
    biology (bi-ol′o-je; the study of life)

27. **Atomic** (adj.)   (R) _____ (S) _____
    atomic (ă-tom′ik; pertaining to an atom)

28. **Molecular** (adj.)   (R) _____ (S) _____
    molecular (mo-lek′u-lar; pertaining to a little mass [molecule])

29. **Peritoneal** (adj.)   (R)_____ (S) _____
    peritoneal (per″i-to″ne′al; pertaining to peritoneum [L. *per*, around + *teinein*, to stretch]
    peritoneal tissue lines the abdominal cavity)

30. **Pleural** (adj.)   (R)_____ (S) _____
    pleural (ploor′al; pertaining to pleura [Gr. "rib," "side"] pleural tissue lines the chest cavity)

ANATOMY AND PHYSIOLOGY

Basic Structure of Matter

Every animal is composed of billions of *organic* (containing carbon) and *inorganic* (noncarbon containing) compounds. All matter is composed of tiny, invisible (to the naked eye) particles called *atoms*. Elements, as we often refer to the basic atomic particles, are each very different. Structurally, each element has a unique atomic structure consisting of a minute, central, positively charged mass *(nucleus)* and "orbiting," negatively charged particles *(electrons)*. They are much like very, very small solar systems, with a "sun" (nucleus) orbited by "planets" (electrons). Have you ever looked at the periodic table of elements (Fig. 3-1) and wondered why the elements are organized and numbered the way they are? The *atomic number* for each element is determined by the number of *protons* (positively charged particles) within the nucleus[3] of an atom. For example, a hydrogen

---

[3]The nucleus of most atoms is composed of both protons and neutrons. Each proton carries a single positive charge, whereas each neutron, being about equal in weight to a proton, carries no electrical charge. (neutr(o)- = neutral)

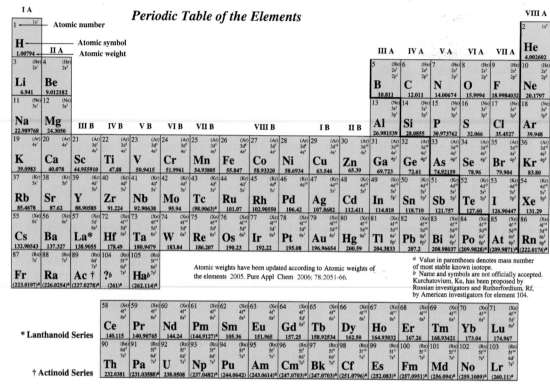

FIGURE 3-1   Periodic table of elements.

atom contains a single proton; therefore, the atomic number of hydrogen is 1. A carbon atom contains six protons and so has the atomic number 6.

Perhaps you've wondered how such tiny entities could possibly be weighed. Well, atoms are not placed on a tiny scale to be weighed. Instead, scientists have discovered how many protons and *neutrons* exist in an atom's nucleus. The approximate, collective weight of these creates the nuclear mass. It is the nuclear mass of the atom that determines the *atomic weight* of the element (see Fig. 3-1). For example, a hydrogen atom contains only one proton and no neutrons. Therefore, its atomic weight is roughly 1.00. In comparison, a carbon atom contains six protons and six neutrons, giving it an atomic weight of approximately 12.0.

What about those electrons that are orbiting the nucleus? The number and the arrangement of the electrons that orbit the nucleus determine all other properties of the element, particularly how it interacts with other elements. Depending on the element, the electrons of an atom are arranged in one or more orbits or "shells" around the nucleus (just like the planets in our solar system

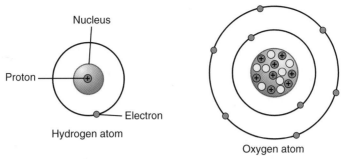

FIGURE 3-2 Atomic structure.

have different orbits). For example, an atom of hydrogen appears as a nucleus orbited by a single electron. Comparatively, an atom of oxygen appears as a nucleus encircled by eight electrons (Fig. 3-2). The number of electrons of an atom equals the number of protons in the nucleus, rendering the atom neutral.

As we just said, the number of electrons is equal to the number of protons in an atom, making it neutral. Being electrically neutral does not mean that a given atom is "stable." The stability of an atom is determined by the number of electrons filling its outermost shell. For elements with atomic numbers 1 through 20, the maximum numbers of electrons that may be held by each shell are as follows:

First shell (closest to the nucleus)   2 electrons
Second shell   8 electrons
Third shell   8 electrons

Elements, like helium, whose outermost shell is filled to capacity are considered stable or *inert*. In comparison, an element like hydrogen is lacking an electron in its outer shell. Therefore, hydrogen atoms are unstable; they will try to bond with other atoms, either gaining or sharing electrons to achieve a stable state. Whenever two or more atoms bond together, they form a new larger particle called a *molecule*. A molecule of hydrogen (H_2) is stable because of the sharing of each atom's single electron. The shared arrangement, in essence, fills the first (outer) shell of each atom (Fig. 3-3). Such a union between atoms is referred to as a *covalent*[4] *bond*. The most common molecule formed with hydrogen is water. Water is composed of two hydrogen atoms plus a single oxygen atom (H_2O). This stable molecule, like hydrogen gas (H_2), also forms by virtue of electron sharing (Fig. 3-4). Water is the most abundant inorganic compound found in the body, making up approximately two thirds or more of the total body mass.

Other molecules are formed through the giving up or taking on of electrons. Sodium chloride is an example of such a molecule. As separate atoms, the sodium atom has one electron in its outer shell, where the chlorine atom has seven electrons in its outer shell. To achieve a stable state, the sodium atom tends to give up the single electron from its outer shell. The chlorine atom, on the other hand,

---

[4]Covalent (ko-va′lent): derived from the prefix co- [together/jointly] + [L. *valere,* to be strong].

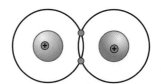

FIGURE 3-3   Hydrogen molecule.

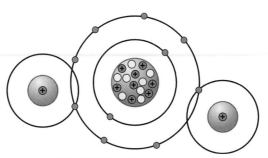

FIGURE 3-4   Water molecule.

must gain an electron to become stable. When these atoms react, the sodium atom gives up the electron to the chlorine atom. Now, however, the electron-proton ratio in each atom is no longer equal (i.e., 1:1). The sodium atom has one more proton than electrons and the chlorine atom has one more electron than protons. This gives a net positive charge to the sodium atom and a net negative charge to the chlorine atom. You've heard the saying, "Opposites attract." Well, these atoms with opposite electrical charges are attracted to each other and are united in an electrovalent bond, known as a sodium chloride molecule (salt) (Fig. 3-5).

Electrolytes are salts, acids, or bases that dissociate (separate) into *ions*[5] in body fluids. Sodium chloride (NaCl) is an example of a salt. When NaCl is dissolved in water, it releases sodium ions (Na^+) and chloride ions (Cl^-). In the body, we refer to these ions as electrolytes. Electrolytes affect many body functions. Salts, like NaCl, tend to attract water, which has an impact on the *hydration*[6] of the body. Other electrolytes, depending on their interaction with hydrogen, form acids and bases. Bases are compounds that combine with hydrogen ions (H^+) in solution, like bicarbonate (HCO_3^-). Acids are compounds that release hydrogen ions in solution. The acid–base balance (pH) of the body is determined by the numbers of hydrogen ions (H^+) versus bicarbonate ions (HCO_3^-). A delicate balance of electrolytes must exist, even at the cellular level, for the body to function properly. Certain electrolytes are critical for very specific body functions. For

---

[5]Ions are electrically charged atoms or molecules in solution. These atoms have become electrically charged by either gaining or losing electrons. Ions with a positive charge are referred to as *cations* and ions with a negative charge are referred to as *anions*.
[6]Hydr(o)- is a combining form meaning "water."

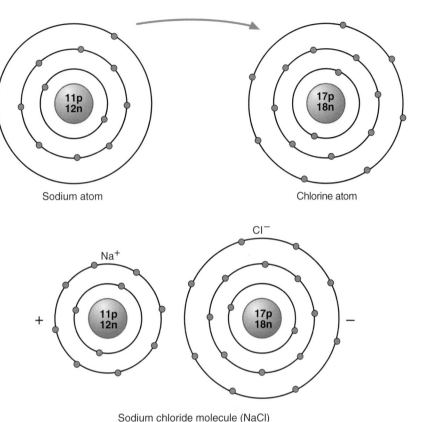

Sodium atom

Chlorine atom

Sodium chloride molecule (NaCl)

FIGURE 3-5 Sodium chloride molecule.

instance, neural impulses occur because of the net exchange of intracellular (K^+) ions and extracellular (Na^+) ions. "For every action, there is an equal and opposite reaction."[7] Consequently, changes in the body, even at the atomic or molecular level, have an effect on the overall function and well-being of the whole animal.

Various molecules combine to form a diverse array of compounds in the body. *Amino acids,* fundamental biologic compounds, are the "building blocks" for proteins. These amino acids are nothing more than large molecules composed of carbon, hydrogen, oxygen, and nitrogen atoms. As various amino acids join together in chains, they form proteins. Most cellular structures are formed from various proteins. The most fundamental molecular compounds for cells are the nucleic acids, which contain phosphorus in addition to C, H, O, and N. The two major types of nucleic acids are *ribonucleic acid* (RNA) and *deoxyribonucleic acid* (DNA). DNA molecules store cellular information in a kind of molecular code, unique to the given cell. For more information regarding cellular anatomy and physiology, refer to Chapter 2. As stated in Chapter 2, cells are the smallest functional units of the body. *En masse,* cells make up the tissues of the body. It is quite a wonder that from individual, seemingly invisible atoms and molecules, they

---

[7]Quote by physicist, Sir Isaac Newton.

combine to form complex, fully unique, functional cells, tissues, and organs. The organized, critically arranged tissues and organs ultimately give us the very visible, tangible, living body of an animal. Amazing when you think about it, isn't it?

Body Tissues

Body tissues are formed by numerous cells. Each of the major tissue types serves a particular function for the organ that it is associated with. The following are major tissue types found in domestic animals. Understanding the structure and function of the various tissues permits us to predict consequences and potential healing time when they are damaged.

Epithelial Tissue

In general, *epithelial tissue* covers all body surfaces, inside and out. It covers all organs, forms the inner lining of body cavities, and lines hollow organs. Epithelial tissue is anchored to underlying connective tissue by a thin basement membrane. The tightly packed structure of epithelium provides an excellent protective barrier for underlying tissues and structures. If epithelial tissue is damaged, it has the capacity to regenerate rapidly to repair the wounded area. Surprisingly, most epithelial tissues do not have a direct blood supply. They receive nourishment by means of nutrients that diffuse from underlying connective tissues.

Epithelial tissues are classified according to the various shapes, arrangements, and functions of their cells. For example, those epithelial tissues composed of single layers of cells are called *simple;* those arranged in layers are called *stratified;* those that appear to be arranged in layers but actually are not are called *pseudostratified*[8]; those composed of thin, flattened cells are called *squamous;* those composed of cube-like cells are called *cuboidal;* and those that are composed of tall, elongated cells are called *columnar.* Each type of epithelium is suited to a particular purpose.

Stratified squamous epithelium is made up of many layers, making it relatively thick (Fig. 3-6). The cells near the surface are flattened. Deeper into the tissue layers (i.e., near the basement membrane), the cells are usually cuboidal in shape. It is in these deeper layers that *mitosis* takes place. As the new cells grow and reproduce, they push the older cells toward the surface. The transitional cells tend to flatten out as they progress toward the surface. When they finally reach the surface, they are true squamous epithelium. Stratified squamous epithelium provides an excellent barrier against *pathogenic*[9] organisms. Areas that contain abundant stratified squamous epithelium include the surface of the skin and the inner surface of the urinary bladder.

Simple squamous epithelium is a thin layer of flattened cells that are interlocked, much like tongue and groove or lap joints used in carpentry (Fig. 3-7). It is designed to permit diffusion of some substances. For instance, simple

---

[8]The prefix pseudo- (su'do) means "false."
[9]Pathogenic is derived from path(o)- [disease] + gen(o)- [producing] + -ic [pertaining to].

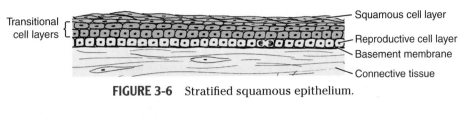

Transitional cell layers

Squamous cell layer
Reproductive cell layer
Basement membrane
Connective tissue

FIGURE 3-6   Stratified squamous epithelium.

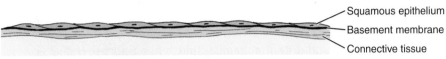

Squamous epithelium
Basement membrane
Connective tissue

FIGURE 3-7   Simple squamous epithelium.

squamous epithelium forms the walls of air sacs in the lungs and the walls of capillaries. Both of these structures must permit diffusion of O_2 and CO_2. Simple squamous epithelium may also be found lining body cavities and vessels. The term *endothelium* is usually used when referring to simple squamous epithelium that lines the interior of blood vessels and lymphatic vessels. Because it is so thin and delicate, simple squamous epithelium is easily damaged.

Simple cuboidal epithelium consists of a single layer of cube-shaped cells (Fig. 3-8). This type of tissue is frequently found in glands and lining the tubules of such organs as the kidneys and the liver. Cuboidal cells generally aid with functions of absorption or secretion. For instance, in glands, these cells are concerned with secretion of glandular products. Along areas of the kidney tubules, cuboidal cells are concerned with absorption of compounds such as water.

Simple columnar epithelium consists of a single layer of cells that are taller than they are wide (Fig. 3-9). It is found in various regions of the body, such as the stomach and intestines. It serves functions similar to those of the cuboidal epithelium. For instance, some columnar epithelial cells of the intestines are very active in the absorption of nutrients, whereas others may be responsible for secreting substances such as mucus.

Pseudostratified columnar epithelium may appear to be layered, but it is not. It appears to be layered because the nuclei of the cells are located at various levels throughout the tissue (Fig. 3-10). Pseudostratified columnar epithelium is commonly found lining certain areas of the body, such as the respiratory tract. Many of these columnar cells are *ciliated*.[10] In the respiratory tract, the cilia help move mucus up and out of the airways.

Connective Tissue

Connective tissue is found throughout the body. It connects structures together, providing support and protection. Unlike epithelial cells, connective tissue cells are farther apart from one another. Between them lies an abundant matrix of

---

[10]Cilia are hair-like projections from the free (exposed) cell wall. They usually provide motion.

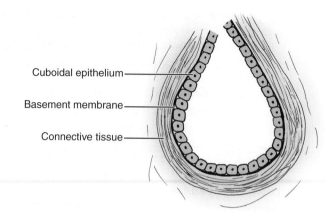

FIGURE 3-8   Simple cuboidal epithelium.

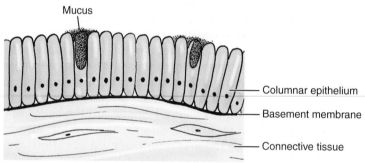

FIGURE 3-9   Simple columnar epithelium.

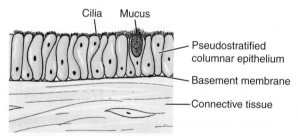

FIGURE 3-10   Pseudostratified columnar epithelium.

fibers or other such substances. Many connective tissues have an abundant blood supply. Types of connective tissue are classified according to their basic structural characteristics. Some of the major types of connective tissue are discussed in this section.

Fibrous connective tissue is a very dense tissue composed of many tightly packed, thick collagen fibers and fine elastic fibers. The collagen fibers are very tough and can withstand extreme forces of pulling. That is why this tissue is crucial in holding bones together (e.g., ligaments) and providing attachments of muscles to bones (e.g., tendons). It is also found in the deeper layers of the skin (i.e., dermis).

Elastic connective tissue is composed primarily of elastic tissue fibers, in addition to some collagenous fibers. As its name implies, it provides elasticity to the structures it forms. It is found predominantly in hollow internal organs and in vessel walls. Elastin is also found in the skin, giving it tremendous flexibility.

Loose connective tissue is a more delicate type of connective tissue. It generally forms thin membranes throughout the body, like the basement membrane that anchors epithelium to underlying tissues. Loose connective tissue provides a loose, flexible attachment of the skin to underlying tissues and organs (e.g., subcutaneous tissue). It is also found between muscles and in other spaces between organs. A specialized form of loose connective tissue is *adipose tissue,* commonly referred to as fat. Specialized cells that make up adipose tissue store fat droplets in their cytoplasm.

Cartilage is a somewhat rigid form of connective tissue. Unlike other types of connective tissue, cartilage does not have a direct blood supply. It receives nutrients from other surrounding connective tissues that do have abundant blood supplies. Cartilage is found in abundance in joints formed between bones. In such areas, the cartilage provides a smooth joint surface, protecting the underlying bone.

Bone is the most dense, rigid type of connective tissue. The hardness of bone results from the presence of minerals and mineral salts in its matrix. Bones provide support for muscles and other body tissues and organs. They provide protection for *viscera*—for example, the rib cage protects the thoracic viscera and the skull protects the brain.

Muscle Tissue

Muscle tissue is subdivided into three different types: *smooth muscle, cardiac muscle,* and *skeletal muscle.* Unlike other types of tissue, muscle tissue has the capacity to contract and relax, changing the given muscle's overall length from one moment to the next. A description of each type of muscle tissue follows.

Smooth muscle (Fig. 3-11) is typically associated with unconscious, involuntary muscular activity. It is found predominantly in the walls of hollow organs, such as the stomach, intestines, blood vessels, and urinary bladder. It is called smooth muscle because its cells lack *striations* (stripes).

Cardiac muscle (Fig. 3-12), like smooth muscle, is also under unconscious, involuntary control. Cardiac muscle is found only in the heart. Its cells are striated and uniquely joined together end to end. These specialized intercellular junctions *(intercalated discs; in"ter-ka'la-ted)* are found only in cardiac muscle and give this muscle extraordinary strength and contractile ability.

Skeletal muscle (Fig. 3-13) is composed of billions of *myocytes* (also called muscle fibers). Each myocyte (Fig. 3-14) has a long, thin, cylindrical shape with rounded ends and numerous nuclei along its length. The rounded ends of the myocytes are attached to fibrous connective tissue. Inside each myocyte are long, thin, thread-like structures called *myofibrils (mi"o-fi'brilz).* These myofibrils are tightly packed and lie parallel to one another, much like the wires within an electrical cord. Unlike wire, however, the myofibrils are very elastic and have

Nuclei

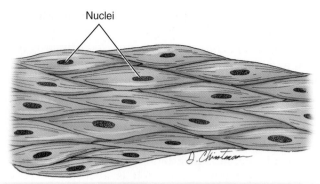

FIGURE 3-11   Smooth muscle tissue.

Intercalated discs   Nuclei

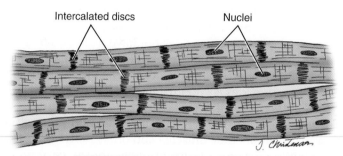

FIGURE 3-12   Cardiac muscle tissue.

Striations   Nuclei

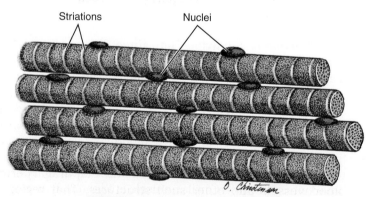

FIGURE 3-13   Skeletal muscle tissue.

tremendous contractile ability. When a myocyte is stimulated by a nerve, the myofibrils inside it synchronously contract. When the nervous stimulation is removed, the myofibrils relax. Numerous muscle fibers are bundled together with fibrous connective tissue. An actual muscle is made up of innumerable bundles of muscle fibers. Muscles are separated from one another by sheets of fibrous connective tissue called *fascia (fash'e-ah)*. The fascia surrounding a muscle extends beyond the ends of the muscle to form the cord-like attachments to the bones (i.e., *tendons*).

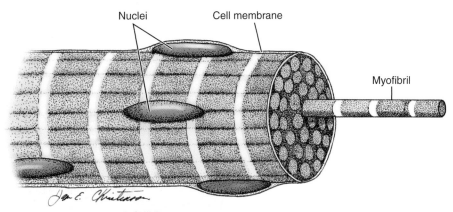

Nuclei   Cell membrane

Myofibril

FIGURE 3-14   Myocyte.

Neural Tissue

Neural tissue is found in the brain, spinal cord, and peripheral nerves. It is composed of nerve cells or *neurons,* which are highly specialized cells responsible for transmitting neuroelectrical impulses. Neurons are supported by other specialized cells and connective tissues. These are discussed in more detail in Chapter 9. Nerves are a collection of bundles of neurons. They transmit impulses to and from the brain and spinal cord and all areas of the body, eliciting various responses from the target organs (e.g., muscle contraction).

Body Cavities

Domestic animals have three principal body cavities (Fig. 3-15). The *cranial vault,* formed by the bones of the cranium, houses the brain. The *thoracic cavity* contains *visceral* components, such as the heart and the lungs. The thoracic cavity is also referred to as the pleural cavity. Finally, the abdominal or peritoneal cavity is the most caudal cavity of the body. *Abdominal viscera* include such organs as the liver, stomach, intestines, and urinary bladder. The thoracic and abdominal cavities are separated by a large muscle called the *diaphragm.* Only a small region of the diaphragm permits passage of major blood vessels and other such structures. That region is called the *hiatus (hi-a'tus).*

Organs and Organ Systems

The body is organized into larger functional collections of tissues and organs. Although each organ system is discussed separately in detail in subsequent chapters, we should remember that all organ systems function interdependently. They each have principal tasks they must carry out, but they must do it without disturbing the normal function of other organ systems. Honestly, as a colleague of mine is so fond of pointing out, the only time body systems can be completely separated

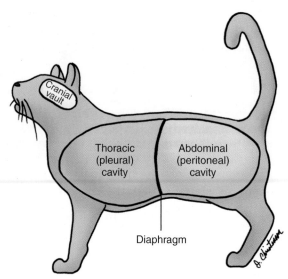

FIGURE 3-15 Principal body cavities of domestic animals.

is on the necropsy[11] table. The specific organ systems and their principal functions (to be discussed later) are summarized in the following list.

1. The *hematopoietic system* is made up of the blood and blood-forming tissues.
2. The *lymphatic system* is composed of a network of vessels and glands that are largely responsible for immunity within the body. It is also responsible for the movement of interstitial[12] fluids back into general circulation.
3. The *musculoskeletal system*, formed of bones, muscles, and connective tissues, provides for the overall structure and movement of the body.
4. The *cardiovascular system*, composed of the heart and blood vessels, provides continual circulation of the blood.
5. The *respiratory system*, consisting of airways running from the nose to the lungs, provides for the needed exchange of gases like O_2 and CO_2.
6. The *neurologic system*, made up of the brain, spinal cord, and peripheral nerves, controls many of the other organ systems with neuroelectrical input.
7. The *alimentary system*, or digestive system, provides for the intake of nutrients for the body and disposal of some wastes.
8. The *urinary system*, including the kidneys and urinary bladder, is also critical for the removal of toxic wastes from the body, as well as the maintenance of water and electrolyte balance.
9. The *reproductive system* provides the means for animals to propagate their species (i.e., reproduce).

---

[11]Necropsy is derived from *necr(o)-* [death] + *-opsy* [viewing]; i.e., an animal's "autopsy."
[12]Interstitial *(in"ter-stish'al)* is derived from *inter-* [between] + *sistere* [to set] + *-al* [pertaining to]. It refers to the spaces between tissues.

10. The *endocrine system,* composed of various glands, provides chemical (hormonal) control over many body functions.
11. The *integumentary system* is made up of the largest organ of the body, the skin, and its associated structures.

Homeostasis

Each of the body's organs/organ systems must carry out specific functions. However, their function must not disturb *homeostasis.* All of the organ systems must function *synergistically* to maintain a balanced, normal state for the body. Whenever a portion of the body deviates from the homeostatic state, disease will result. As stated earlier, the various body systems each are discussed in detail later in this text. Although diseases may be discussed in relation to a given body system, one must remember that disease in any one body system will, to one degree or another, have an impact on the rest of the body. Fortunately, the body has built-in mechanisms that attempt to correct abnormalities, to bring the whole body back into a state of homeostasis. At times, these mechanisms may be efficient enough to provide for the *symbiotic* relationship between domestic animals and other organisms. For example, in the digestive tract of an animal are many *commensal (kŏ-men'sal,* cf. symbiotic) microorganisms, such as bacteria. The digestive tract provides an environment suitable to support life for the bacteria, while the bacteria aid in the digestion of food for the animal without causing disease. If these same bacteria were somehow to gain entry to areas of the body other than the digestive tract, disease would likely result. Veterinary professionals must acquire knowledge of normal physiology, as well as *pathophysiology.* The understanding of how domestic animals function in health and disease will guide the medical decisions and therapies given to veterinary patients. Our ultimate goals are to restore and to maintain homeostasis in our patients.

SELF-TEST

Using the previous information in this chapter, complete the following crossword puzzle using the most appropriate medical term(s).

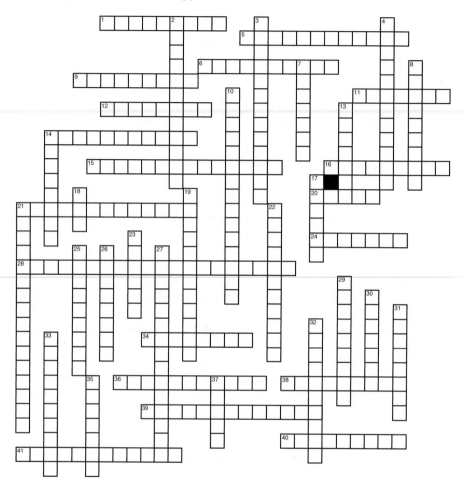

ACROSS

1   The body system whose glands exert hormonal control over other organs and tissues
5   Pertaining to the space between tissues
6   The digestive system
9   The condition or state of water content in the body, influenced by salts, like NaCl
11   A compound that contains carbon
12   Two or more atoms bonded together
14   A compound, such as salt, that dissociates into ions in body fluids
15   The body system made up of the heart and blood vessels
16   The relationship in which two organisms live together, mutually benefiting each other

20	Stable elements, like helium and argon, whose outermost shell is filled to capacity with electrons
21	A chart of elements, containing each element's symbol, atomic number, and atomic weight (2 words)
24	The body system containing the kidneys and bladder
28	DNA (2 words)
34	A type of molecular bond in which two atoms share an electron
36	The balanced, stable state of the body
38	A compound that does not contain carbon
39	The body system responsible for blood formation
40	Body cavity containing the digestive viscera; cf. peritoneal cavity
41	The body cavity that houses the brain (2 words)

DOWN

2	The body system that permits males and females of a species to bear young
3	The body system containing the largest organ of the body, the skin
4	The process of disease production
7	A specialized type of loose connective tissue composed of cells that store fat in their cytoplasm
8	The state of working together
10	RNA (2 words)
13	A muscle cell
14	A small, almost weightless, negatively charged particle that is in constant motion around the nucleus of an atom
17	The region of the diaphragm through which major vessels pass between the pleural and peritoneal cavities
18	An electrically charged atom or molecule in solution
19	Pertaining to nerve study
21	A type of columnar epithelium that gives the false impression of being layered but it is not
22	The body system made up of the airways and lungs
23	A positively charged nuclear atomic particle
25	The body system that provides for immunity and the movement of interstitial fluids
26	Pertaining to organs
27	The body system made of bones and muscles
29	The study of disease
30	A nuclear atomic particle that has neither a positive nor a negative charge but adds to the atomic weight
31	Pertaining to the thorax or chest
32	Complex, fundamental molecules of carbon, oxygen, hydrogen, and nitrogen that are referred to as the building blocks of proteins (2 words)
33	Pertaining to epithelium
35	Another name for the thoracic cavity
37	Tiny, invisible particles, from which all matter is made

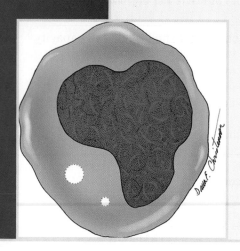

CHAPTER 4

The Hematopoietic System

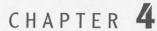

GOALS AND OBJECTIVES

By the conclusion of this chapter, the student will be able to:

1. Recognize common root words, prefixes, and suffixes related to blood.
2. Divide simple and compound words into their respective parts.
3. Recognize, correctly pronounce, and appropriately use common medical terms related to blood.
4. Demonstrate an understanding of the composition of blood.
5. Recognize basic morphologic characteristics of normal blood cells.
6. Demonstrate an understanding of the basic physiology of hematopoiesis and the function of each major constituent of the blood, including hemostasis and specific cell types.
7. Demonstrate a basic understanding of hematology, including the clinical determination of the packed cell volume (PCV), total protein (TP), and morphologic evaluation of blood smears.
8. Recognize common red blood cell shape changes.

INTRODUCTION TO RELATED TERMS

Divide each of the following terms into its respective parts ("R," root; "P," prefix; "S," suffix; "CV," combining vowel).

1. **Hematology** (n.)   (R) _____ (CV) _____ (S) _____
   hematology (hēm'ah-tol"o-je; the study of blood)

2. **Morphology** (n.)   (R) _____ (CV) _____ (S) _____
   morphology (mor-fol'o-je; the study of form)

3. **Erythrocyte** (n.)   (P) _____ (CV) _____ (S) _____
   erythrocyte (e-rith'ro-sīt; a red cell; clinically refers to red blood cells)

4. **Reticulocyte** (n.)   (R) _____ (CV) _____ (S) _____
   reticulocyte (re-tik′u-lo-sĭt″; a "net" cell; clinically refers to a young red blood cell
   containing remnant ribosomes and endoplasmic reticulum)

5. **Polychromasia** (n.)   (P) _____ (R) _____ (S) _____
   polychromasia (pol″e-kro-ma′ze-ah; a condition of many colors; clinically refers
   to erythrocytes with varied staining qualities)

6. **Anisocytosis** (n.)   (P) _____ (CV) _____ (R) _____
                                   (CV) _____ (S) _____
   anisocytosis (an-e″so-si-to′sis; a condition of unequal cells; clinically refers to size
   variations of red blood cells)

7. **Anemia** (n.)   (P) _____ (R) _____ (S) _____
   anemia (ah-ne′me-ah; a condition without blood; clinically refers to a deficiency
   of erythrocytes and/or hemoglobin)

8. **Pancytopenia** (n.)   (P) _____ (R) _____ (CV) _____ (S) _____
   pancytopenia (pan″si-to-pe′ne-ah; a deficiency of all cells; clinically refers to a deficiency
   of all blood cells)

9. **Leukocyte** (n.)   (P) _____ (CV) _____ (S) _____
   leukocyte (lu′ko-sīt; a white cell; clinically refers to white blood cells)

10. **Leukopenia** (n.)   (P) _____ (CV) _____ (S) _____
    leukopenia (lu″ko-pe′ne-ah; a deficiency of white; clinically refers to a deficiency of white
    blood cells)

11. **Leukocytosis** (n.)   (P) _____ (CV) _____ (R) _____
                                    (CV) _____ (S) _____
    leukocytosis (lu″ko-si-to′sis; a condition of white cells; clinically refers to increased
    numbers of white blood cells)

12. **Neutropenia** (n.)   (P) _____ (CV) _____ (S) _____
    neutropenia (nu″tro-pe′ne-ah; a deficiency of neutrophils; clinically refers to decreased
    numbers of neutrophilic leukocytes in the blood)

13. **Basophilic** (adj.)   (P) _____ (CV) _____ (R) _____ (S) _____
    basophilic (ba-so-fil′ik; pertaining to blue affinity; clinically refers to things that stain
    readily with basic or blue dyes)

14. **Eosinophilia** (n.)   (P) _____ (CV) _____ (R) _____ (S) _____
    eosinophilia (e″o-sin″o-fil′e-ah; a condition of red affinity; clinically refers to increased
    numbers of eosinophilic leukocytes in the blood)

15. **Lymphocytosis** (n.)   (R) _____ (CV) _____ (R) _____
                                     (CV) _____ (S) _____
    lymphocytosis (lim″fo-si-to′sis; a condition of lymph cells; clinically refers to increased
    numbers of lymphocytic leukocytes in the blood)

16. **Monocytosis** (n.)   (P) _____ (R) _____ (CV) _____ (S) _____
    monocytosis (mon″o-si-to′sis; a condition of one cell; clinically refers to increased numbers
    of monocytic leukocytes in the blood)

17. **Polymorphonuclear** (adj.)   (P) _____   (R) _____   (CV) _____
    (R) _____   (S) _____
    polymorphonuclear (pol″e-mor″fo-nu′kle-ar; pertaining to a multishaped nucleus)

18. **Thrombocyte** (n.)   (R) _____   (CV) _____   (S) _____
    thrombocyte (throm′bo-sīt; a clot cell; clinically refers to blood platelets)

19. **Hemostasis** (n.)   (R) _____   (CV) _____   (S) _____
    hemostasis (he″mo-sta′sis; the process of blood stoppage [i.e., the process of clotting])

20. **Thrombus** (n.)   (R) _____   (S) _____
    thrombus (throm′bus; a clot)

21. **Phagocyte** (n.)   (R) _____   (CV) _____   (S) _____
    phagocyte (fag′o-sīt; an eating cell; clinically refers to leukocytes that ingest foreign organisms and particles)

22. **Macrophage** (n.)   (P) _____   (CV) _____   (S) _____
    macrophage (mak′ro-faj; a large eater; clinically refers to phagocytic leukocytes found wandering outside the bloodstream, in the tissues of the body)

23. **Anticoagulant** (n.)   (P) _____   (R) _____   (S) _____
    anticoagulant (an″ti-ko-ag′u-lant; one that is against clotting; clinically refers to any chemical agent that prevents clotting of blood)

24. **Hemolysis** (n.)   (R) _____   (CV) _____   (S) _____
    hemolysis (he-mol′ĭ-sis; the process of destroying blood; clinically refers to lysis or breakage of erythrocytes)

25. **Hemorrhage** (n.)   (R) _____   (CV) _____   (S) _____
    hemorrhage (hem′or-ij; blood escaping; i.e., bleeding)

26. **Hematoma**[1] (n.)   (R) _____   (S) _____
    hematoma (he″mah-to′mah; a blood swelling; clinically refers to a localized accumulation of blood between tissues or tissue layers, due to a break in a blood vessel)

27. **Hematocrit** (n.)   (R) _____   (CV) _____   (S) _____
    hematocrit (he-mat′o-krit; to separate blood)

28. **Megakaryocyte** (n.)   (P) _____   (R) _____   (CV) _____   (S) _____
    megakaryocyte (meg″ah-kar′e-o-sīt; a large nucleated cell; clinically refers to a cell found in the bone marrow that contains a very large nucleus and from which platelets are formed)

29. **Poikilocytosis** (n.)   (R) _____   (CV) _____   (R) _____
    (CV) _____   (S) _____
    poikilocytosis (poi″kĭ-lo-si-to′sis; a condition of varied/irregular cells; clinically refers to varied shapes of erythrocytes)

30. **Hypoproteinemia** (n.)   (P) _____   (R) _____   (R) _____   (S) _____
    hypoproteinemia (hi″po-pro″tĭ-ne′me-ah; a condition of deficient protein of the blood; below normal plasma proteins)

---

[1]Note that the suffix -oma usually denotes the presence of a tumor. The suffix -oma is thought to have been originally adapted from the Greek word *onkoma,* meaning "a swelling." In the case of the word hematoma, the suffix meaning is derived from this early interpretation.

31. **Lipemia** (n.)   (R) _____ (R) _____ (S) _____
    lipemia (li-pe'me-ah; a condition of fat blood; clinically refers to an excess of fats or lipids in the blood, giving a milky appearance to the blood and plasma)

32. **Leukemia** (n.)   (P) _____ (R) _____ (S) _____
    leukemia (lu-ke'me-ah; a condition of white blood; clinically refers to malignancy of the blood-forming tissues, resulting in excessive numbers of abnormal leukocytes in the blood)

33. **Bilirubinemia** (n.)   (R) _____ (R) _____ (S) _____
    bilirubinemia (bil"ĭ-roo-bĭ-ne'me-ah; a condition of bilirubin blood; bilirubin is a bile pigment produced by the breakdown of hemoglobin in erythrocytes; bilirubinemia indicates excesses of bilirubin in the circulating blood)

34. **Icteric** (adj.)   (R) _____ (S) _____
    icteric (ik-ter'ik; pertaining to icterus; jaundice)

35. **Rubriblast** (n.)   (R) _____ (CV) _____ (R) _____
    rubriblast (roo'brĭ-blast; a red germ ["seed"]; clinically refers to the youngest form of erythrocytes, found only in the bone marrow)

36. **Prorubricyte** (n.)   (P) _____ (R) _____ (CV) _____ (S) _____
    prorubricyte (pro-roo'brĭ-sīt; an early red cell; clinically refers to a very young erythrocyte that is found in the bone marrow, the next stage of red cell development after the rubriblast)

37. **Rubricyte** (n.)   (R) _____ (CV) _____ (S) _____
    rubricyte (roo'brĭ-sīt; a red cell; clinically refers to a young erythrocyte)

38. **Metarubricyte** (n.)   (P) _____ (R) _____ (CV) _____ (S) _____
    metarubricyte (met"ah-roo'brĭ-sīt; a changed red cell; clinically refers to a young erythrocyte that is about to discharge its nucleus; it is the most frequently observed nucleated red blood cell in circulating blood)

39. **Myelocyte** (n.)   (R) _____ (CV) _____ (S) _____
    myelocyte (mi'ĕ-lo-sīt; a marrow cell; clinically refers to immature leukocytes that are generally found only in the bone marrow)

40. **Metamyelocyte** (n.)   (P) _____ (R) _____ (CV) _____ (S) _____
    metamyelocyte (met"ah-mi'-lo-sīt"; an after/changed marrow cell; clinically it is an immature leukocyte [neutrophil] that may be seen in peripheral blood in a patient with overwhelming disease)

41. **Prothrombin** (n.)   (P) _____ (R) _____ (S) _____
    prothrombin (pro-throm'bin; a before clot; clinically refers to clotting Factor II, which is a precursor to thrombin in the clotting cascade)

42. **Fibrinogen** (n.)   (R) _____ (CV) _____ (R) _____
    fibrinogen (fi-brin'o-jen; fiber producing; clinically refers to clotting Factor I, which is the precursor to fibrin [the protein fibers that form in a clot])

43. **Spherocyte** (n.)   (R) _____ (CV) _____ (S) _____
    spherocyte (sfe'ro-sīt; a ball cell; clinically it is an erythrocyte that is round rather than discoid, lacking a zone of central pallor)

44. **Stomatocyte** (n.)   (R) _____ (CV) _____ (S) _____
    stomatocyte (sto'mah-to-sīt; a mouth cell; clinically it is a poikilocytic erythrocyte that appears to have a "smiley face" centrally in the cell)

45. **Keratocyte** (n.)   (R) _____ (CV) _____ (S) _____
    keratocyte (ker'ah-to-sīt"; a horn cell; clinically it is a poikilocytic erythrocyte that appears to have horns)

46. **Echinocyte** (n.)   (R) _____ (CV) _____ (S) _____
    echinocyte (e-ki'no-sīt; a hedgehog cell; clinically it is a poikilocytic erythrocyte that appears spiney like a hedgehog)

47. **Acanthocyte** (n.)   (R) _____ (CV) _____ (S) _____
    acanthocyte (a-kan'tho-sīt; a thorn cell; clinically it is a poikilocytic erythrocyte that has multiple [usually only a few] irregularly placed projections)

48. **Schizocyte** (cf. schistocyte) (n.)   (R) _____ (CV) _____ (S) _____
    schizocyte (skiz'o-sīt; a divided cell); schistocyte (skis'to-sīt; a split cell; clinically both refer to a poikilocytic erythrocyte that has been torn into fragments)

49. **Myelodysplasia** (n.)   (R) _____ (CV) _____ (P) _____
                                     (R) _____ (S) _____
    myelodysplasia (mi"-ĕ-lo-dis-pla'se-ah; a condition of marrow malformation/poor development)

HEMATOPOIETIC ANATOMY AND PHYSIOLOGY

Whole Blood

Blood is composed of a liquid component *(plasma)* and a cellular component. If whole blood, mixed with an *anticoagulant,* were left to stand in a tube over a period of time, these two major components would separate (Fig. 4-1). The heavier cellular component containing *erythrocytes, leukocytes,* and *thrombocytes* would settle in the tube. The transparent plasma would be left at the top of the tube. The erythrocytes, being the heaviest of the cells, would settle to the bottom, while the leukocytes and thrombocytes would form a thin layer between the erythrocytes and the plasma. This thin layer of leukocytes and thrombocytes is often referred to as the *"buffy coat."* In clinical practice, the settling of cells is accelerated by the use of a *centrifuge* (sen-trĭ-fūj'). Whole blood is placed in a *hematocrit tube;* a clay plug in one end of the tube prevents the blood from escaping. The hematocrit tube is then placed into a centrifuge and spun at a very high rate of speed. The centrifugal force quickly forces the cells to the bottom (plugged end) of the hematocrit tube. The spun sample is removed from the centrifuge and measured. The measurement from the bottom to the top of the column of erythrocytes is called the *packed cell volume* (PCV; Fig. 4-2). The PCV, recorded as a percentage, is the percentage of erythrocytes compared with the total sample volume in the hematocrit tube (Fig. 4-3).

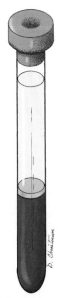

FIGURE 4-1   Whole blood components.

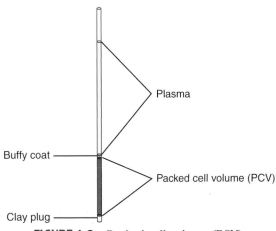

FIGURE 4-2   Packed cell volume (PCV).

Plasma is predominantly composed of water. Dissolved and suspended in that water are many proteins, lipids, sugars, and electrolytes. The concentration of these dissolved particles may be determined in many ways. One of the most frequently used tests is for the determination of *total protein* (TP). Because proteins are building blocks for cells, the concentration of plasma proteins reflects the general well-being of the body. Evaluation of the TP is simple. The column of plasma contained in a spun hematocrit tube is used for this determination. The plasma is placed on an instrument called a *refractometer* (re"frak-tom'et-er; so called because it uses the refraction of light through the sample to determine

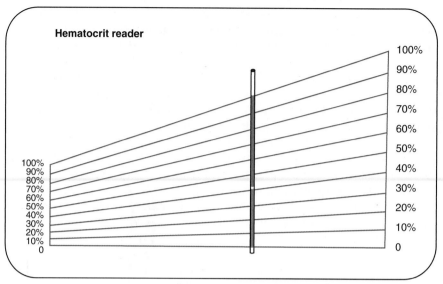

FIGURE 4-3   Spun hematocrit reading (PCV 40%).

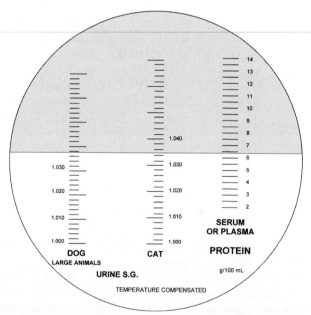

FIGURE 4-4   Total protein determination with a refractometer (TP 6.4 g/dL).

the concentration of all particles in a solution. Since the refractometer cannot distinguish between actual proteins versus other particles, some would refer to this instrument's determination as "Total Solids" or TS. For the purpose of this discussion, we'll refer to the end result as the TP). The greater the concentration of particles, the more the light will be refracted or bent. The TP is read where the light intersects a calibrated scale within the instrument (Fig. 4-4). Because the refractometer relies on refraction of light to measure plasma proteins, large extraneous elements that alter light refraction through the plasma will result in erroneous results. Some elements that may alter light refraction include free *hemoglobin* (he-mo-glo'bin) and lipids.

Plasma should be as free of these "contaminants" as possible, to ensure the accuracy of tests conducted. Consequently, whole blood specimens must be carefully handled during and after collection to prevent *hemolysis*. *Hemolyzed* specimens may render many test results invalid. Hemolyzed specimens may be quickly recognized because of the variable red discoloration of the plasma. The degree of discoloration depends on the amount of *hemoglobin* that is released into the plasma from destroyed erythrocytes. *Lipemic* samples, whose plasma appears cloudy and white, tend to hemolyze more easily. The plasma of lipemic, hemolyzed samples will appear cloudy and pink. Special processing of such a sample may be required to remove some of the lipids and to minimize hemolysis. If the sample cannot be analyzed because of the presence of the lipemia and hemolysis, another sample may need to be collected. Lipemia can be avoided in many cases by simply collecting blood specimens after the patient has fasted for an appropriate period of time. Finally, a plasma sample may appear *icteric,* because of *bilirubinemia*. Bilirubinemia may be indicative of serious disease processes, including intravascular hemolysis or liver disease. One must be aware of species differences with regard to plasma characteristics, especially if *icterus* is thought to be present. Horses, for example, tend to normally have a degree of yellow coloration to their plasma. This may make gross detection of icteric plasma difficult in equine patients.

Plasma analyses and the PCV are valuable pieces of laboratory data for determining the health or disease state of veterinary patients. Quantitation of erythrocyte, leukocyte, and thrombocyte numbers, as well as evaluation of their *morphology,* is also of great diagnostic value. This is where hematology can be exciting.

Blood Cells

Most of the blood cells are formed in the bone marrow by a process known as *hematopoiesis*. In general, only the more mature cells are found in the circulating blood. Those mature cells in normal domestic animals are the focus of the discussion in this chapter.

Erythrocytes originate in the bone marrow from *rubriblasts*. The kidney produces a hormone called *erythropoietin* that stimulates the bone marrow to produce erythrocytes. While in the bone marrow, the developing red blood cells are nuclear. They include, in order of maturity, the *prorubricyte,* the *rubricyte,* and the *metarubricyte,* with the metarubricyte being the most mature of those in the bone marrow. Just before being released from the bone marrow, the metarubricytes discard their nuclei. Therefore, erythrocytes in the circulating blood of most domestic animals are anuclear, biconcave, discoid cells (Fig. 4-5). The youngest of these in circulation may still contain portions of their rough endoplasmic reticulum; consequently they are called *reticulocytes*.

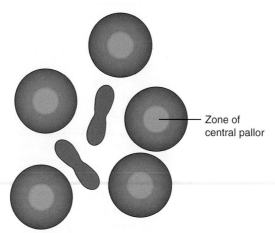

Zone of
central pallor

FIGURE 4-5   Erythrocytes in circulating blood.

Erythrocytes contain a protein compound called hemoglobin that is essential for the transport of oxygen and some carbon dioxide. The primary role of erythrocytes is to transport oxygen to the tissues of the body. A secondary role is to remove carbon dioxide from the tissues; however, most CO_2 is dissolved in the plasma for transport. It is the hemoglobin, when bound with oxygen, that gives the cells their red coloration. Hemoglobin when bound to carbon dioxide exhibits a darker bluish coloration, which may be seen grossly through the vessels and the skin of animals.

Laboratory *morphologic* evaluation of blood cells is important in determining the overall health status of the body. This morphologic evaluation is accomplished through making a smear of the patient's blood on a glass microscopic slide. *Eosinophilic* and *basophilic* stains are then applied to the dried blood smear to enhance morphologic characteristics of the cells. Mature erythrocytes accept the eosinophilic stains and, therefore, appear red on a blood smear. Less mature, newly released erythrocytes are somewhat larger *(macrocytic)* than fully mature erythrocytes and may stain with a slightly basophilic hue in addition to the red. This staining characteristic is reported clinically as *polychromasia*. *Anisocytosis* would also be noted in such a patient, as a result of the size variation between mature and immature erythrocytes (Fig. 4-6). *Polychromasia* and *reticulocytes* are indicative of the bone marrow's responsiveness. Special stains are required for reticulocyte counts, because routine staining of blood smears will not reveal the ribosomes and endoplasmic reticulum of these cells (Fig. 4-7). However, these young cells will appear *polychromatophilic* with routine staining. For any *anemic* patient (due to *hemorrhage* or *myelodysplasia*), the presence of polychromasia and reticulocytes are critical prognostic[2] observations. If they are present, the clinician will know that there is still a portion of functional bone marrow capable of responding to the body's needs.

---

[2]Prognostic from [Gr. *prognosis,* foreknowledge]; a prognosis is a forecast of an expected outcome.

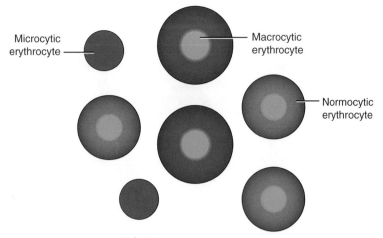

FIGURE 4-6   Anisocytosis.

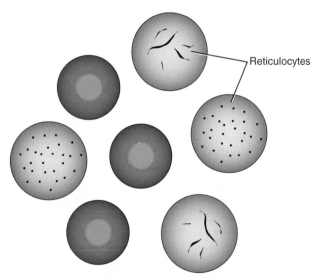

FIGURE 4-7   Reticulocytes.

Many different types of leukocytes are produced by the bone marrow. All are larger than erythrocytes. The three *granulocytes* are the *neutrophil,* the *basophil,* and the *eosinophil.* They are referred to as "granulocytes" because they each contain many cytoplasmic granules. Each specific cell name indicates the staining characteristics of the cytoplasmic granules of the cell type. The neutrophil is so named because its granules do not readily accept stain, giving them a neutral coloration. Basophils contain basophilic cytoplasmic granules. Last, eosinophils contain many eosinophilic cytoplasmic granules. In most domestic animals, the neutrophils make up the largest portion of the circulating leukocytes. *Agranular*[3] leukocytes are the *monocyte* and the *lymphocyte.* Each

[3]Agranular: A- (without) + granul(o)- + -ar; pertaining to without granules.

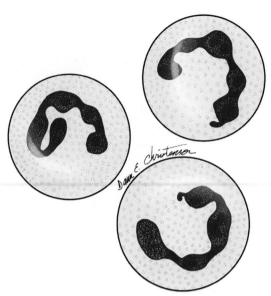

FIGURE 4-8   Neutrophils.

of these different leukocytes plays a somewhat different role in the fighting of disease.

Morphologically, **neutrophils** are *polymorphonuclear* (Fig. 4-8). That is to say, the nucleus of the neutrophil tends to take many shapes, but is usually very linear, curved, and somewhat lobulated. The nuclear chromatin of a mature neutrophil is very condensed, giving it a characteristic dark purple staining. The cytoplasm and granules are colorless to a very slight pink hue. This makes it difficult to visualize clearly distinct granules in the neutrophil, especially if the microscope is improperly illuminated. Neutrophils are important in ridding the body of foreign invaders. Their cytoplasmic granules contain potent enzymes, thus giving the neutrophil powerful phagocytic capabilities. Because of their important disease-fighting role, neutrophils tend to be the predominant leukocyte in many domestic animals.

The other important phagocyte is the **monocyte.** The monocyte is the largest of the leukocytes (Fig. 4-9). The nucleus tends to be large and potentially multilobed, with a very loose, lightly basophilic staining chromatin pattern. The abundant cytoplasm of the monocyte is a homogeneous, light grayish color. Although monocytes may contain vacuoles, this is a very unreliable criterion for cell identification. Functionally, both monocytes and neutrophils can slip through blood vessel walls to provide phagocytic services out in the tissues of the body. Once these cells have left the circulating blood, they are referred to as *macrophages*.

Eosinophils have only marginal phagocytic abilities. Like the neutrophils, they are polymorphonuclear. However, the eosinophil's nucleus characteristically stains lighter than that of the neutrophil. The eosinophilic staining granules are important in allergic reactions (Fig. 4-10). **Basophils** are morphologically similar to neutrophils and eosinophils. The basophilic staining

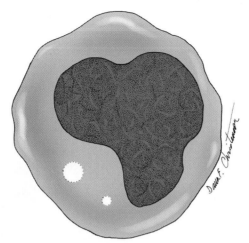

FIGURE 4-9   Monocyte.

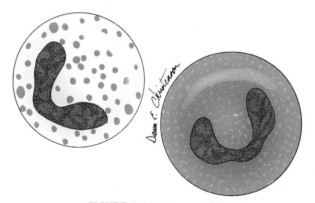

FIGURE 4-10   Eosinophils.

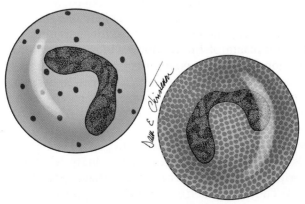

FIGURE 4-11   Basophils.

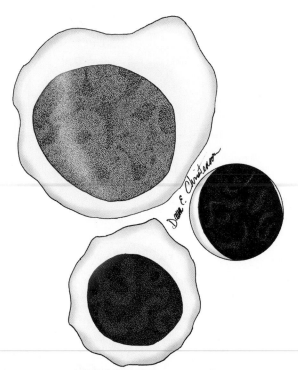

FIGURE 4-12   Lymphocytes.

granules of basophils are also important in allergic reactions (Fig. 4-11). Generally, basophils have fewer cytoplasmic granules than the other granulocytes, and their cytoplasm stains lightly basophilic.

Lymphocytes, depending on their age, may range in size from just smaller than a monocyte to just larger than an erythrocyte (Fig. 4-12). The younger the lymphocyte, the larger it is, and the older the lymphocyte, the smaller it is, with very little cytoplasm. The nuclear morphology tends to be round to ovoid, with varying degrees of chromatin density. The condensation and dark, basophilic staining qualities of the nucleus increase with the age of the lymphocyte. The cytoplasm is usually colorless, but may have a thin basophilic rim around its outer edges. Lymphocytes are important for body immunity and the production of *antibodies*. Antibodies are specialized proteins that, when attached to foreign invaders, help the body recognize and rid itself of the invaders. Antibodies and immunity will be discussed more in Chapter 5. In many ruminants, such as cattle and sheep, lymphocytes tend to predominate the leukocytic series.

Thrombocytes, or *platelets,* are actually nuclear fragments of large, specialized cells *(megakaryocytes)* that are found in the bone marrow. These fragments, in the peripheral blood, generally appear as mottled, lavender-staining objects (Fig. 4-13). They are much smaller than erythrocytes. As their name implies, thrombocytes are important for clot formation.

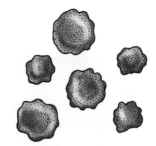

FIGURE 4-13   Thrombocytes.

Hemostasis

Hemostasis is the process by which *hemorrhage* is stopped. This happens in several stages. First, immediately after a blood vessel is injured, the smooth muscle in that vessel constricts. This constriction makes the lumen of the vessel much smaller, thereby slowing the flow of blood from the wound. The thrombocytes tend to stick to exposed connective tissues (collagen) surrounding the vessel. Platelets have kind of a "mob mentality." Once a few of them are activated, they'll get a whole crowd of platelets excited and activated. Soon, many platelets find themselves stuck to the edges of the wound and to each other, forming what is called a *platelet plug*. Until the platelet plug is formed, blood from a superficial vessel may ooze out under the intact skin, creating a *hematoma*. Once a stable platelet plug is formed, hemorrhage at the site stops. The plug alone is somewhat fragile and may be dislodged easily. Therefore, many of the plasma proteins (clotting factors), specifically designed for coagulation, also combine and form a strong matrix of fibers that secures the platelet plug at the wound site. Tissue *thromboplastins* are important for activating another concurrent portion of the coagulation cascade. Tissue thromboplastins are substances released from damaged cells. The more tissue damage, the more thromboplastins are released and the more explosive the coagulation. This is one big reason why crushing injuries don't tend to bleed as much as "clean" cuts. Twelve clotting factors in all are involved in the coagulation process. Whether stimulated by activated thrombocytes, by exposure to collagen and thromboplastins, or by stasis of blood flow, clotting factors are like dominoes. Knock over the first domino, and the sequence of falling won't end until the last domino falls. Well, in a normal animal, once the coagulation cascade is set in motion, it doesn't stop until a fibrin clot is formed. Most clotting factors are identified by number. A few, like prothrombin and fibrinogen, are named. As their names imply, these are the last couple of "dominoes" to "fall" before the thrombus is formed. The most abundant clotting factor in plasma is *fibrinogen*. The ultimate *thrombus* that is formed contracts with the healing wound and is dissolved over time.

These same clotting mechanisms can be used to our advantage in the laboratory. Many blood chemistry tests cannot be run on plasma or whole blood. For such tests, the whole blood specimen is placed into a plain (i.e., not containing anticoagulant) blood tube. The sample is left undisturbed for a period of time, permitting it to clot. As the plasma proteins coagulate, they trap all of the cells in the sample in the clot. The final clot can be easily removed from the sample. Any remaining cells can be centrifuged out, leaving the transparent liquid called *serum*. This serum may now be used for numerous serum chemistry tests. If one were to compare the TP of serum with that of plasma, serum would contain far less protein than the plasma. This makes sense, because many of the proteins (clotting factors) have been removed from the serum as a result of the clot formation.

Disease

Various diseases have different effects on the whole body, including the hematopoietic system. In general, one would expect the body to respond to the presence of pathogenic organisms by producing sufficient numbers of leukocytes to fight the invaders. Therefore, in many instances overwhelming numbers of white blood cells are released from the bone marrow, creating a *leukocytosis*. Once the pathogenic organisms are removed from the body, leukocyte numbers in the circulating blood return to normal. Some diseases, such as *feline panleukopenia,* make the body incapable of producing sufficient numbers of leukocytes to defend against the pathogenic organism. Cats with this disease cannot defend against the panleukopenia virus, and, because of the insufficient numbers of leukocytes, they cannot defend against secondary invading organisms such as bacteria. Other disease entities may affect only one specific cell type. For this reason, differential counts of the various cell types are important diagnostic tools. Concurrent changes in the numbers of the different leukocyte types may be indicative of specific disease conditions. Where a *neutropenia* with an accompanying *lymphocytosis* may indicate one disease, an *eosinophilia* and an accompanying *monocytosis* may indicate another. In simply looking at the neutrophil, much can be revealed about the significance of the disease state and the body's ability to appropriately respond to that disease. A mature neutrophilia may result from stress during the blood collection or be an early response to disease. If a disease begins to overwhelm the body and consume excessive numbers of mature neutrophils, immature neutrophils such as *bands*[4] and *metamyelocytes* may be released too early from the marrow. This is called a *"left shift."* (It is so called because as one looks at a chart showing the maturation sequence of neutrophils, myeloblasts are shown on the far left progressing to mature neutrophils on the far right.) The relationship of mature versus immature neutrophils in circulation offers prognostic information for the patient. Too many metamyelocytes with too few mature neutrophils may indicate that the patient is losing his battle with the disease. This inappropriate left shift could be likened to sending boys off to fight a man's war. *Myeloblasts* should never be seen in circulation. If seen, this finding usually indicates *leukemia*.

---

[4]A band is an immature neutrophil recognized by its linear nucleus with parallel sides and loose, lightly staining chromatin.

Neutrophil Maturation Sequence

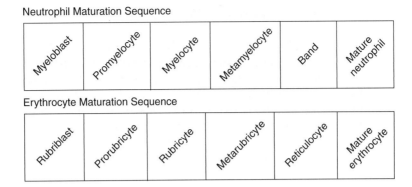

Myeloblast	Promyelocyte	Myelocyte	Metamyelocyte	Band	Mature neutrophil

Erythrocyte Maturation Sequence

Rubriblast	Prorubricyte	Rubricyte	Metarubricyte	Reticulocyte	Mature erythrocyte

Erythrocytes are also important indicators of disease conditions within veterinary patients. One would expect to see decreased numbers of erythrocytes on a blood smear from a patient with a *hemolytic anemia* or a patient with *hemorrhagic anemia*. Morphologically, the erythrocytes seen in the two types of anemia are quite different. Polychromasia and anisocytosis may be present in both types of anemia. However, the *poikilocytosis* (Fig. 4-14) present in the hemolytic anemia distinguishes it from a hemorrhagic anemia. Poikilocytosis, as well as bilirubinemia, are often a characteristic of hemolytic anemias. *Spherocytosis* is frequently observed in hemolytic anemias. Spherocytes result from macrophages in the spleen repairing damaged or diseased erythrocytes. *Schizocytes* are a common fragmentation change, resulting from the erythrocytes literally being ripped and torn by *fibrin* strands in the vasculature. This could be an indication of a severe *coagulopathy* and may warrant testing for *prothrombin, thrombin, fibrinogen,* and other essential clotting factors. *Keratocytosis* too may indicate a coagulopathy. However, keratocytes may also form from oxidative changes to the cell membrane or as an artifactual change to the anticoagulant EDTA.[5] Prekeratocytes are frequently referred to as "blister cells," because of the large pseudovacuole that forms just before the horn-like projections of the keratocyte. *Acanthocytosis,* with their 2 to 10 blunt, finger-like projections, may indicate a lipoprotein disorder. *Stomatocytes* may be a normal

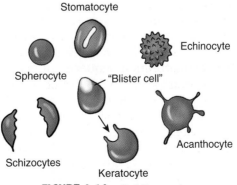

FIGURE 4-14 Poikilocytosis.

[5]EDTA means ethylenediaminetetraacetic acid.

macrocytic change due to the excessive cellular membrane of newly released erythrocytes. However, stomatocytosis in the absence of polychromasia may indicate a systemic problem, such as liver disease. Although *echinocytes* are often an artifactual change, they may also result from venomous snake bites. Recognizing these differences is important not only for determining a specific diagnosis but also for determining appropriate medical management of the patient. The medical management of these anemic patients is markedly different. It is through hematology that many diseases are identified, with painstaking gathering of minute clues that may be found only in the blood. Many of these clues can be detected only through microscopic evaluation of a peripheral blood smear.

SELF-TEST

Using the previous information in this chapter, complete the following crossword puzzle using the most appropriate medical term(s). Do not use abbreviations.

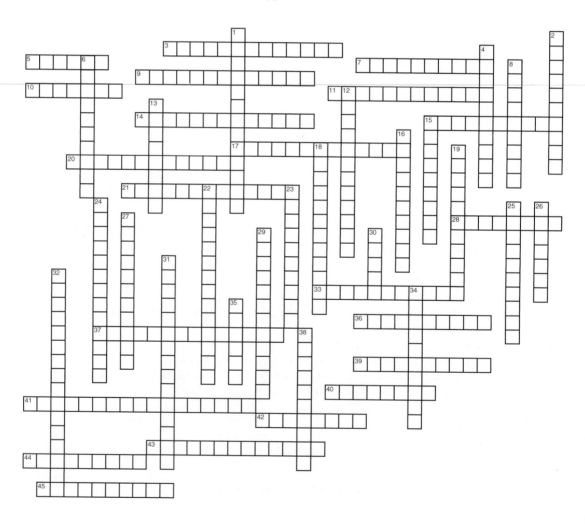

ACROSS

3	A chemical that prohibits clotting
5	The liquid component of whole blood that is made up predominantly of water
7	Bleeding
9	A condition of increased numbers of lymphocytes
10	Jaundiced
11	A deficiency of all cells
14	An immature erythrocyte nearly ready to lose its nucleus
15	Pertaining to a large cell
17	The cell from which platelets are formed
20	A deficiency of monocytes
21	The process of blood production
28	Malignancy of white blood cells
33	A clot cell
36	A granulocyte whose granules stain red
37	The hormone that stimulates bone marrow production of erythrocytes
39	An erythrocyte stem cell
40	A clot
41	Pertaining to a multishaped nucleus
42	A granulocyte whose granules stain blue
43	Excessive bilirubin in circulating blood
44	A white cell
45	A granulocyte whose granules do not readily accept stain

DOWN

1	Multiple staining qualities of erythrocytes
2	A "ball" cell
4	The study of blood
6	The study of form
8	The layer in a PCV tube that contains leukocytes and platelets (2 words)
12	Size variation of erythrocytes
13	A swelling of blood; for instance, under the skin
15	A marrow cell
16	To separate blood
18	An erythrocyte with remnants of its rough endoplasmic reticulum
19	A cell with granules
22	Shape changes of erythrocytes
23	A split cell; a fragmentation change of a red blood cell
24	An instrument that determines quantities of dissolved particles in solution by refraction, as in determining TP (TS)
25	The process of stopping bleeding
26	State of fatty blood
27	A red cell
29	An immature erythrocyte found in the bone marrow as the next stage of maturation beyond the stem cell
30	The liquid component of blood left over after the blood has clotted

31	Deficient blood protein
32	The percent of erythrocytes per total sample volume (3 words)
34	An instrument used to rapidly spin specimens to separate sample components
35	A condition of deficient erythrocytes
38	The protein within erythrocytes that transports oxygen

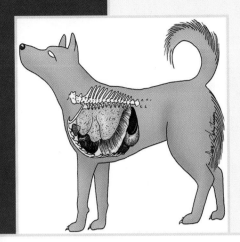

CHAPTER 5

The Lymphatic System

GOALS AND OBJECTIVES

By the conclusion of this chapter, the student will be able to:

1. Recognize common root words, prefixes, and suffixes related to the lymphatic system.
2. Divide simple and compound words into their respective parts.
3. Recognize, correctly pronounce, and appropriately use common medical terms related to the lymphatic system.
4. Demonstrate an understanding of the basic anatomy and physiology of the lymphatic system.
5. Demonstrate an understanding of the lymphatic system as it relates to edema formation.
6. Demonstrate an understanding of the basic role of the lymphatic system in immunity.

INTRODUCTION TO RELATED TERMS

Divide each of the following terms into its respective parts ("R," root; "P," prefix; "S," suffix; "CV," combining vowel).

1. **Lymphadenopathy** (n.)   (R) _____ (R) _____ (CV) _____ (S) _____
   lymphadenopathy (lim-fad″ĕ-nop′ah-the; disease of the lymph glands; often refers to enlarged lymph nodes)

2. **Splenic** (adj.)   (R) _____ (S) _____
   splenic (splen′ik; pertaining to the spleen)

3. **Lymphangitis** (n.)   (R) _____ (R) _____ (S) _____
   lymphangitis (lim″fan-ji′tis; inflammation of lymph vessels)

4. **Lymphocyte** (n.)   (R) _____ (CV) _____ (S) _____
   lymphocyte (lim′fo-sīt; a lymph cell)

5. **Splenomegaly** (n.)   (R) _____ (CV) _____ (S) _____
   splenomegaly (splĕ"no-meg'ah-le; a condition of splenic enlargement)

6. **Interstitial** (adj.)   (P) _____ (R) _____ (S) _____
   interstitial (in"ter-stish'al; pertaining to between tissues; cf. intercellular)

7. **Macrophage** (n.)   (P) _____ (CV) _____ (S) _____
   macrophage (mak'ro-faj; a large eater; clinically refers to large phagocytic cells)

8. **Phagocytosis** (n.)   (R) _____ (CV) _____ (R) _____ (S) _____
   phagocytosis (fag"o-si-to'sis; the process of cellular eating)

9. **Pathogenic** (adj.)   (R) _____ (CV) _____ (R) _____ (S) _____
   pathogenic (path-o-jen'ik; pertaining to disease production)

10. **Tonsillectomy** (n.)   (R) _____ (S) _____
    tonsillectomy (ton"sĭ-lek'to-me; cutting out the tonsils; clinically interpreted as surgical removal of the tonsils)

11. **Tonsillitis** (n.)   (R) _____ (S) _____
    tonsillitis (ton"sĭ-li'tis; inflammation of the tonsils)

12. **Lymphoid** (adj.)   (R) _____ (S) _____
    lymphoid (lim'foid; resembling lymph)

13. **Lymphoma** (n.)   (R) _____ (S) _____
    lymphoma (lim-fo'mah; a lymph tumor; a general term referring to a cancerous [usually malignant] disorder of lymphoid tissue)

14. **Immunogenic** (adj.)   (R) _____ (CV) _____ (R) _____ (S) _____
    immunogenic (im"u-no-jen'ik; pertaining to exemption producing; i.e., something that stimulates immunity; cf. antigenic [anti(body)+gen(o)-+-ic])

15. **Immunoglobulin** (n.)   (R) _____ (CV) _____ (R) _____ (S) _____
    immunoglobulin (im"u-no-glob'u-lin; an exempt globule/"blob"; i.e. an antibody)

16. **Inflammation** (n.)   (R) _____ (S) _____
    inflammation (in"flah-ma'shun; act of setting on fire; inflamed tissue is characterized by pain, heat, redness, swelling, and loss of function)

17. **Erythematous** (adj.)   (R) _____ (S) _____
    erythematous (er-ĭ-them'ah-tus; pertaining to "flush upon the skin," i.e., redness)

18. **Hyperemia** (n.)   (P) _____ (R) _____ (S) _____
    hyperemia (hi"per-e'me-ah; a condition of excessive blood; clinically this is an engorged area that appears reddened)

19. **Algesia** (n.)   (R) _____ (S) _____
    algesia (al-je'ze-ah; a condition of pain)

LYMPHATIC ANATOMY AND PHYSIOLOGY

General

The lymphatic system is composed of the tonsils, spleen, thymus (thi'mus), numerous glands, vessels, and cells that provide the body with *immunity* (resistance to disease) and destroy *pathogens*. The lymphatic system is also important for the constant transport of fluid (lymph) from the interstitial spaces to the general circulating blood.

Tonsils

The tonsils are made up of *lymphoid* tissue, but they are not referred to as lymph nodes. Anatomically, the two tonsils are located in the throat (one tonsil on each side, near the base of the tongue; Fig. 5-1). Unless a disease process is present to create *tonsillitis,* they are usually contained (hidden) within the *tonsillar crypts* in the throat. Therefore, during physical examination of a normal patient, the tonsils may not be visible. For those animals with persistent tonsillitis, such that it interferes with swallowing or breathing, a *tonsillectomy* may be performed.

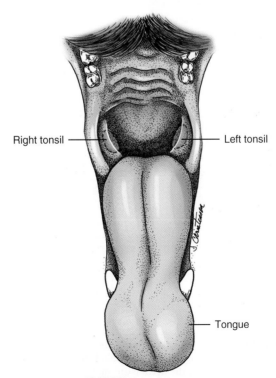

Right tonsil ———   ——— Left tonsil

——— Tongue

FIGURE 5-1   Tonsils.

Spleen

The spleen is a large, tongue-shaped organ located in the left craniodorsal abdominal cavity, closely associated with the stomach and protected by the caudal rib cage (Fig. 5-2). On routine physical examination, the spleen is not palpable in the abdomen unless *splenomegaly* exists. The spleen is very important for filtration of the blood. It is a highly vascular organ that contains many macrophages. *Splenic macrophages* repair or remove damaged red blood cells from circulation. The splenic macrophages are also very important for *phagocytosis* of *pathogenic* organisms found in the blood. In addition to filtration, the spleen also serves as a very important storage area for red blood cells. During times of hemorrhage or increased need for greater oxygen transport in the body, the spleen will eject some of its stored blood back into circulation.

Thymus

The thymus is a glandular lymphoid organ located in the *mediastinum*[1] of the cranioventral thoracic cavity (see Fig. 5-2). The thymus is extremely important for the maturation of specialized lymphocytes. The lymphocytes that mature

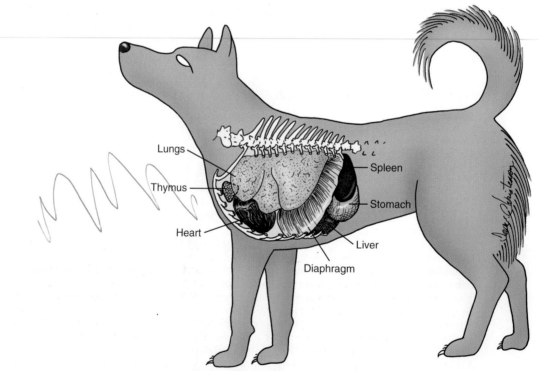

FIGURE 5-2   Thymus and spleen in situ (left ribs removed).

[1]Mediastinum (me″de-as-ti′num; n.); the mediastinum is a tissue found in the thoracic cavity that divides that cavity into right and left halves; mediastinal lymph nodes are located in multiple sites throughout the mediastinum. For more information regarding the mediastinum, see Chapter 8, "The Respiratory System."

in the thymus are critical for the production of *immunoglobulins* or *antibodies*. Antibodies are specialized proteins that help the body recognize *pathogenic* organisms, so that macrophages can destroy the *pathogens*. This process of literally turning pathogens into "useable food" for the macrophages is called *opsonization.*[2] Therefore, the thymus plays an integral role in the maintenance of immunity for the body. Interestingly, the thymus is quite large in young, developing animals. As animals age, the size and function of the thymus diminish. Consequently, the immune capabilities of very young and of geriatric animals is compromised. The very young have not yet produced sufficient amounts of immunoglobulins, and geriatric animals no longer have the capacity to maintain sufficient antibody levels. This leaves these patients very susceptible to disease. Immunity will be discussed in more detail later in this chapter.

Lymph Nodes and Vessels

Lymph glands (also called lymph nodes) are located throughout the body. Many of them are named by virtue of the region of the body in which they are located. For example, lymph nodes located in the axillary region are called axillary lymph nodes.[3] Those peripheral lymph nodes that are clinically important for physical examinations in small animal medicine are the axillary lymph nodes, the mandibular lymph nodes,[4] the cervical lymph nodes,[5] the prescapular lymph nodes,[6] the popliteal lymph nodes,[7] and the superficial inguinal lymph nodes[8] (Fig. 5-3). The mandibular, prescapular, and popliteal lymph nodes should always be palpated during a physical examination of a small animal patient. Although palpation of the axillary, cervical, superficial inguinal, and mesenteric

---

[2]Opsonization [op″so-ni-za′shun; n., Gr. *opsonein,* "to buy victuals"; victuals are "useable food"] Opsonization turns pathogens into useable food by making them recognizable and able to be captured and phagocytized, through the attachment of immunoglobulins.

[3]Axillary (ak′sĭ-lar″e; adj., pertaining to the axilla); the axilla, also referred to as the "armpit" in humans, is that ventral region where the forelimb adjoins the thoracic wall; axillary lymph nodes are those lymph glands located deep in the tissues of the axilla.

[4]Mandibular (man-dib′u-lar; adj., pertaining to the mandible); the mandible is the lower jaw bone; mandibular lymph nodes are located caudoventral to the mandible.

[5]Cervical (ser′vĭ-kal; adj., pertaining to the neck); cervical lymph nodes are located bilaterally, deep in the musculature of the dorsolateral neck.

[6]Prescapular (pre-skap′u-lar; adj., pertaining to before the scapula); prescapular lymph nodes are located craniomedial to the shoulder joint. For more information regarding the scapula and the shoulder joint, see Chapter 6, "The Musculoskeletal System."

[7]Popliteal (pop-lit′e-al, pop″lĭ-te′-al; adj., pertaining to the "ham" ["ham" is acquired from the semimembranosus/semitendinosus muscles of the caudal thigh]); popliteal lymph nodes are located caudal to the stifle (femorotibial) joint. For more information regarding the stifle joint, see Chapter 6, "The Musculoskeletal System."

[8]Inguinal (ing′gwĭ-nal; adj., pertaining to the inguen [groin]); the inguen is that ventral region where the hindlimb adjoins the abdominal wall; superficial inguinal lymph nodes are located deep in the tissues of the inguen.

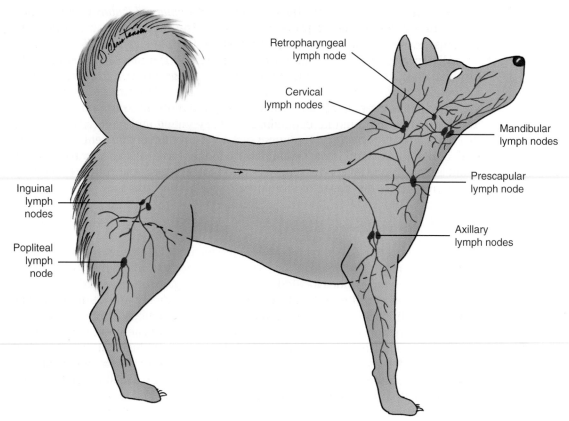

FIGURE 5-3 Superficial lymph nodes.

lymph nodes[9] should be attempted, they may be felt only if *lymphadenopathy* is present. Retropharyngeal lymph nodes[10] cannot be palpated. However, they are of clinical importance for pathologists, especially when looking for postmortem[11] evidence of diseases like tuberculosis. Many other lymph nodes are present throughout the thoracic cavity (mediastinal lymph nodes). Obviously, the rib cage prohibits palpation of these latter glands. Lymphadenopathy of mediastinal nodes may be detected radiographically, if significant enlargement is present.

Lymph nodes are small, glandular structures that are partly responsible for the production of lymphocytes. Connected by an intricate network of lymphatic

---

[9]Mesenteric (mes"en-ter'ik; adj., pertaining to the mesentery); the mesentery is a tissue found in the abdominal cavity that provides support and attachments for the abdominal viscera; mesenteric lymph nodes are located in multiple sites throughout the mesentery. (See Fig. 12-16.) For more information regarding the mesentery, see Chapter 12, "The Alimentary System."

[10]Retropharyngeal (re"tro-fah-rin'je-al; adj., *retro-* "backward, behind" +*pharyng(o)-* "throat" +*-al;* pertaining to behind the throat); the retropharyngeal lymph nodes are found deep in the tissues of the throat and filter lymphatic fluid from the nasal and oral cavities, pharynx, and ear.

[11]Postmortem (pōst-mor'tem; n., adj., [L. after death]).

vessels, the lymph nodes are responsible for filtration of lymphatic fluid. Macrophages located in the lymph nodes phagocytize pathogenic organisms from the lymphatic fluid. It should be noted that, unlike blood, lymphatic fluid does not flow in response to pressure within the lymphatic system. Lymphatic fluid is passively absorbed from the interstitium into the lymphatic vessels. Gravity and movement of the muscles and other tissues that closely approximate the lymphatic vessels force the fluid to flow passively. Unidirectional (one-way) valves within the vessels keep the fluid flowing in one direction (arrows, see Fig. 5-3). Ultimately, lymphatic fluid flows until it finds its way to the general circulating blood. Most of the lymphatic fluid of the body will enter the bloodstream via the thoracic duct. Generally, lymphatic fluid is a transparent, colorless, watery substance. However, mesenteric lymphatic fluid, following a meal, will appear cloudy and white. This is due to the lipids (fats) absorbed from digestion. Ultimately, this fat-laden lymphatic fluid will flow into general circulation, resulting in *lipemia*.

Edema

All of the tissues of the body are bathed in interstitial fluid. This fluid is constantly percolating through the tissues. It originates predominantly from capillaries (cap-ĭ-lar-ēz). Capillaries are the smallest blood vessels of the body, made up of simple squamous endothelium. The capillary structure facilitates diffusion of some molecules (O_2 and CO_2) and minor, normal "leakage" of fluid from the bloodstream. The constant replenishment of interstitial fluid ensures cellular respiration and nutritional support for even the most remote tissues of the body.

Excessive accumulation of interstitial fluid is clinically referred to as edema (ĕ-de′mah; [L. *oidema,* "swelling"]). If the lymphatic system is diseased in some way (e.g., lymphadenopathy or lymphangitis), it may not be able to accommodate the routine production and flow of the interstitial fluid. Absorption of the fluid into the lymphatic vessels may be impaired, or flow of lymphatic fluid within those vessels may be significantly impaired because of obstruction. In either case, interstitial fluid builds up and is clinically recognized as edema. One should realize that many other mechanisms may contribute to edema formation. Some of those mechanisms include lymphatic disease, changes in osmotic[12] pressures (e.g., hypoproteinemia—a condition of low protein in the blood), changes in hydrostatic pressures (e.g., pulmonary [lung] edema and/or *ascites*[13] due to congestive heart failure), and inflammation due to tissue trauma. Often, edema results from a combination of causative factors. Knowledge of the lymphatic system's function may be very useful clinically for the prevention of or reduction of edema.

---

[12]Osmosis (oz-mo′sis; n., [Gr. *osmos,* "impulsion"]); osmosis is the movement of water across a semipermeable membrane, from an area of low particle numbers to an area of high particle numbers. In essence, water moves to dilute an area of high particle concentration.
[13]Ascites [ah-si′tēz; n., L. *askites,* "bag"] Ascites is an accumulation of fluid in the peritoneal (abdominal) cavity.

Inflammation

Inflammation is a normal physiologic response to disease or injury. When tissues are injured, chemicals are released from the damaged cells. These inflammatory mediators stimulate a cascade of events in the injured area. Locally, *hyperemia* from vasodilation will occur, resulting in a very *erythematous* appearance and increased heat in the area. Increased blood flow will provide a ready supply of oxygen and nutrients, as well as easy access for phagocytes (such as neutrophils and monocytes). Increased cellular activity for debridement and repair of the area will also contribute to the localized increased heat. With added heat, the capillaries will become more permeable and leak excessively into the interstitium. This *edematous* fluid will serve to dilute *cytotoxic*[14] agents, as well as provide some protective cushioning of the area. Of course, nerve endings will be stimulated, resulting in *algesia*. The algesic effect is often the single most important protective mechanism, leading to decreased use and guarding of the injured area. So, the cardinal signs of inflammation that result are erythema, heat, edema, algesia, and loss of function.

Immunity

Immunogenic responses (i.e., active immunity) create a variety of *immunoglobulins*. Generally, lymphocytes produce IgG (immunoglobulin G) in response to exposure to *pathogens*. IgG is often referred to as a "good" antibody, by virtue of the way it provides protection for the body. As mentioned earlier, very young animals are not yet immune-competent. Therefore, they must rely on "passive immunity," in which IgG from the mother is passed to her offspring via her milk (colostrum[15]). These immunoglobulins will persist for various periods of time in the youngster. It is because of these maternal antibodies that we repeat immunizations at standard intervals in young animals. We do not know in each individual how long the maternal antibodies will persist. They must decrease enough so that the vaccine exposure will render an immunogenic response. Plus, repeated exposure to the *antigen* in the vaccine at an appropriate time will stimulate an *anamnestic*[16] response, for better active immunity. Depending on the animal and the disease, many newborns will be protected via passive immunity for several weeks to even a few months. Woe to the newborn who does not receive or absorb these maternal antibodies. That would be likened to sending someone blindfolded into a raging military battle, with no weapons and no body armor. Not only can the individual not protect himself, but he cannot even see to recognize the enemy. Risk of death in such a situation would be very high, just as it is for the newborn who does not receive maternal antibodies. That is why it is critical for all newborns to suckle within 12 hours of birth.

---

[14]Cytotoxic [sīt″o-toks′ic; adj., *cyt(o)*- cell + *tox(o)*- poison + -*ic* pertaining to].

[15]Colostrum (ko-los′trum; [L.]; the first milk produced by the dam that contains maternal antibodies).

[16]Anamnestic [an″am-nes′tik; adj., Gr. *anamnesis,* a recalling/memory]; in an anamnestic response, the immune system recalls the antigen from previous exposures and rebounds to a higher level of immunoglobulin production and immunity.

Immunity, when actively functioning in an appropriate manner, is very beneficial. There are times, however, when lymphocytes begin to recognize certain parts of the body as "foreign." As a result, *autoantibodies*[17] are produced and the targeted tissue will ultimately be destroyed. *Autoimmune hemolytic anemia* is a good example of such an occurrence. In this immune-mediated syndrome, erythrocytes are *opsonized*. In fact, so much erythrocyte-targeted IgG will present that *agglutination*[18] will be visible, often both microscopically and macroscopically (grossly) in a blood sample. This is a huge diagnostic clue for the veterinarian. Unfortunately, the *opsonization* and the resulting hemolysis may quickly become life-threatening. Treatment for autoimmune disorders, such as this, requires the administration of *immunosuppressive*[19] drugs. On one hand, the treatment stops the body's self-destruction. On the other hand, the treatment may make the animal highly susceptible to infectious diseases. This level of immunosuppression is not unlike that of *oncology*[20] patients being treated for diseases such as *lymphoma*. In either case, such patients must be carefully managed to minimize their risk of exposure to infectious diseases.

IgE is yet another immunoglobulin that is typically associated with allergic responses. Allergies or *hypersensitivity*[21] reactions develop over time and multiple exposures. In a classic, type I hypersensitivity reaction (e.g., pollen allergy) the individual is *"sensitized"* to the *allergen*.[22] In the sensitization process, excessive amounts of IgE are produced. The IgE "arms" mast cells[23] of the body. Once fully "armed," when reexposed to the allergen in what is called a *"challenge"* exposure, if two IgE molecules are bridged by the allergen, the mast cell will release its inflammatory mediators (principally histamine). Acute (rapid) inflammation will develop in the area. In humans with pollen allergies, these mast cells tend to predominate in the mucous membranes of the nasal passages and eyes. In animals, however, mast cells are most abundant in the skin. Rather than sneezing, animals will develop very erythematous, *pruritic*[24] skin. Some allergens can produce very complex, intense, persistent reactions. For example, a dog or cat hypersensitive to flea saliva will have a very intense *dermatitis*[25] that may last 3 months from one flea bite. *Antihistamines* tend not to be very effective in treating allergies in veterinary patients. So, if the allergen cannot be eliminated

---

[17]Autoantibody [aw″to-an′tĭ-bod″e; n., *auto-* prefix meaning "self"; autoantibodies are immunoglobulins that target components of the body itself.

[18]Agglutination [ah-gloo″tĭ-na′shun; n., L. *agglutinatio,* "gluing"]; immune-mediated diseases may "glue" erythrocytes together with immunoglobulins. When this happens, the red blood cells appear in irregular, grape-like clusters. Marked agglutination can be seen grossly.

[19]Immunosuppressive [im″u-no-su-pres′iv; adj., cf. immunodepression]; pertaining to immunity suppression or depression.

[20]Oncology [ong-kol′o-je; n., Gr. *onkos* "mass" (aka tumor) + *-logy* "the study of"] Oncology patients are cancer patients.

[21]Hypersensitivity [hi″per-sen′sĭ-tiv″ĭ-te; adj., *hyper-* "excessive" + sensitivity] Hypersensitivity reactions are exaggerated, allergic responses to foreign agents.

[22]Allergen [al′er-jen; n., *allergy* + *gen* "to produce"; an allergy producer].

[23]A mast cell is a cell with histamine-containing cytoplasmic granules that is found in abundance in the skin, airways, and digestive tract and plays a pivotal role in allergic reactions.

[24]Pruritic [proo-rit′ik; adj., L. *prurire,* "to itch"; pertaining to an itch] Note, this is the adjective form of the word. Pruritus is the noun.

[25]Dermatitis [der″mah-ti′tis; n., *dermat(o)-* "skin" + *-itis* "inflammation of"].

from the environment or avoided, *hyposensitization*[26] therapy may be warranted. Through this therapy, very low doses of the allergen are given at prescribed intervals. The dose is enough to stimulate an IgG immunogenic response, but not enough to challenge and stimulate an *allergenic* reaction. In so doing, the body is retrained to produce IgG appropriately, rather than IgE. Mast cells are no longer armed. Therefore, the allergen-histamine reaction cannot occur. The patient is effectively desensitized to the specific allergen.

Of course, the most serious of all hypersensitivity reactions is *anaphylaxis*. In an *anaphylactic* reaction, all mast cells of the body release histamine *en masse*. Where are all of these mast cells? Predominantly, mast cells will be found in the skin, airways, and digestive tract. Now, imagine acute, profound inflammation developing in all of these areas simultaneously with each area vasodilating and developing extreme edematous fluids. With so much fluid lost to the interstitium, very rapidly there will not be sufficient circulating blood volume to sustain life. Additionally, nerve endings stimulated in the airways will result in muscular contraction and constriction of the small airways. Even the throat itself can become so edematous that the individual cannot breathe. With an inability to breathe and insufficient blood volume to maintain blood pressure for vital organs, death rapidly results.

---

[26]Hyposensitization [hi″po-sen″sĭ-ti-za′shun; n., *hypo-* "below, deficient"; the process of making deficient sensitivity; aka desensitization].

SELF-TEST

Using the previous information in this chapter, complete the following crossword puzzle using the most appropriate medical term(s). Do not use abbreviations, unless specifically requested.

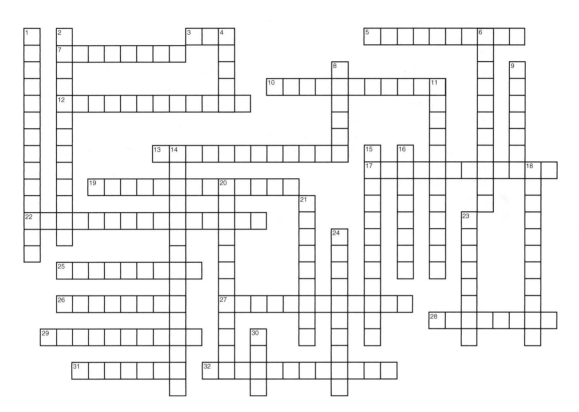

ACROSS

3	Abbreviation for immunoglobulin E
5	An immune memory response that renders heightened immunity
7	The study of tumors
10	A life-threatening hypersensitivity reaction
12	Pertaining to between tissues
13	An adjective meaning redness
17	The process of cellular eating
19	Immune-mediated "gluing" together of erythrocytes into grape-like clusters
22	A disease of lymph glands
25	The lymph nodes found caudal to the femorotibial joint
26	The lymph nodes found in the "armpit"
27	The body's response to injury that is characterized by redness, heat, swelling, pain, and loss of function
28	Resembling lymph

29	A large phagocytic cell
31	Pain
32	Inflammation of lymph vessels

DOWN

1	An antibody
2	Surgical removal of the tonsils
4	Swelling
6	Inflammation of the tonsils
8	The lymphoid structure in which lymphocytes mature that is found in the mediastinum
9	An accumulation of edematous fluid in the peritoneal cavity
11	Enlargement of the spleen
14	Pertaining to behind the throat
15	The process by which pathogens are made ready for phagocytosis (i.e., turned into useable food)
16	A disease producer
18	Synonym for antigenic
20	An immunoglobulin that targets a component of the body itself
21	A condition of excessive blood (i.e., engorged with blood)
23	A tumor of lymphoid tissue
24	Inflammation of the skin
30	Prefix meaning below or deficient

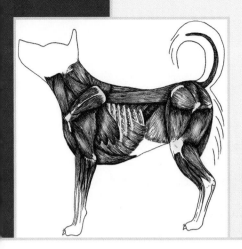

CHAPTER 6

The Musculoskeletal System

GOALS AND OBJECTIVES

By the conclusion of this chapter, the student will be able to:

1. Recognize common root words, prefixes, and suffixes related to the musculoskeletal system.
2. Divide simple and compound words into their respective parts.
3. Recognize, correctly pronounce, and appropriately use common medical terms related to the musculoskeletal system.
4. Recognize major bones and joints of domestic animals.
5. Translate/compare musculoskeletal anatomy of dogs with horses and cattle.
6. Recognize the parts of a bone.
7. Demonstrate a basic understanding of bone growth and repair.
8. Demonstrate an understanding of joint anatomy and function.
9. Recognize major muscle groups and common intramuscular injection sites of domestic animals.
10. Recognize common types of traumatic fractures.

INTRODUCTION TO LIMB ANATOMY

Limb Anatomy

The musculoskeletal system is composed of numerous muscles and bones. The bones provide support for muscles and other tissues of the body. They also provide protection for vital organs, such as the brain and thoracic viscera. Many joints of the body are named using the names of the bones that form the joint (articulate). Figure 6-1 identifies many of the bones of the canine limbs. Review the illustration and the descriptions that follow to familiarize yourself with canine limb anatomy before completing the word exercises of this introductory section.

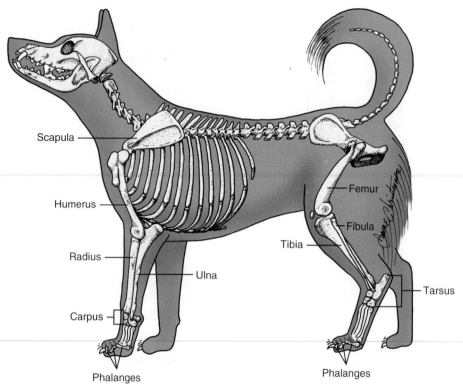

FIGURE 6-1   Bones of the canine limbs.

Scapula (skap'u-lah)

The scapula is a flat bone that is the most proximal bone of the forelimb. The thin, bony ridge found on its lateral surface is referred to as the spine of the scapula. The distal end of the scapula articulates with the humerus to form the shoulder joint.

Humerus (hu'mer-us)

The humerus is a long bone of the proximal forelimb (i.e., brachium[1]). The proximal end of the humerus articulates with the scapula to form the shoulder joint. The distal end of the humerus articulates with the radius and ulna bones to form the elbow joint.

Radius (ra'de-us)

The radius is a long bone of the forelimb (i.e., antebrachium[2]). The radius lies on the cranial aspect of the antebrachium. The proximal end of the radius articulates with the humerus to form, in part, the elbow joint. The distal end of the radius articulates with the bones of the carpus.

---

[1]Brachium (bra'ke-um; [L. *brachium,* "arm"]); the proximal portion of the forelimb between the shoulder and elbow joints.
[2]Antebrachium (an"te-bra'ke-um; [ante- "before," + brachium]); the portion of the forelimb between the elbow and carpal joints.

Ulna (ul'nah)

The ulna is a long bone of the antebrachium. The ulna lies on the caudal aspect of the antebrachium. The proximal end of the ulna articulates with the humerus to form, in part, the elbow joint. On the caudal aspect of its proximal end, the ulna has a large, bony protuberance or process, the olecranon (o-lek'rah-non), which forms the point of the elbow. The distal end of the ulna articulates with the bones of the carpus.

Carpus (kar'pus)

The carpus is a joint of the distal forelimb. It is composed of numerous small, short bones. The proximal border of the carpus articulates with the radius and ulna.

Phalanx (fa'lanks)

A phalanx is a small bone of the foot. Each digit (dij'it; toe) is composed of three phalanges (fah-lan'jēz).

Femur (fe'mur)

The femur is a long bone of the proximal hindlimb (i.e., thigh). The proximal end of the femur articulates with the pelvis to form the hip. On the lateral aspect of the proximal femur is a large, bony protuberance called the greater trochanter (tro-kan'ter). The distal end of the femur articulates with the tibia to form the stifle (sti'ful) joint.

Tibia (tib'e-ah)

The tibia is a long bone of the hindlimb (i.e., crus[3]). The proximal end of the tibia articulates with the femur to form the stifle joint. The distal end of the tibia articulates with the tarsus.

Fibula (fib'u-lah)

The fibula is a thin, long bone of the crus. It lies lateral to the tibia. The proximal end of the fibula, in most domestic animals, falls just short of the stifle joint. The distal end of the fibula articulates with the tarsus.

Tarsus (tahr'sus)

The tarsus is a joint of the distal hindlimb. It is composed of numerous small, short bones. The proximal border of the tarsus articulates with the tibia and fibula.

INTRODUCTION TO RELATED TERMS

Divide each of the following terms into its respective parts ("R," root; "P," prefix; "S," suffix; "CV," combining vowel).

1. **Scapulohumeral** (adj.)   (R) _____ (CV) _____ (R) _____ (S) _____
   scapulohumeral (skap"u-lo-hu'mer-al; pertaining to the scapula and humerus; anatomically refers to the shoulder joint)

2. **Humeroradioulnar** (adj.)   (R) _____ (CV) _____ (R) _____
   (CV) _____ (R) _____ (S) _____
   humeroradioulnar (hu"mer-o-ra"de-o-ul'nar; pertaining to the humerus, radius, and ulna; anatomically refers to the elbow joint)

---

[3]Crus [L.] "leg," old reference to the lower leg (i.e., rear leg in animals).

3. **Carpal** (adj.)   (R) _____   (S) _____
   carpal (kar'pal; pertaining to the carpus)

4. **Metacarpal** (adj.)   (P) _____   (R) _____   (S) _____
   metacarpal (met"ah-kar'pal; pertaining to beyond/after the carpus; anatomically refers
   to the portion of the distal forelimb that lies between the carpus and the phalanges)

5. **Metacarpophalangeal** (adj.)   (P) _____   (R) _____   (CV) _____
                                        (R) _____   (CV) _____   (S) _____
   metacarpophalangeal (met"ah-kar"po-fah-lan'je-al; pertaining to the metacarpus and
   phalanges; anatomically refers to any joint formed by a metacarpal bone and a phalanx)

6. **Interphalangeal** (adj.)   (P) _____   (R) _____(CV) _____   (S) _____
   interphalangeal (in"ter-fah-lan'je-al; pertaining to between the phalanges; anatomically refers
   to those joints formed by phalanges)

7. **Coxofemoral** (adj.)   (R) _____   (CV) _____   (R) _____   (S) _____
   coxofemoral (kok"so-fem'o-ral; pertaining to the hip and femur; anatomically refers to the hip joint)

8. **Femorotibial** (adj.)   (R) _____   (CV) _____   (R) _____   (S) _____
   femorotibial (fem"o-ro-tib'e-al; pertaining to the femur and tibia; anatomically refers to the
   stifle joint)

9. **Tarsal** (adj.)   (R) _____   (S) _____
   tarsal (tahr'sal; pertaining to the tarsus)

10. **Metatarsal** (adj.)   (P) _____   (R) _____   (S) _____
    metatarsal (met"ah-tar'sal; pertaining to beyond/after the tarsus; anatomically refers
    to that portion of the distal hindlimb that lies between the tarsus and the phalanges)

11. **Metatarsophalangeal** (adj.)   (P) _____   (R) _____   (CV) _____
                                        (R) _____   (CV) _____   (S) _____
    metatarsophalangeal (met"ah-tar"so-fah-lan'je-al; pertaining to the metatarsus and
    phalanges; anatomically refers to any joint formed by a metatarsal bone and a phalanx)

12. **Cervical** (adj.)   (R) _____   (S) _____
    cervical (ser'vĭ-kal; pertaining to the neck)

13. **Intervertebral** (adj.)   (P) _____   (R) _____   (S) _____
    intervertebral (in"ter-ver'tĕ-bral, in"ter-ver-te'bral; pertaining to between vertebrae[4];
    anatomically refers to the joints formed between the bones of the spinal column)

14. **Lumbosacral** (adj.)   (R) _____   (CV) _____   (R) _____   (S) _____
    lumbosacral (lum"bo-sa'kral; pertaining to the lumbus and sacrum; anatomically refers
    to the joint formed by the last lumbar vertebra and the sacrum)

15. **Coccygeal** (adj.)   (R) _____   (CV) _____   (S) _____
    coccygeal (kok-sij'e-al; pertaining to the coccyx; anatomically refers to the tail)

16. **Epaxial** (adj.)   (P) _____   (R) _____   (S) _____
    epaxial (ep-ak'se-al; pertaining to upon the axis; anatomically refers to the region along
    the dorsal vertebral column)

---

[4]Vertebra (ver'tĕ-brah), singular; vertebrae (ver'tĕ-brā), plural.

17. **Intercostal** (adj.)   (P) _____ (R) _____ (S) _____
    intercostal (in″ter-kos′tal; pertaining to between ribs; anatomically refers to the spaces found between ribs)

18. **Costochondral** (adj.)   (R) _____ (CV) _____ (R) _____ (S) _____
    costochondral (kos″to-kon′dral; pertaining to rib cartilage; anatomically refers to the cartilage that connects the bony ribs to the sternum)

19. **Sternal** (adj.)   (R) _____ (S) _____
    sternal (ster′nal; pertaining to the sternum)

20. **Epiphysis** (n.)   (P) _____ (R) _____
    epiphysis (e-pif′ĭ-sis; to grow upon; anatomically refers to the end of a long bone, usually covered with cartilage; pl. epiphysēs)

21. **Metaphysis** (n.)   (P) _____ (R) _____
    metaphysis (me-taf′ĭ-sis; to grow beyond; anatomically refers to the wider portion of the shaft of a long bone that is found at each end and is adjacent to the epiphysis; pl. metaphysēs)

22. **Diaphysis** (n.)   (P) _____ (R) _____
    diaphysis (di-af′ĭ-sis; to grow between; anatomically refers to the shaft of a long bone; pl. diaphysēs)

23. **Periosteal** (adj.)   (P) _____ (R) _____ (S) _____
    periosteal (per″e-os′te-al; pertaining to around bone; anatomically refers to the periosteum, a specialized connective tissue that covers the outer surfaces of all bones)

24. **Endosteum** (n.)   (P) _____ (R) _____ (S) _____
    endosteum (en-dos′te-um; within bone; anatomically it is the specialized tissue membrane that covers the interior surfaces of all bones)

25. **Synovial** (adj.)   (P) _____ (R) _____ (S) _____
    synovial (sĭ-no′ve-al; pertaining to with [egg]; anatomically refers to the synovia, a thick, transparent fluid that is found in joints and resembles egg whites)

26. **Arthritis** (n.)   (R) _____ (S) _____
    arthritis (ar-thri′tis; inflammation of a joint)

27. **Myositis**[5] (n.)   (R) _____ (S) _____
    myositis (mi″o-si′tis; inflammation of muscle)

28. **Orthopedic** (adj.)   (R) _____ (CV) _____ (R) _____ (S) _____
    orthopedic (or″tho-pe′dik; pertaining to straightening a child; clinically refers to the correction of deformities of the musculoskeletal system)

29. **Flexion** (n.)   (R) _____ (S) _____
    flexion (flek′shun; the act of bending)

30. **Extension** (n.)   (P) _____ (R) _____ (S) _____
    extension (ek-sten′shun; the act of out-stretching)

---

[5]Myositis: note that the root myos- is derived from [Gr. *myos,* muscle]. In general, the combining form used to indicate muscle is my(o)-.

31. **Abduction** (n.)   (P) _____ (R) _____ (S) _____
    abduction (ab-duk'shun; the act of abducting; to draw away; ab- = away)

32. **Adduction** (n.)   (P) _____ (R) _____ (S) _____
    adduction (ah-duk'shun; the act of adducting; to draw toward; ad- = toward)

33. **Circumduction** (n.)   (P) _____ (R) _____ (S) _____
    circumduction (ser"kum-duk'shun; the act of circumducting; to draw around)

34. **Intramuscular** (adj.)   (P) _____ (R) _____ (S) _____
    intramuscular (in"trah-mus'ku-lar; pertaining to within muscle; clinically refers to a route
    of medication administration in which medication is injected into a muscle mass)

35. **Osteoblast** (n.)   (R) _____ (CV) _____ (S) _____
    osteoblast (os"te-o-blast'; a bone "seed"; this is a germinal cell responsible for deposition
    of calcium for bone formation)

36. **Osteoclast** (n.)   (R) _____ (CV) _____ (S) _____
    osteoclast (os"te-o-klast'; a bone "breaker"; this is a cell responsible for remodeling
    and resorption of bone)

37. **Intramedullary** (adj.)   (P) _____ (R) _____ (S) _____
    intramedullary (in"trah-med'u-lar"e; pertaining to within the marrow)

38. **Panosteitis** (n.)   (P) _____ (R) _____ (S) _____
    panosteitis (pan-os'te-i"tis; inflammation of all bone; i.e., inflammation of all parts
    of the bone)

39. **Spondylopathy** (n.)   (R) _____ (CV) _____ (S) _____
    spondylopathy (spon"di-lop'ah-the; a disease of the vertebrae [spine])

40. **Osteomyelitis** (n.)   (R) _____ (CV) _____ (R) _____ (S) _____
    osteomyelitis (os"te-o-mi"ah-li'tis; inflammation of the bone and marrow)

MUSCULOSKELETAL ANATOMY AND PHYSIOLOGY

Bone Anatomy

Bones come in many different shapes and sizes: long, short, flat, sesamoid, and
irregular. Long bones are generally found in extremities. Short bones are found
in joints, like the *carpus* and *tarsus*. Flat bones are found in the skull, pelvis, scapula, and ribs. A *fossa*[6] is a depressed area that is often found on flat bones, like
the scapula, providing a contoured area in which muscle can nestle. Vertebrae
would be classified as irregular bones. Sesamoid bones are so called because
they resemble sesame seeds. Sesamoid bones are found near joints, like the
patella (pah-tel'ah; "knee cap"), which is associated with the stifle. Sesamoid
bones, like the patella lying in the femoral *trochlear*[7] groove (Fig. 6-2), act like a

---

[6]Fossa [fos'ah; L. "trench"].
[7]Trochlear [trok'le-ar; L. *trochlearis,* "pulley"].

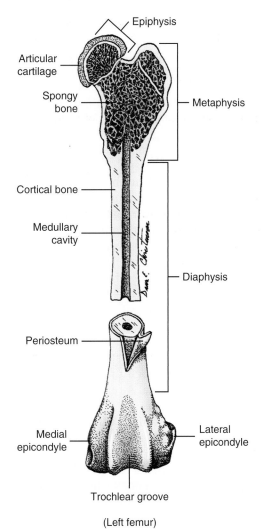

Epiphysis

Articular cartilage

Spongy bone

Metaphysis

Cortical bone

Medullary cavity

Diaphysis

Periosteum

Medial epicondyle

Lateral epicondyle

Trochlear groove

(Left femur)

FIGURE 6-2 Bone anatomy.

wheel in a pulley system, guiding the forces applied to tendons in the vicinity. For the following anatomic discussion, a long bone is used because it is easier to demonstrate specific anatomic structures.

Long bones are divided into three major regions: the epiphysis, the metaphysis, and the diaphysis (see Fig. 6-2). The epiphyses are found at the very ends of a long bone. The epiphysis is usually the portion of the bone that is covered with *articular* (joint) cartilage. The diaphysis is the shaft of a long bone. The metaphysis is found between the epiphysis and the diaphysis, providing a gradual, broadening transition between the two.

The wall of the diaphysis is composed of tightly compact (cortical) bone. Cortical bone is extremely dense and strong, to withstand forces of bending. The cortical bone of the diaphysis forms a central canal called the medullary cavity, which contains the bone marrow. The metaphyses and epiphyses are covered by a thin layer of cortical bone. Under the cortical bone of the metaphyses and epiphyses, however, is a network of numerous thin, irregular, branching, *osseous*[8] plates and interconnecting spaces. Because it looks like a sponge, it has been called spongy bone. Unlike a sponge, however, spongy bone is very strong and designed to withstand natural compression forces (much like steel trusses in architectural structures). The spaces found in spongy bone help reduce the overall weight of the bone and, in the metaphyses, provide space for additional marrow. The medullary cavity and the spaces of the spongy bone are lined with a connective tissue membrane called the *endosteum*. The vascularity of the medullary cavity and the spongy bone of the metaphysis make them useful for *intraosseous*[9] fluid administration, particularly when peripheral vessels cannot be accessed. Covering the entire bone, except for the articular cartilage on the epiphyses, is a tough connective tissue membrane called the *periosteum*. Also found predominantly over the metaphysis and at various points along the diaphysis are various sized *tubercles* and *tuberosities*.[10] These raised, rough areas of the bone are sites of attachment for ligaments and tendons. Shown in Figure 6-2 are two such sites—the medial and lateral *epicondyles*.[11]

Bone Growth

Bones in a developing fetus start off as layers of fibrous connective tissue and cartilage. Eventually, much of the connective tissue and cartilage is replaced with hard, calcified bone. After birth, the bones continue to grow until the animal reaches maturity.

In a young, growing animal, the epiphyses are demarcated from the metaphyses by growth plates (epiphyseal plates; Fig. 6-3). The epiphyseal plate is made up of cartilage and *osteoblasts*. During the growth process, osteoblasts of the epiphyseal plates deposit calcified bone, causing the bone to grow in length. Periosteal osteoblasts deposit calcified bone, causing the bone to grow in width. On reaching maturity, the epiphyseal plate is incorporated into the spongy bone of the epiphysis and metaphysis.

Fractures and Fracture Repair

A fracture (frak'tūr) is the breakage of a bone. Many different types of fractures occur for many different reasons. Trauma is the most frequent cause of fractures. Every fracture falls into one of two major categories: (1) simple fracture, one that is contained within the skin and soft tissues; or (2) compound fracture, one that is open to the environment through a penetrating soft tissue wound. (Compound fractures are at grave risk of infection. The inflammation associated

---

[8]Osseous [os′e-us; L. "bone," "bony"].
[9]Intraosseous [in″trah-os′e-us; intra- "within" + osseous "bone"].
[10]Tubercle and tuberosity [L. tuber "a swelling," "protuberance" (i.e., "bump"). In skeletal anatomy, tubercle is generally used to refer to small bumps, whereas tuberosity generally refers to larger bumps on bones].
[11]Epicondyle [ep″ĭ-kon′dīl; epi- "upon" + L. *condylos,* "knuckle"].

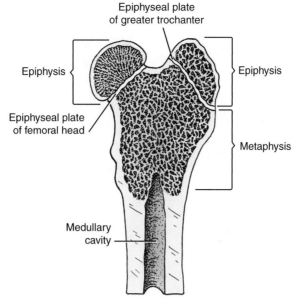

Epiphyseal plate
of greater trochanter

Epiphysis

Epiphysis

Epiphyseal plate
of femoral head

Metaphysis

Medullary
cavity

FIGURE 6-3   Epiphyseal plates.

with such an event may rapidly involve the entire bone. *Panosteitis* and osteomyelitis are far more painful than the fracture itself. That is why compound fractures require immediate, aggressive management by the veterinary health care team. A complication like osteomyelitis is also why strict adherence to principles of sterility is so important in orthopedic surgery.) Within these two categories, fractures are specifically named by the nature of the bone breakage. Figure 6-4 illustrates five of the common types of fractures in domestic animals:

Fissured fracture
   An incomplete break, parallel to the longitudinal (length) axis of the bone.
Greenstick fracture
   An incomplete break, involving predominantly one side of the bone, created by a bending force. It was so named because of the way it resembles the breakage of a young, supple, green twig. This type of fracture is common in young animals.
Transverse fracture
   A complete break that occurs perpendicular (at right angles) to the longitudinal axis of the bone.
Comminuted fracture
   A complete break that results in numerous bony fragments.
Oblique fracture
   A complete break that occurs at an angle oblique to the longitudinal axis of the bone.

Within days of a fracture occurring, cells that produce fibrocartilage (fi″bro-kar′tĭ-lij, a specialized type of cartilage) and bone infiltrate the area (Fig. 6-5).

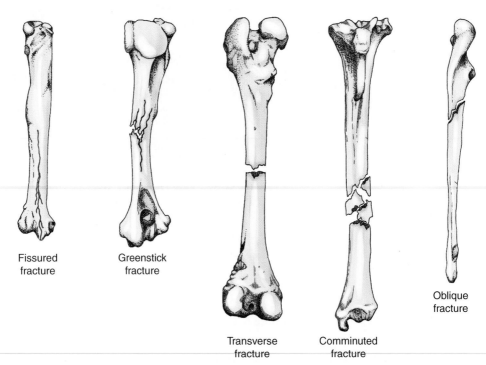

Fissured
fracture

Greenstick
fracture

Transverse
fracture

Comminuted
fracture

Oblique
fracture

FIGURE 6-4 Common traumatic fractures.

Most of these cells originate from the periosteum and the endosteum. Fibrocartilage and bone deposited at the fracture site provide the initial, but unstable, union between the broken ends of the bone. The fibrocartilage matrix eventually is replaced by calcified bone. Orthopedic support devices, such as *intramedullary* pins, are often warranted to stabilize the fracture site during these early stages of repair. Osteoblasts continue to deposit spongy bone until all of the fibrocartilage is replaced. Once the fibrocartilage has been replaced by bone, it is referred to as a bony callus. Bone continues to be deposited and reorganized until the fracture site is fully healed. Osteoclasts remodel the callus, removing excess bone and fragments from the fracture site.

Joints

A joint is formed wherever two or more bones meet. Joints differ structurally and functionally. Some joints are completely immobile and intended purely to hold opposing bones together, like those of the skull. *Intervertebral* joints are designed to allow minimal flexibility of the spinal column, protecting the spinal cord within each vertebral foramen and the spinal nerves where they exit through the intervertebral foramina (Fig. 6-6). A unique feature of intervertebral joints is the intervertebral discs that act as small shock absorbers along the spinal column. An intervertebral disc is found between each of the adjoining vertebral bodies, except between the first and second cervical vertebrae. Note that the "shock absorption" capacity of the intervertebral discs is enhanced by their

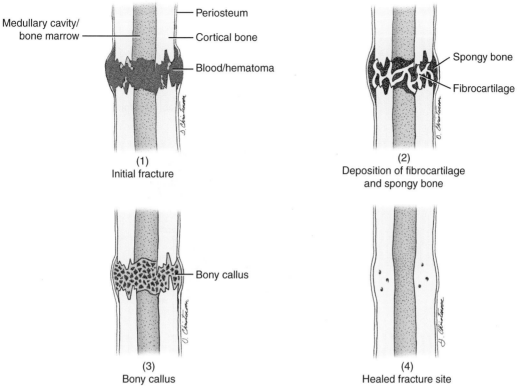

FIGURE 6-5   Fracture repair.

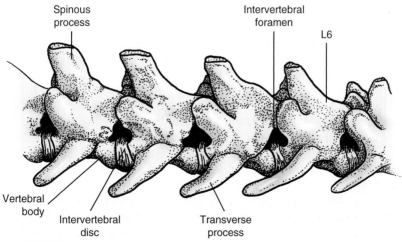

FIGURE 6-6   Spinal anatomy: left lateral view of lumbar vertebrae.

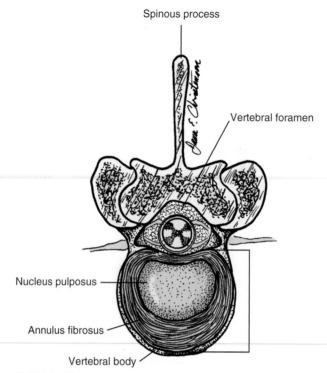

Spinous process

Vertebral foramen

Nucleus pulposus

Annulus fibrosus

Vertebral body

FIGURE 6-7   Spinal anatomy: transverse spinal section.

structure (i.e., gelatinous, nucleus pulposus contained within the fibrocartilage of the annulus fibrosus) (Fig. 6-7). Certain dog breeds are predisposed to *spondylopathies,* such as intervertebral disc disease (IVDD). The neurologic consequences of this disease will be discussed in Chapter 9, "The Neurologic System." Finally, synovial joints are those found in the limbs of domestic animals (Fig. 6-8).

The epiphyses of the bones in a synovial joint are covered with a layer of articular cartilage. It is designed to resist wear and produce minimal friction when the joint is moved. The joint is fully enclosed by a tubular joint capsule. Made of very tough, fibrous connective tissue, the joint capsule not only encloses the joint cavity, it also helps prevent the articular surfaces of the bones from being pulled apart. *Ligaments* also play a major role in holding the bones together and minimizing movement. They are composed of bundles of fibrous connective tissue. Filling the joint cavity is a transparent, viscous fluid called synovial fluid. The synovial fluid acts as a lubricant for the articular surfaces. In arthritic conditions, articular cartilage will wear abnormally, such that the synovial fluid can no longer provide sufficient lubrication. Movement of the affected joint will become difficult and painful.

Action or movement within a synovial joint depends on the bones that form it. For hinged joints, like the elbow, only *flexion* and *extension* are possible. *Rotation* (twisting around an axis) is made possible by pivot joints like those found between the head and neck, as well as the lumbosacral joint. For a ball and socket

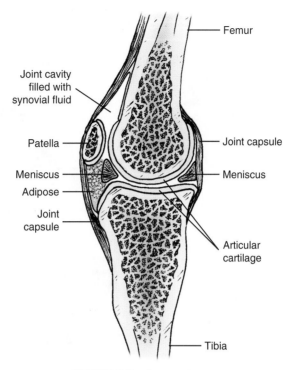

Femur

Joint cavity
filled with
synovial fluid

Patella

Meniscus

Adipose

Joint
capsule

Joint capsule

Meniscus

Articular
cartilage

Tibia

FIGURE 6-8   Synovial joint.

joint like the hip, multiple movements are possible, including *adduction, abduction,* and *circumduction.* If joint range of motion (ROM) is requested for diagnostic or therapeutic reasons, the anatomic structure and natural movements of each joint involved must be considered to carry out the medical order fully and correctly. See Figure 6-9 for schematic illustrations of various joint movements.

Comparative Skeletal Anatomy

Horses and ruminants (cattle, sheep, and goats) differ from dogs and cats not just because they are much larger. The skeletal structure of horses and ruminants have evolved quite differently, particularly in the limbs, to support their massive weight. Refer to Figures 6-10 through 6-15 for a comparative look at the canine, equine, and bovine species. Beginning with the skull, notice the difference in the orbital structure. The dog's orbit is incomplete, making it relatively easy to "pop" an eye out with somewhat minimal trauma. In horses and ruminants, the orbit must be fractured for this to occur. Dental differences will be discussed in Chapter 12, "The Alimentary System." Moving into the cervical area, horses and ruminants have a prominent suspensory apparatus called the ligamentum nuchae[12] designed to support the massive weight of their heads. The

---

[12]Ligamentum nuchae (lig″ah-men′tum nu′ka); in Latin, ligament comes from *ligare,* "to bind." Ligaments "bind" bones to one another. Also in Latin, *nucha* refers to the "scruff" of the neck.

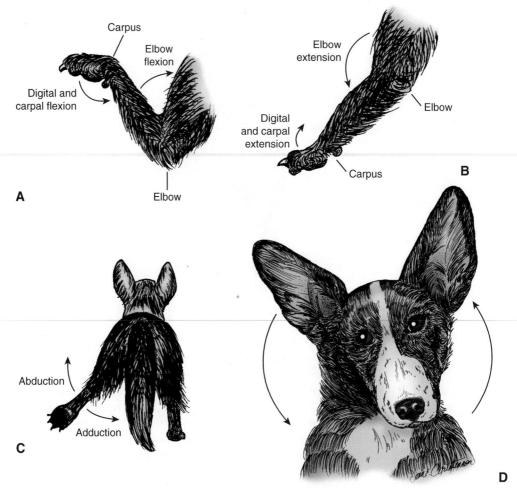

FIGURE 6-9   Joint movements. **A,** Flexion of the elbow and carpus. **B,** Extension of the elbow and carpus. **C,** Adduction and abduction of the rear limb. **D,** Rotation of the head.

thickest portion of this structure runs from the skull to the thoracic vertebrae and provides the dorsal border of the lateral neck intramuscular (IM) injection site. Notice that there is also a laminar portion that connects to each of the cervical vertebrae.

In comparing the forelimb of horses and ruminants with that of a dog, beginning proximally, the scapula and humerus appear quite similar. It is not until a point distal to the *humeroradioulnar* joint that the anatomy begins to differ significantly. In the dog, the radius and ulna are separate bones, the radius being the most cranial of the two. In large animals, the radius and ulna are fused. The carpus of each of the animals is very similar, with numerous carpal bones, including an accessory carpal bone on the palmar aspect of the joint. Distal to the carpus, the most significant differences are observed. A normal dog stands

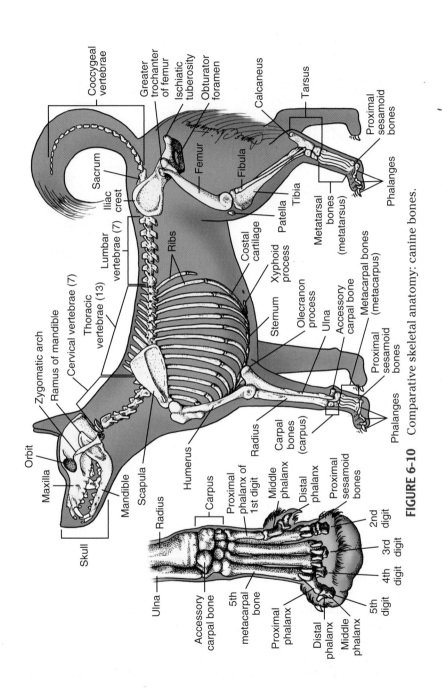

FIGURE 6-10 Comparative skeletal anatomy: canine bones.

Coccygeal vertebrae

Greater trochanter of femur

Ischiatic tuberosity

Obturator foramen

Calcaneus

Tarsus

Proximal sesamoid bones

Phalanges

Sacrum

Femur

Fibula

Tibia

Patella

Metatarsal bones (metatarsus)

Iliac crest

Lumbar vertebrae (7)

Ribs

Costal cartilage

Xyphoid process

Metacarpal bones (metacarpus)

Proximal sesamoid bones

Phalanges

Thoracic vertebrae (13)

Cervical vertebrae (7)

Sternum

Olecranon process

Ulna

Accessory carpal bone

Zygomatic arch

Ramus of mandible

Proximal phalanx of 1st digit

Middle phalanx

Distal phalanx

Proximal sesamoid bones

Orbit

Maxilla

Mandible

Scapula

Humerus

Radius

Carpal bones (carpus)

Radius

2nd digit

3rd digit

4th digit

5th digit

Skull

Ulna

Accessory carpal bone

Carpus

5th metacarpal bone

Proximal phalanx

Distal phalanx

Middle phalanx

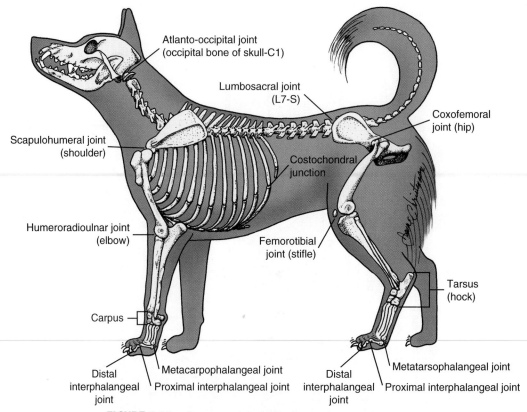

Atlanto-occipital joint
(occipital bone of skull-C1)

Lumbosacral joint
(L7-S)

Coxofemoral
joint (hip)

Scapulohumeral joint
(shoulder)

Costochondral
junction

Humeroradioulnar joint
(elbow)

Femorotibial
joint (stifle)

Tarsus
(hock)

Carpus

Distal
interphalangeal
joint

Metacarpophalangeal joint

Proximal interphalangeal joint

Distal
interphalangeal
joint

Metatarsophalangeal joint

Proximal interphalangeal joint

FIGURE 6-11   Comparative skeletal anatomy: canine joints.

on four of five digits. Digits are numbered in the dog from medial (#1) to lateral (#5). The first digit is vestigial[13] on the medial aspect of the metacarpus and is not used to bear weight. This is frequently referred to as the dewclaw. Each of the weight-bearing digits has associated with it three phalanges and a metacarpal bone. The horse, on the other hand, stands on only one digit! If compared with the dog, the horse is actually standing on the third digit. The third metacarpal bone of the horse has become massive to support weight. The vestigial second and fourth metacarpal bones are fused to the third metacarpal bone on the palmaromedial and palmarolateral aspects of the bone. Ruminants differ slightly from the horse, in that they stand on two digits (third and fourth). The phalanges of ruminants form separate toes, but the metacarpal bones are fused, with the fifth metacarpal being just a vestigial remnant. The proximal sesamoid bones of horses and ruminants are quite apparent near the palmar aspect of the *metacarpophalangeal* joint. They help support the large ligaments and tendons of the distal limb, as does(do) the distal sesamoid bone(s), found cradled behind the distal phalanx. The distal phalanx of large animals cannot

[13]Vestigial (ves-tij'e-al; pertaining to a vestige); rudimentary.

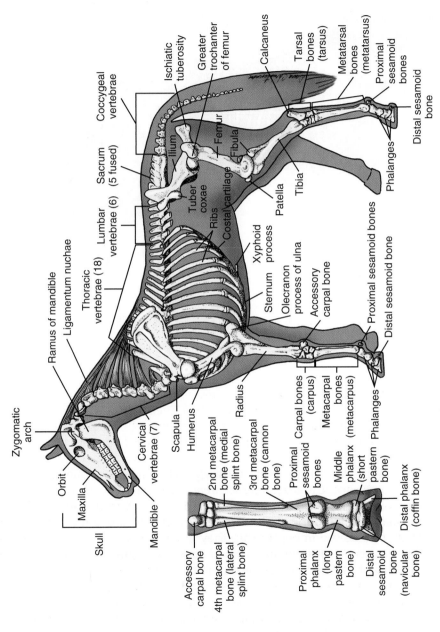

FIGURE 6-12 Comparative skeletal anatomy: equine bones.

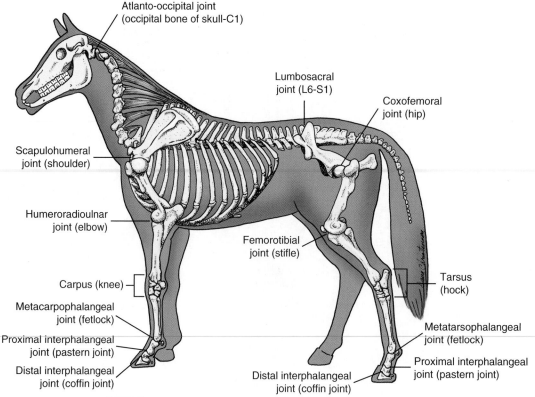

Atlanto-occipital joint
(occipital bone of skull-C1)

Lumbosacral
joint (L6-S1)

Coxofemoral
joint (hip)

Scapulohumeral
joint (shoulder)

Humeroradioulnar
joint (elbow)

Femorotibial
joint (stifle)

Carpus (knee)

Tarsus
(hock)

Metacarpophalangeal
joint (fetlock)

Metatarsophalangeal
joint (fetlock)

Proximal interphalangeal
joint (pastern joint)

Proximal interphalangeal
joint (pastern joint)

Distal interphalangeal
joint (coffin joint)

Distal interphalangeal
joint (coffin joint)

FIGURE 6-13   Comparative skeletal anatomy: equine joints.

be seen, except radiographically, because it is found in the hoof. (In the dog, the distal phalanx is found in the claw.) Even the distal interphalangeal joint is difficult to visualize in horses and ruminants because of the hoof wall. The proximal interphalangeal joint, on the other hand, is quite easy to see and to palpate.

The next skeletal area in which major differences are found between horses, ruminants, and the dog is in the rear. The pelvic structural differences are discussed first here. In the dog, the ilium is a wing-like portion of the pelvis that is oriented in a sagittal plane. The horse and the ruminant have an ilium, too; however, in these animals, it is as though the ventral border of the ilium has been twisted laterally and dorsally. That is why the most prominent osseous protuberance on a large animal ilium is not the iliac crest, like in the dog. The most prominent osseous protuberance of an equine, bovine, caprine, or ovine ilium is the *tuber coxae*.[14] The proximal hindlimbs of all these animals are similar. They each have a femur and a patella that is associated with

---

[14]Tuber coxae (tu-ber koks′a), derived from [L. *tuber,* a swelling or protuberance] and [L. *coxa,* "hip"].

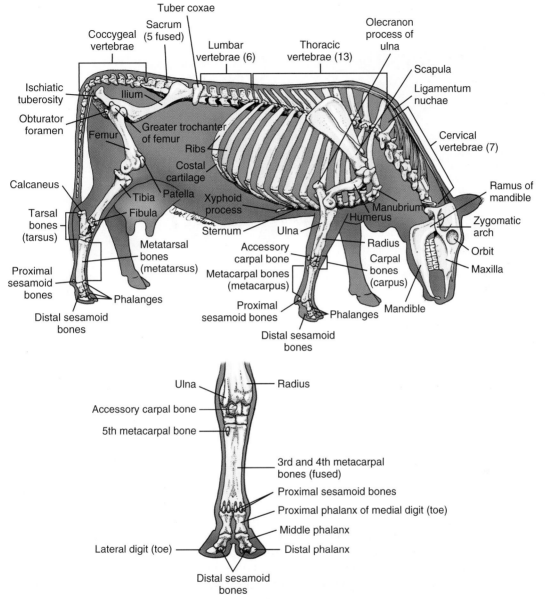

FIGURE 6-14   Comparative skeletal anatomy: bovine bones.

the *femorotibial* joint. Distal to that joint, differences begin to appear. Horses and ruminants have only a vestigial fibula, near the proximal end of the tibia (horse) and near the distal tibia (ruminants). Much of the fibula has been fused to and is indiscernible from the tibia. The tarsus of each of these animals is very similar. They have multiple tarsal bones, including the calcaneus (kal-ka′ne-us), which is the largest, rearmost tarsal bone. Distal to the tarsus,

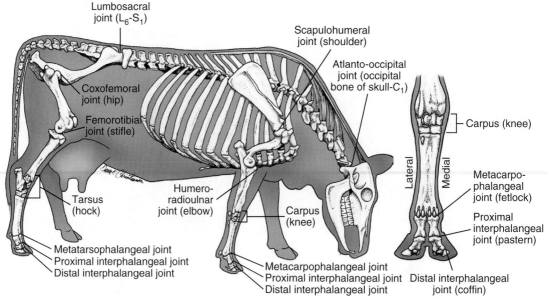

FIGURE 6-15   Comparative skeletal anatomy: bovine joints.

differences between the dog and the horse/ruminant are similar to those in the forelimb. The horse stands on the third *metatarsal* bone, with the second and fourth metatarsal bones vestigial and fused to the third. Ruminants stand on fused third and fourth metatarsal bones. The phalanges and sesamoid bones are arranged just as they are in the forelimb. The dog still bears weight on digits two through five. The first digit is frequently absent in the hindlimbs of normal dogs and cats.

Muscle Anatomy and Activity

Muscles in this chapter are discussed by functional muscles or muscle groups (for details regarding muscle tissue, refer to Chapter 3, "Muscle Tissue"). Because the muscles are firmly attached to the bones by *tendons,* it is by virtue of muscle activity (i.e., contraction and relaxation) that joints are moved. Refer to Figures 6-16 through 6-18 for major extremity extensor and flexor muscles and muscle groups. (Some superficial muscles have been removed in the canine and equine illustrations for better visualization of individual muscles and muscle groups. All superficial muscles are in place in the bovine illustration for comparison.) Notice that each major joint has opposing muscles associated with it. So, with regard to joints and their associated muscles, "for every action there is an equal and opposite reaction."[15]

---

[15]Quote by physicist, Sir Isaac Newton.

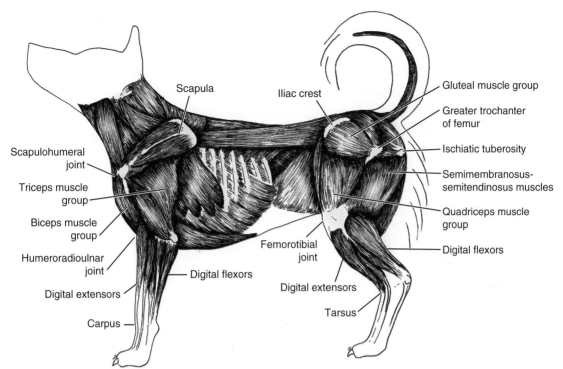

FIGURE 6-16   Canine comparative muscular anatomy (Note: superficial muscles removed).

Muscle groups of the limbs, shown in Figures 6-16 through 6-18, are as follows:

Biceps (bi'seps) muscle group
Flexor of the humeroradioulnar joint; located cranial to the humerus.
Triceps (tri'seps) muscle group
Extensor of the humeroradioulnar joint; located caudal to the humerus.
Digital extensor muscles of the forelimb
Extend the carpus and the digits; located cranial to the radius and ulna.
Digital flexor muscles of the forelimb
Flex the carpus and the digits; located caudal to the radius and ulna.
Gluteal (gloo'te-al) muscle group
Serves in part for flexion of the coxofemoral joint and abduction of the hindlimb; located between the ilium, sacrum, and proximal femur.
Quadriceps (kwod'rĭ-seps) muscle group
Extensor of the femorotibial joint; located cranial to the femur.
Semimembranosus-semitendinosus muscle group
Flexor of the femorotibial joint; located caudal to the femur.
Digital extensor muscles of the hindlimb (predominantly the cranial tibial muscle)
Extend the digits and flex the tarsus; located cranial to the tibia.
Digital flexor muscles of the hindlimb (predominantly the gastrocnemius [gas"trok-ne'me-us] muscle)
Flex the digits and extend the tarsus; located caudal to the tibia.

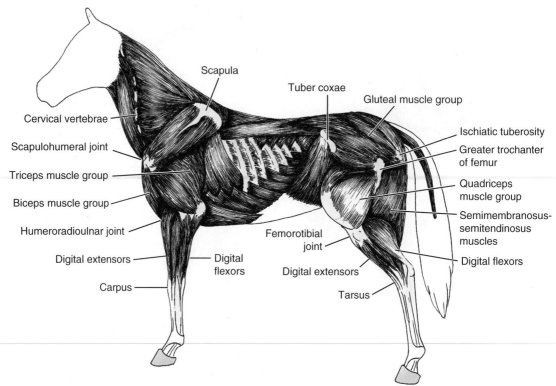

FIGURE 6-17   Equine comparative muscular anatomy (Note: superficial muscles removed).

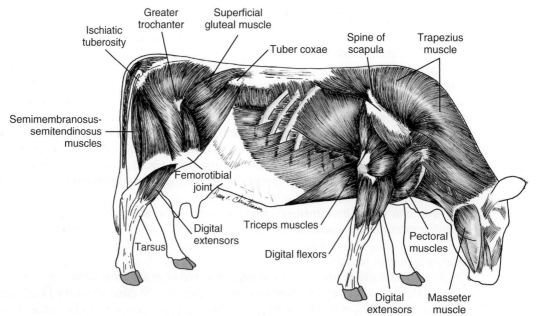

FIGURE 6-18   Bovine comparative muscular anatomy (Note: superficial muscles included).

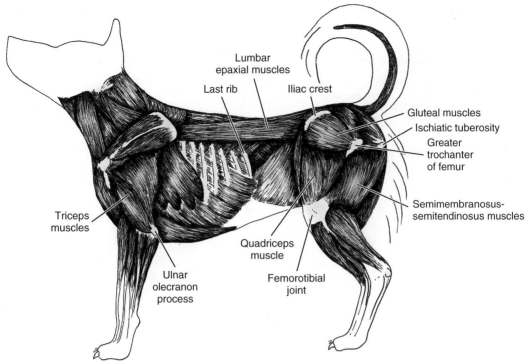

FIGURE 6-19   Common canine intramuscular injection sites.

Common Intramuscular Injection Sites

IM injections are frequently used for medication administration. Because muscles have significant blood supply, they provide relatively rapid absorption of injected agents. It is important that students have a working knowledge of the muscle sites that provide suitable locations for IM injections. Refer to Figures 6-19 through 6-21 for the common IM injection sites used in veterinary medicine. Compare these illustrations with the skeletal illustrations to define the osseous landmarks for each site. It is very important to locate and maintain isolation of a muscle group using its osseous landmarks whenever an IM injection is administered.

The following list gives each IM injection site, along with its respective osseous landmarks and the species in which it is most frequently used.

Lateral neck muscles
Used predominantly in adult horses and cattle, the lateral neck muscles are bordered by the ligamentum nuchae (dorsally), the scapula (caudally), and the cervical vertebrae (ventrally). This injection site should be avoided in young animals, because it may interfere with nursing.

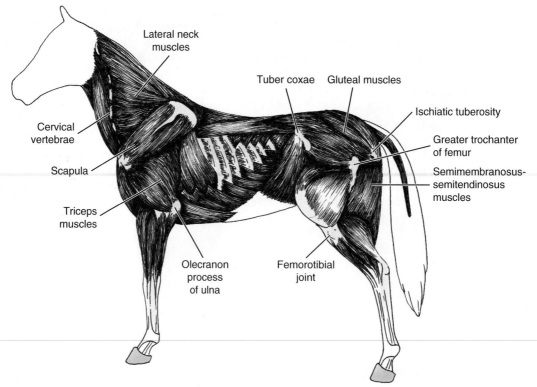

FIGURE 6-20   Common equine intramuscular injection sites.

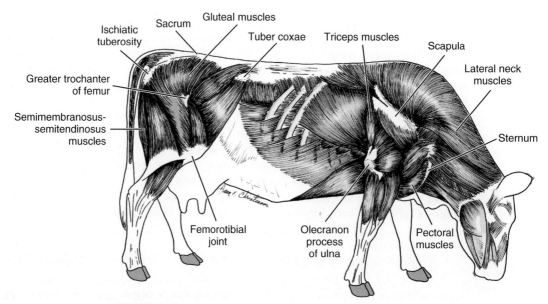

FIGURE 6-21   Common bovine intramuscular injection sites.

Lumbar epaxial muscles

Used predominantly in companion animals (i.e., dogs and cats), the lumbar epaxial muscles are bordered by the caudal rib (cranially), the spinous processes of the lumbar vertebrae (medially), and the iliac crest (caudally).

Gluteal muscles

As used in horses and ruminants, the gluteal muscles are bordered by the sacrum (medially), the tuber coxae (cranially), the greater trochanter of the femur (laterally), and the ischiatic tuberosity[16] (caudally). As used in companion animals, the gluteal muscles are bordered by the sacrum (medially), the iliac crest (cranially), and the greater trochanter of the femur (laterally). The ischiatic tuberosity is often helpful in locating the greater trochanter of the femur, but otherwise is not a functional osseous landmark for this injection site in dogs and cats.

Quadriceps muscles

Used predominantly in companion animals, the quadriceps muscles are bordered by the coxofemoral joint (proximally), the femur (caudally), and the femorotibial joint (distally).

Semimembranosus-semitendinosus muscles

Used in both large and small animal medicine, the semimembranosus and semitendinosus muscles are bordered by the ischiatic tuberosity (proximally), the femur (cranially), and the femorotibial joint (distally). It should be noted that a major nerve (the sciatic nerve[17]) passes through this muscle group just caudal to the femur. Damage to this nerve could result in paralysis of that limb. Therefore, students should not attempt to use this muscle group for IM injections in dogs and cats until they have been appropriately instructed in the safe use of the site.

When little muscle mass is available because of poor condition or size of the animal, other muscle groups that may be used are the triceps (all animals) and the pectoral muscles (bilaterally on the cranioventral chest of horses and ruminants). These are typically not used until all other sites have been exhausted.

Please note that muscles associated with breathing will be discussed and shown in Chapter 8, "The Respiratory System."

---

[16]Ischiatic tuberosity (is"ke-at'ik, ish"e-at'ik; pertaining to the ischium); the ischium is the most caudal portion of the pelvis; the ischiatic tuberosity is a caudolateral osseous protuberance of the ischium.

[17]Sciatic nerve (si-at'ik); this nerve and its branches supply motor function to the semimembranosus-semitendinosus muscle group, the digital flexors, and the digital extensors of the hindlimb.

SELF-TEST

Using the previous information in this chapter, complete the following crossword puzzle using the most appropriate medical term(s). Do not used abbreviations or common names, unless specifically requested.

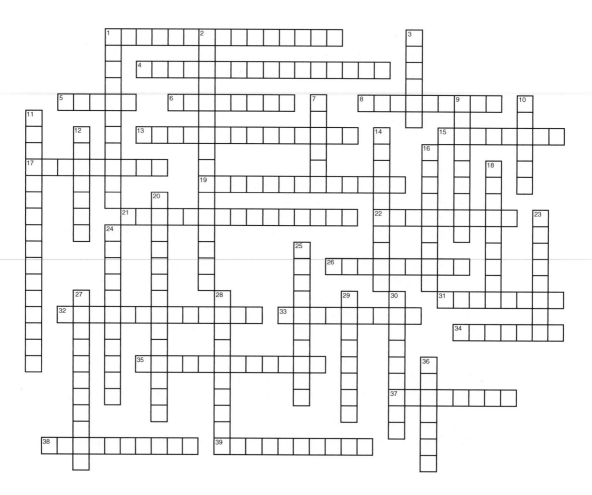

ACROSS

1	A joint formed by two bones of the toe
4	The dorsal border of the lateral neck IM injection site (2 words)
5	The digit on which a horse bears weight
6	The vertebrae of the neck
8	The membrane that lines the wall of the medullary cavity
13	A foramen through which a spinal nerve passes
15	A band of connective tissue that joins one bone to another
17	The act of drawing a limb away from the body
19	Within muscle
21	The gelatinous center of an intervertebral disc (2 words)

22	Inflammation of a joint
26	The act of drawing a limb toward the body
31	Those vertebrae associated with the chest cavity
32	The junction between the osseous rib and its associated cartilage
33	Vertebrae of the tail
34	The sesamoid bone of the stifle
35	The stifle joint
37	A muscle group that outstretches a joint
38	The muscle of the cranial thigh
39	A fracture type in which numerous bone fragments occur

DOWN

1	The space found between ribs
2	The elbow joint
3	The connective tissue that attaches muscle to bone
7	The "knee" of the horse
9	The end of a long bone covered by articular cartilage
10	A muscle group that reduces the angle of the joint
11	The joint formed by the skull and the first vertebra of the neck
12	The IM injection site of the dog bordered by the sacrum, iliac crest, and greater trochanter
14	The portion of the hindlimb immediately distal to the hock
16	The shaft of a long bone
18	Common name for the distal sesamoid bone of the horse
20	The shoulder joint
23	Pertaining to the viscous, egg-white-like fluid that lubricates joints
24	Inflammation of all bone
25	A specialized cell that deposits calcium for bone formation
27	The hip joint
28	A surgical procedure used to correct a musculoskeletal deformity
29	Inflammation of muscle
30	The largest bone of the tarsus
36	Common name for the metacarpophalangeal joint of the horse

ANATOMY CHALLENGE

On each of the diagrams provided (Figs. 6-22 through 6-24), identify as many of the bones and joints as you can within a timed period. Try to allow only 10 minutes per diagram. Each blank has been numbered so that you may find the correct answers in the answer key for this section.

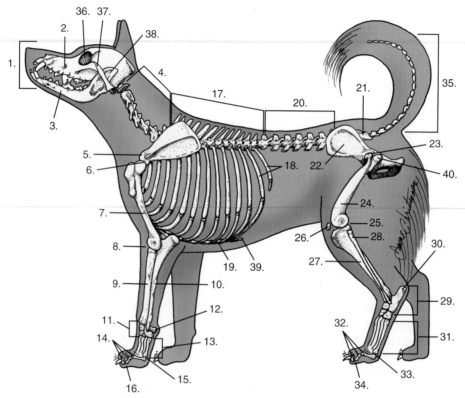

FIGURE 6-22   Canine anatomy challenge.

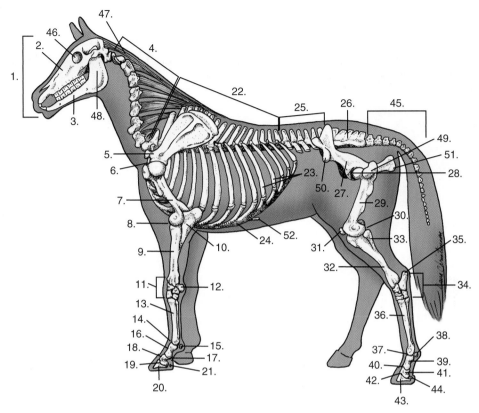

FIGURE 6-23   Equine anatomy challenge.

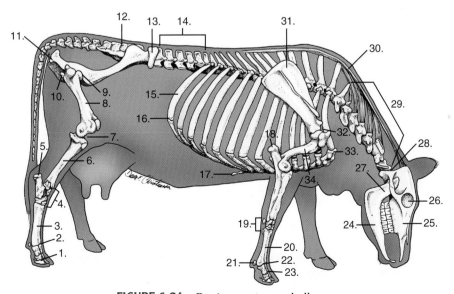

FIGURE 6-24   Bovine anatomy challenge.

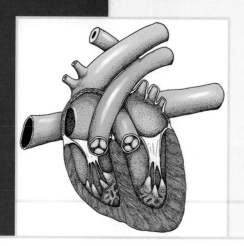

CHAPTER 7

The Cardiovascular System

GOALS AND OBJECTIVES

By the conclusion of this chapter, the student will be able to:

1. Recognize common root words, prefixes, and suffixes related to the cardiovascular system.
2. Divide simple and compound words into their respective parts.
3. Recognize, correctly pronounce, and appropriately use common medical terms related to the cardiovascular system.
4. Demonstrate an understanding of cardiovascular anatomy.
5. Recognize common pulse points and phlebotomy sites in domestic animals.
6. Trace the blood flow of an adult animal sequentially through a complete cycle.
7. Demonstrate a basic understanding of cardiovascular physiology with regard to blood flow, the cardiac cycle (systole and diastole), heart sounds, and electrocardiography.
8. Demonstrate familiarity with common cardiac diseases.

INTRODUCTION TO RELATED TERMS

Divide each of the following terms into its respective parts ("R" root, "P" prefix, "S" suffix, "CV," combining vowel).

1. **Cardiac** (adj.) (R) _____ (S) _____
   cardiac (kar'de-ak; pertaining to the heart)

2. **Cardiologist** (n.) (R) _____ (CV) _____ (R) _____
   (S) _____
   cardiologist (kar-de-ol'o-jist; one who specializes in heart study; a doctor specializing in heart disease and treatment)

3. **Pericardial** (adj.)   (P) _____ (R) _____ (S) _____
   pericardial (per"ĭ-kar'de-al; pertaining to surrounding the heart; anatomically refers
   to the tissue membrane that surrounds the heart, called the pericardium)

4. **Epicardium** (n.)   (P) _____ (R) _____ (S) _____
   epicardium (ep"ĭ-kar'de-um; upon the heart; anatomically refers to the thin, most
   superficial tissue layer of the heart)

5. **Myocardial** (adj.)   (R) _____ (CV) _____ (R) _____ (S) _____
   myocardial (mi"o-kar'de-al; pertaining to muscle of the heart)

6. **Endocardium** (n.)   (P) _____ (R) _____ (S) _____
   endocardium (en"do-kar'de-um; within the heart; anatomically refers to the thin tissue
   layer that lines the interior of the heart)

7. **Atrial** (adj.)   (R) _____ (S) _____
   atrial (a'tre-al; pertaining to an atrium; anatomically the atria are two of the four chambers
   within the heart)

8. **Ventricular** (adj.)   (R) _____ (S) _____
   ventricular (ven-trik'u-lar; pertaining to a ventricle; anatomically the ventricles are two
   of the four chambers within the heart)

9. **Atrioventricular** (adj.)   (R) _____ (CV) _____ (R) _____ (S) _____
   atrioventricular (a"tre-o-ven-trik'u-lar; pertaining to an atrium and a ventricle)

10. **Aortic** (adj.)   (R) _____ (S) _____
    aortic (a-or'tik; pertaining to the aorta; anatomically the aorta is the main artery leading
    from the heart)

11. **Pulmonic** (adj.)   (R) _____ (S) _____
    pulmonic (pul-mon'ik; pertaining to the lungs)

12. **Arterial** (adj.)   (R) _____ (CV) _____ (S) _____
    arterial (ar-te're-al; pertaining to an artery or arteries)

13. **Arteriole** (n.)   (R) _____ (CV) _____ (S) _____
    arteriole (ar-te're-ōl; a small artery)

14. **Venous** (adj.)   (R) _____ (S) _____
    venous (ve'nus; pertaining to a vein or veins)

15. **Venule** (n.)   (R) _____ (S) _____
    venule (ven'ūl; a small vein)

16. **Phlebotomy** (n.)   (R) _____ (CV) _____ (S) _____
    phlebotomy (flĕ-bot'o-me; the cutting of a vein; clinically refers to the puncture of a vein
    with a needle for the withdrawal of blood)

17. **Phlebitis** (n.)   (R) _____ (S) _____
    phlebitis (flĕ-bi'tis; inflammation of a vein)

18. **Cardiomyopathy** (n.)   (R) _____ (CV) _____ (R) _____
                                    (CV) _____ (S) _____
    cardiomyopathy (kar"de-o-mi-op'ah-the; a disease of heart muscle)

19. **Electrocardiogram** (n.)   (R) _____ (CV) _____ (R) _____
                                        (CV) _____ (S) _____

   electrocardiogram (e-lek"tro-kar'de-o-gram; a recording of electricity of the heart;
   clinically referred to as an ECG, the electrocardiogram is a graphic tracing of the heart's
   electrical activity)

20. **Echocardiogram** (n.)   (R) _____ (R) _____ (CV) _____ (S) _____

   echocardiogram (ek"o-kar'de-o-gram; a recording of echoes of the heart;
   clinically refers to the use of ultrasonic waves to record the anatomy and
   motion of the heart)

21. **Angiogram** (n.)   (R) _____ (CV) _____ (S) _____

   angiogram (an'je-o-gram; a recording of vessels; clinically refers to a radiographic
   procedure in which radiopaque dye is injected into the vasculature for better visualization
   of the vessels)

22. **Intravenous** (adj.)   (P) _____ (R) _____ (S) _____

   intravenous (in"trah-ve'nus; pertaining to within a vein; clinically often refers to a route
   of medication administration)

23. **Perivascular** (adj.)   (P) _____ (R) _____ (S) _____

   perivascular (per"ĭ-vas'ku-lar; pertaining to around a vessel)

24. **Bradycardia** (n.)   (P) _____ (R) _____ (S) _____

   bradycardia (brād"ĕ-kar'de-ah; a condition of a slow heart, i.e., heart rate)

25. **Tachycardia** (n.)   (P) _____ (R) _____ (S) _____

   tachycardia (tak"ĕ-kar'de-ah; a condition of a rapid heart, i.e., heart rate)

26. **Systolic** (adj.)   (R) _____ (S) _____

   systolic (sis-tol'ik; pertaining to contraction; clinically refers to the phase of the cardiac
   cycle when the myocardium is contracting)

27. **Diastolic** (adj.)   (R) _____ (S) _____

   diastolic (di"ah-stol'ik; pertaining to expansion; clinically refers to the phase of the cardiac
   cycle when the myocardium is relaxed, allowing the chambers to expand)

28. **Asystole** (n.)   (P) _____ (R) _____

   asystole (a-sis'to-le, ah"sis'to-le; absence of contraction; clinically refers to the absence
   of cardiac activity)

29. **Stenosis** (n.)   (R) _____ (CV) _____ (S) _____

   stenosis (ste-no'sis; a condition of narrowing)

30. **Cardiomegaly** (n.)   (R) _____ (CV) _____ (S) _____

   cardiomegaly (kar"de-o-meg'ah-le; enlargement of the heart)

31. **Hypertrophy** (n.)   (P) _____ (R) _____

   hypertrophy (hi-per'tro-fe; excessive development)

32. **Interatrial** (adj.)   (P) _____ (R) _____ (S) _____

   interatrial (in"ter-a'tre-al; pertaining to between the atria)

33. **Interventricular** (adj.)   (P) _____ (R) _____ (S) _____

   interventricular (in"ter-ven-trik'u-lar; pertaining to between the ventricles)

34. **Arrhythmia** (n.)   (P) _____ (R) _____ (S) _____
    arrhythmia (a-rith′me-ah, ah-rith′me-ah; a condition without rhythm)

35. **Vasoconstriction** (n.)   (R) _____ (CV) _____ (R) _____ (S) _____
    vasoconstriction (vas″o-kon-strik′shun; the process of vessel constricting)

36. **Vasodilation** (n.)   (R) _____ (CV) _____ (R) _____ (S) _____
    vasodilation (vas″o-di-la′shun; the process of vessel dilating)

37. **Sphygmomanometer** (n.)   (R) _____ (CV) _____ (R) _____
    (CV) _____ (S) _____
    sphygmomanometer (sfig″mo-mah-nom′ĕ-ter; measurer of pulse pressure; clinically refers
    to an instrument used to measure blood pressure)

38. **Endocarditis** (n.)   (P) _____ (R) _____ (S) _____
    endocarditis (en″do-kar-di′tis; inflammation within the heart; truly it is inflammation of the
    endocardium)

39. **Thrombosis** (n.)   (R) _____ (CV) _____ (S) _____
    thrombosis (throm-bo′sis; a condition of a clot; typically this refers to clot formation
    somewhere within the vasculature)

40. **Thrombophlebitis** (n.)   (R) _____ (CV) _____ (R) _____ (S) _____
    thrombophlebitis (throm″bo-flĕ-bi′tis; inflammation and clotting of a vein)

41. **Hypotension** (n.)   (P) _____ (R) _____ (S) _____
    hypotension (hi″po-ten′shun; a state or condition of below normal "pressure" [L. *tensio,*
    "stretch"]; clinically this refers to abnormally low blood pressure)

42. **Hypertensive** (adj.)   (P) _____ (R) _____ (S) _____
    hypertensive (hi″per-ten′siv; pertaining to excessive "pressure"; clinically this refers to
    abnormally high blood pressure)

43. **Hypovolemia** (n.)   (P) _____ (R) _____ (R) _____ (S) _____
    hypovolemia (hi″po-vo-le′me-ah; a state or condition of below normal volume of blood;
    clinically this refers to abnormally low circulating blood volume)

44. **Ischemia** (n.)   (R) _____ (R) _____ (S) _____
    ischemia (is-ke′me-ah; a condition of suppression of blood; clinically this refers to
    diminished blood flow to a part of the body)

45. **Infarction** (n.)   (R) _____ (S) _____
    infarction (in-fark′shun; [L. *infarciere,* "to stuff in"] the act of "stuffing"; clinically this refers
    to acute obstruction of vasculature, often due to an embolus,[1] resulting in interruption of
    arterial blood supply to the area)

46. **Inotropic** (adj.)   (R) _____ (R) _____ (S) _____
    inotropic (in″o-trop′ik; pertaining to fiber influence; in cardiology, inotropic agents
    influence the strength of myocardial contraction)

---

[1]Embolus: em′bo-lus; [Gr. *embolos,* "plug"]; a clot or other type of plug carried by circulation and forced into
a small vessel, resulting in obstruction of the vessel.

CARDIOVASCULAR ANATOMY AND PHYSIOLOGY

Cardiac Anatomy

The heart is located in the ventral chest cavity, between the third and seventh ribs for most domestic animals (Fig. 7-1). The heart is designed to pump blood throughout the body. So, it is very muscular and is made up of a series of chambers and valves.

The heart is enveloped by the *pericardial* sac. Anatomically, when the pericardial sac is removed, the next tissue layer of the heart exposed is the *epicardium* (Fig. 7-2). The epicardium is the thin, most superficial epithelial tissue of the heart proper. It serves to produce a thin, proteinaceous fluid that prevents friction between the epicardium and the pericardial sac. Beneath the epicardium is the *myocardium* (see Chapter 3, the section entitled "Muscle Tissue," for details regarding myocardial tissue). The interior of the cardiac chambers is lined with endocardium, an endothelial tissue.

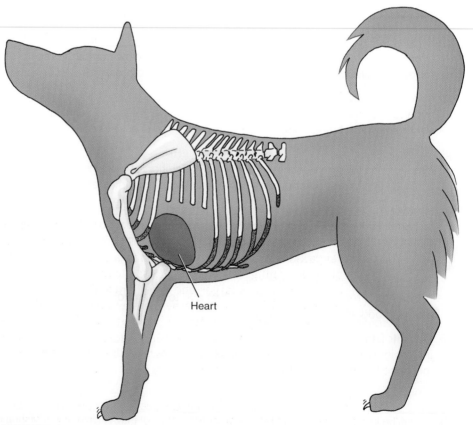

Heart

FIGURE 7-1   Heart position in the thoracic cavity (ribs 4-7 partially removed).

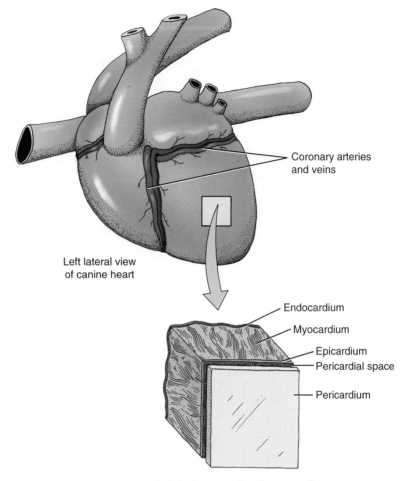

Left lateral view
of canine heart

Coronary arteries
and veins

Endocardium
Myocardium
Epicardium
Pericardial space
Pericardium

Full thickness cardiac tissue specimen

FIGURE 7-2   Cardiac tissues.

The heart is divided into four chambers (Fig. 7-3). The smallest, least muscular of the chambers are the atria. The atria are located near the base of the heart.[2] They are separated into right and left chambers by a wall, the *interatrial* septum.[3] Venous blood returning to the heart enters the atria first.

The ventricles are the larger and more muscular of the cardiac chambers. They are separated from one another by the *interventricular* septum and are separated from the atria by valves. The right chambers are separated by the right *atrioventricular* valve, and the left chambers are separated by the left atrioventricular valve. These two valves are open during the filling phase of the heart and closed during ventricular *systole* (sis′to-le). During ventricular

---

[2]The base of the heart is found on the dorsal aspect. The great vessels of the heart (vena cavae, aorta, pulmonary arteries, and pulmonary veins) are clustered at the base of the heart.
[3]Septum (sep′tum; [L. "wall"]).

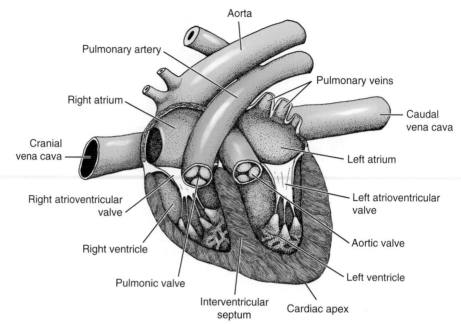

FIGURE 7-3   Cardiac chambers and valves (schematic left-lateral view of canine heart).

systole, the blood is forced from the ventricles through two other valves. Blood from the right ventricle passes through the *pulmonic* valve and blood from the left ventricle passes through the *aortic* valve. These valves close during *diastole* (di-as'to-le). Because blood from the left ventricle must travel farther through the body, the myocardium making up the walls of that chamber is much thicker. It is the myocardium of the left ventricle that forms the cardiac apex (a'peks).

Vasculature

Arteries are thick-walled, muscular vessels that carry blood away from the heart to other areas of the body. The basic structure of an artery is a series of layers (Fig. 7-4). The innermost arterial layer is composed of endothelial cells. These cells, much like those that make up the endocardium, provide a very smooth intra-arterial surface for the blood to flow through. The endothelium is supported by a layer of elastic and fibrous connective tissues. Surrounding these tissues is a very thick layer of smooth muscle, which makes up the bulk of the arterial wall. This smooth muscle is very important for changing the diameter of the vessel lumen.[4] When the smooth muscle contracts, the diameter of the arterial lumen is reduced *(vasoconstriction)*. Conversely, when the smooth muscle is relaxed, the diameter of the arterial lumen is increased in size *(vasodilation)*. Arterioles, with far less smooth muscle, experience similar lumen changes. The activities of vasoconstriction and vasodilation play a significant role in the regulation of

---

[4]Lumen (lu'men; the cavity within a tubular structure).

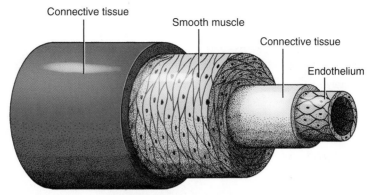

Connective tissue

Smooth muscle

Connective tissue

Endothelium

FIGURE 7-4   Arterial wall.

blood pressure and other physiologic activities, such as temperature regulation. By either increasing or decreasing vessel lumen size, resistance to blood flow is either increased or decreased, and thereby blood pressure is increased or decreased. Enveloping all of the layers of the arterial wall is a thick layer of elastic and fibrous connective tissues. The connective tissues of the arterial wall provide strength to withstand the forces of high blood pressure (inherent to arteries). They also provide great elasticity, permitting the arteries to stretch in accommodation to the increased blood volumes associated with ventricular systole.

The largest artery of the body is the aorta. It originates from the left ventricle, arches shortly after leaving the heart, and then courses caudally along the dorsum of the animal. It terminates at the final arterial branches that supply the hindlimbs. All major arteries of the body originate from the aorta, with the exception of the coronary (kor′ŏ-na-re) arteries, which supply the heart itself, and the pulmonary arteries, which supply the lungs. The size of the arteries progressively becomes smaller the farther away from the heart they are. Many of the peripheral arteries can be used clinically as pulse points. By palpating over a peripheral artery, the pulsation created by the heart pumping the blood can be felt. For each contraction of the heart, a peripheral pulse should be felt. Figures 7-5 and 7-6 show the common pulse points in domestic animals. (If you are unfamiliar with some of the anatomic landmarks cited for these vessels, refer to Chapter 6, "The Musculoskeletal System.") Note that most peripheral vessels are bilaterally symmetrical.

The following are common pulse points of domestic animals. Each artery has been listed, with a brief description of its location and species specificity for use, where applicable.

Sublingual (sub-ling′gwal) artery
   The sublingual artery is located on the ventral midline of the tongue. It is a commonly used pulse point in anesthetized animals.
Facial (fa′shal) artery
   The facial artery is frequently used as a pulse point in horses and cattle. Three branches are easily palpated: the transverse branch courses along the zygomatic arch, just caudal to the lateral canthus of the eye; another branch

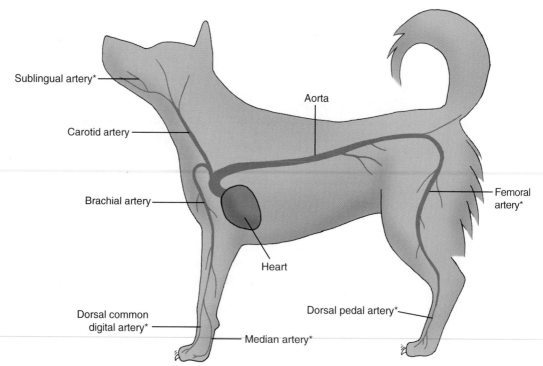

FIGURE 7-5 Major canine arteries and pulse points. (The asterisk [*] denotes common pulse points for dogs and cats.)

courses over the ventrocaudal mandible, usually palpable in a small notch below the ramus of the mandible; this latter branch actually continues over the lateral maxilla to form the lateral nasal artery.

Carotid (kah-rot'id) artery

The carotid artery lies in the ventrolateral neck, lateral to the trachea (windpipe). This artery may be difficult to palpate in most domestic animals, especially those that are heavily muscled.

Median artery

The median artery is located near the midline of the palmar aspect of the metacarpus. It is readily palpated in dogs and cats.

Dorsal common digital (dij'ĭ-tal) artery

The dorsal common digital artery is located on the dorsal aspect of the metacarpus, coursing across the metacarpus at a mediolateral oblique angle. It is easily palpated in dogs and cats.

Medial and lateral digital arteries

The medial and lateral digital arteries are located on the palmar (plantar) aspect of the proximal phalanges. The medial branch is located near the palmaromedial (plantaromedial) aspect of the limb, whereas the lateral branch is located near the palmarolateral (plantarolateral) aspect of the limb. These arteries, found in all four limbs, are used as pulse points in horses.

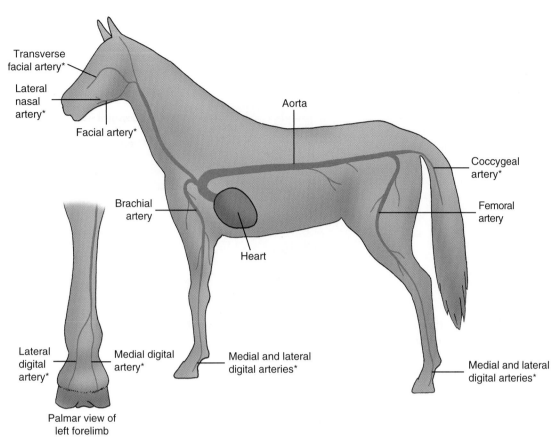

FIGURE 7-6 Major equine arteries and pulse points. (The asterisk [*] denotes common pulse points of horses and cattle.)

Brachial (bra'ke-al) artery

The brachial artery lies on the medial aspect of the proximal forelimb (i.e., medial to the humerus). This artery may be difficult to palpate in heavily muscled companion animals. Therefore, its use as a pulse point is limited. It is, however, a very important pressure point for the control of hemorrhage in a forelimb.

Femoral (fem'or-al) artery

The femoral artery lies on the medial aspect of the proximal hindlimb (i.e., medial to the femur). It is probably the most frequently used pulse point in dogs and cats. Like the brachial artery, the femoral artery serves as an important pressure point for the hindlimb. Do not attempt to use this artery in horses or cattle.

Medial and lateral digital arteries

The lateral digital arteries lie in the distal limbs, on the lateral aspect of the metatarsus and metacarpus. The medial digital arteries lie in the distal limbs, on the medial aspect of the metatarsus and metacarpus. They are used for pulse determination in horses.

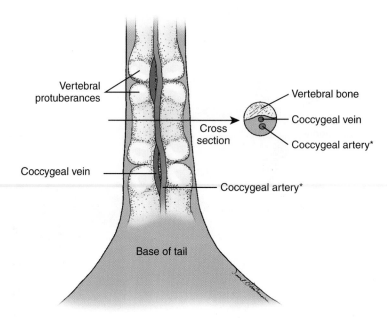

FIGURE 7-7   Coccygeal artery and vein. (The asterisk [*] denotes common equine and bovine pulse point.)

Dorsal pedal artery
> The dorsal pedal artery is located on the dorsal midline of the metatarsus. It is frequently used for pulse and blood pressure determination in dogs and cats.

Coccygeal (kok-sij'e-al) artery
> The coccygeal artery (Fig. 7-7) is located on the ventromidline of the tail. It is most easily palpated in horses and cattle at the proximal third of the tail. It is the most frequently used pulse point in cattle.

Veins (vānz) are vessels that carry blood to the heart. Structurally, veins are much thinner and less muscular than arteries (Fig. 7-8). The interior surfaces of veins are lined with endothelium, just like the arteries. In contrast, however, because the blood flowing through veins is under far less pressure than arterial blood, *intravenous* unidirectional valves keep the blood flowing one way. The smooth muscle and connective tissue layers are arranged similarly to arteries, but with less bulk. Because smooth muscle is present in venous walls, veins too have the capacity to vasoconstrict and vasodilate, contributing to the regulation of blood pressure, temperature, and so forth.

The largest vein of body is the vena cava, which is divided into cranial and caudal portions. The cranial vena cava collects blood from the head and the cranial body, and the caudal vena cava collects blood from the abdomen and caudal body. Both the cranial and caudal vena cavae deposit blood into the right atrium. Most other major veins of the body (with the exception of coronary and pulmonary veins) ultimately deposit their blood into the cranial and caudal vena cavae. Pulmonary veins carry blood from the lungs to the left atrium.

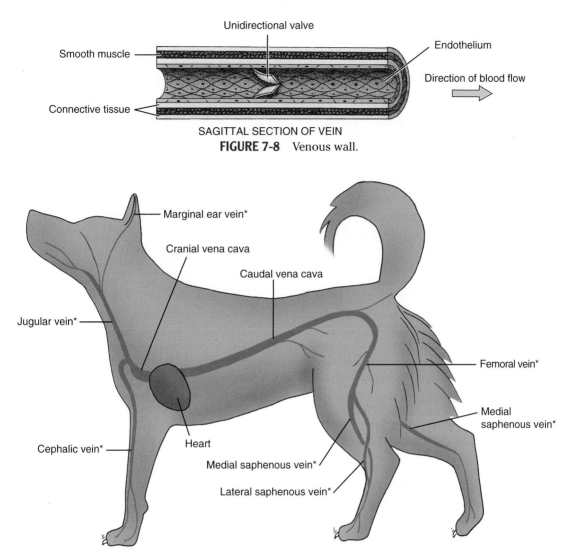

Smooth muscle

Connective tissue

Unidirectional valve

Endothelium

Direction of blood flow

SAGITTAL SECTION OF VEIN

FIGURE 7-8 Venous wall.

Marginal ear vein*

Cranial vena cava

Caudal vena cava

Jugular vein*

Femoral vein*

Medial
saphenous vein*

Cephalic vein*

Heart

Medial saphenous vein*

Lateral saphenous vein*

FIGURE 7-9 Major canine veins and phlebotomy sites. (The asterisk [*] denotes common phlebotomy sites for dogs and cats.)

Veins have thin walls, are under less pressure than arteries, and carry blood to the heart for redistribution throughout the body. For those reasons, they are frequently used for blood collection and administration of intravenous (IV) medications. Some medications are too caustic to come in contact with most tissues of the body. Such medications must be given intravenously, using a large vein for quick dilution of the agent. If a portion of a caustic medication were given *perivascularly,* tissues in that area may become inflamed, die, and slough (sluf) from the body. Appropriate *aseptic* technique must be observed for *phlebotomy* and administration of IV medications to prevent the development of *phlebitis* or *thrombophlebitis*. Figures 7-9 and 7-10 show the common phlebotomy sites in domestic animals.

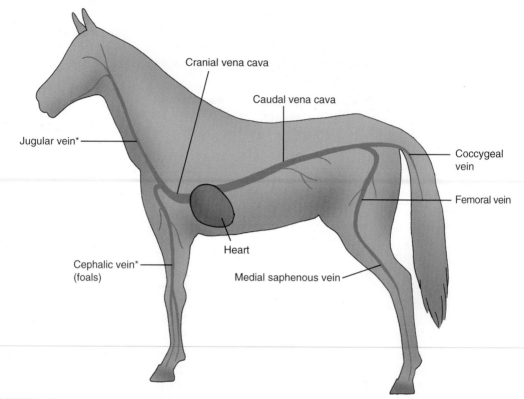

FIGURE 7-10 Major equine veins and phlebotomy sites. (The asterisk [*] denotes common phlebotomy sites for horses.)

The following is a list of each phlebotomy site, including anatomic landmarks and those species in which it is most frequently used.

Cephalic (sĕ-fal'ik) vein
> The cephalic vein is located on the craniomedial aspect of the forelimb, between the elbow and the carpus. It is the most frequently used phlebotomy site in dogs and cats. It is an alternative site in horses, particularly foals.

Jugular (jug'u-lar) vein
> The jugular vein is located in the ventrolateral neck, lateral to the trachea, in the jugular furrow. It is frequently used for collection of large volumes of blood from all domestic animals. It is very important to use the middle third of this vein. Cranially near the mandible and caudally near the thoracic inlet, the jugular vein lies very near the carotid artery and the vagus nerve. Penetration of either of those structures could have serious, even lethal, effects.

Marginal ear vein
> The marginal ear vein is located at the margins of the ear pinna (flap). It is frequently used in rabbits, pigs, and flop-eared dogs (e.g., Basset Hounds).

Lateral saphenous (sah-fe'nus, să'fĕ-nus) vein

> The lateral saphenous vein is located on the lateral aspect of the hindlimb. It courses across the distal, lateral tibia at a craniocaudal-distoproximal oblique angle. It is frequently used in dogs and cats and is an alternative site in horses, particularly foals.

Medial saphenous vein

> The medial saphenous vein is located on the medial aspect of the distal hindlimb and courses medial to the tibia between the tarsus and the femorotibial joint. It is used frequently in cats and dogs.

Femoral vein

> The femoral vein is located on the medial aspect of the proximal hindlimb, medial to the femur. It is used most frequently in cats and sometimes in dogs.

Coccygeal vein

> The coccygeal vein is located on the ventral midline of the tail. It is frequently used at its proximal aspect in cattle. Note in Figure 7-7 how it weaves with the coccygeal artery over the osseous protuberances of the vertebrae. Because of the close proximity of these vessels, it is possible to inadvertently collect an arterial sample. If this occurs, prolonged pressure must be applied to the site, to prevent hematoma formation.

Capillaries (kap'ĭ-lar″ēz) are the smallest, thinnest-walled vessels of the cardiovascular system. Capillaries are so small that blood cells literally have to squeeze through the lumen single file. They are minute, yet critically important, connections between arterioles and venules. Structurally, capillaries have no smooth muscle surrounding them. In fact, they are for all practical purposes merely an extension of the endothelial lining from adjoining vessels, supported by a thin basement membrane. This thin structure of the capillary wall, the tiny gaps found between the endothelial cellular membranes, and the pores in the cellular membranes make capillaries very permeable to blood gases, like oxygen and carbon dioxide. Their structure also makes them naturally "leaky." This is how water can naturally seep out from the bloodstream and percolate through the interstitium, eventually to be absorbed into lymphatic vessels (see Chapter 5). In the presence of inflammation, capillary permeability increases, resulting in edema. (Events like this will be discussed further in the Pathophysiology and Disease section.) It should also be noted that the thin walls of capillaries permit visualization of the color of the blood within them. Mucous membranes are packed with capillaries. So, on physical examination, we always evaluate mucous membrane color. Of course, remember that the quality and intensity of mucous membrane color can be significantly influenced by arterial supply to the capillary bed (vasoconstriction will render pale coloration), blood gas concentrations (especially oxygen and carbon dioxide), and the quantity and quality of erythrocytes present. Frightened, anemic, and hypoxic patients can all have pale mucous membranes, but for very different reasons.

Blood Flow

It is essential that the flow of blood throughout the body be a consistent, never-ending process. The constant movement of the blood helps prevent *thrombosis*, delivers oxygen and other nutrients to body tissues, and removes wastes from

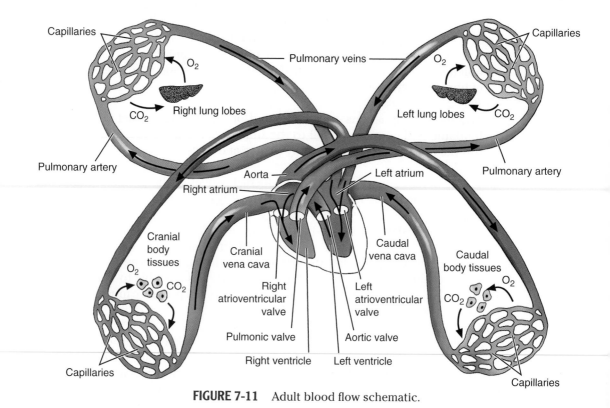

FIGURE 7-11   Adult blood flow schematic.

body tissues. The entire cardiovascular system was designed for one-way flow of blood. If a pair of red blood cells were followed through one circuit in an adult animal, the sequence of events would be as follows (Fig. 7-11). Let's begin in the vena cavae. We will follow one cell through the caudal vena cava and the other cell through the cranial vena cava. They will meet in the right atrium; from there they flow through the right atrioventricular valve (commonly called the tricuspid valve), into the right ventricle, through the pulmonic valve, and into the pulmonary artery. The blood at this time is carrying very little oxygen and large quantities of carbon dioxide. To make the appropriate gas exchanges in the lungs, we must go through a gradual transition of pulmonary arteries and arterioles to reach the capillaries, where gas exchange takes place. As we squeeze through the pulmonary capillaries, we will pick up a new supply of oxygen and eliminate carbon dioxide (Fig. 7-12). We exit the capillaries into pulmonary venules, then flow into pulmonary veins and into the left atrium of the heart. From the left atrium we pass through the left atrioventricular valve (commonly called the mitral or bicuspid valve), into the left ventricle, through the aortic valve, and into the aorta. In the systemic circulation, we carry our fresh supply of oxygen through a series of arteries, arterioles, and capillaries. In the systemic capillaries, oxygen is delivered to the tissues, carbon dioxide and other wastes are picked up (Fig. 7-13), and we return by way of the systemic venules and

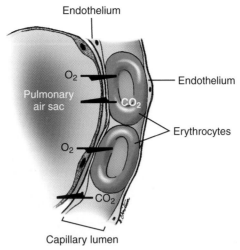

FIGURE 7-12   Pulmonary capillary.

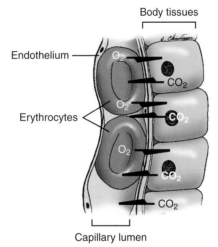

FIGURE 7-13   Tissue capillary.

veins to the vena cavae. The thoracic duct is the principle lymphatic vessel that delivers lymphatic fluid to the vena cava (see Chapter 5). So, all of the water that seeped out of our porous capillaries eventually makes its way back into general circulation. Figure 7-14 summarizes the blood flow circuit discussed.

Cardiac Cycle

The cardiac cycle is the activity that the heart engages in to create a heart-beat. It is a series of synchronous events. Throughout the cardiac cycle, pressures within the heart and in general circulation rise and fall. During *diastole,*

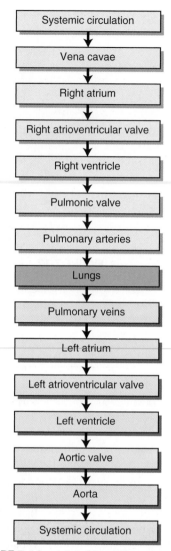

FIGURE 7-14   Adult blood flow summary.

the myocardium is relaxed, permitting the atria and the ventricles to fill with blood. The atrioventricular valves are open and pressures in the system are relatively low during diastole. Near the end of the filling phase, the atria contract (atrial *systole*), forcing as much blood as possible into the ventricles. On being engorged with blood, the ventricles contract (ventricular systole). At the beginning of ventricular systole, the pressure within the ventricles rises sharply. The increased pressure forces the atrioventricular valves to close and, with nowhere else to go, the blood forces open and rushes through the pulmonic and aortic valves. When ventricular systole is complete, the heart again enters into its diastolic phase and the aortic and pulmonic valves close.

Blood pressure is influenced by a number of variables, including blood volume, vasoconstriction, vasodilation, and cardiac output. Cardiac output is the sum of cardiac rate plus cardiac stroke volume.[5] Blood pressure can be measured by the use of a *sphygmomanometer*. The cuff of the sphygmomanometer is placed over a peripheral artery and inflated enough to occlude the artery completely. The air pressure within the cuff is gradually released to the point where blood begins to flow through the artery again. The reading taken at this moment is referred to as the *systolic* pressure. The air continues to be released from the cuff until blood flow through the artery can no longer be detected. The reading taken at this moment is referred to as the *diastolic* pressure. Blood pressure readings are recorded in millimeters of mercury (mm Hg), as systolic over diastolic. The two numbers reflect the pressures exerted by the blood on the vasculature during ventricular systole and diastole. Capillary refill time (CRT) is a simple, cursory indicator of blood pressure and cardiac output. To evaluate the CRT of a patient, firm digital pressure is applied momentarily to an accessible mucous membrane, such as the gums in the mouth. Observing the site, the CRT is timed in seconds to see how rapidly the tissue reperfuses with blood. A prolonged CRT indicates poor cardiac output and *hypotension*. The quality of pulses can also be an indicator of cardiac output and blood pressure. In a normal animal, pulses should be palpable in most peripheral arteries. Assuming that the heart is beating and that no *infarction* has occurred, failure to feel a pulse in a large, peripheral artery may indicate significant hypotension (<50 mm Hg systolic pressure). In a hypotensive state such as that, blood pressure must be improved quickly. If it is not, crucial organs, like the kidneys, will begin to fail. Pressure may be improved many ways, including the use of positive *inotropic* agents and/or administration of IV fluids to improve cardiac output.

Heart Sounds

Normal heart sounds are created by the synchronous closure of the valves. The sounds generated are much like those created by slamming a door. The heart sounds can be divided into a first heart sound (lub) and a second heart sound (dup). The first heart sound is produced by the closure of the atrioventricular valves, and the second heart sound is created by closure of the aortic and pulmonic valves. During a single cardiac cycle, both the first and the second heart sounds are generated; they mark the beginning and the end of each cycle.

Abnormal heart sounds are usually created either by asynchronous closure of the valves, by splashing of blood into a large chamber, or by turbulent blood flow creating audible vibrations. Asynchronous closure of valves may be heard as split heart sounds (lub-d-dup). The splashing of blood into the ventricles, when the atrioventricular valves open, may create a third heart sound (lub dup dup).

---

[5]Cardiac stroke volume is the volume of blood pumped (each time) during ventricular systole.

In an animal like a horse, whose ventricles are naturally large, generation of such a third heart sound may be normal. In most companion animals, however, a third heart sound may be indicative of *dilatory cardiomyopathy*. The abnormal heart sounds produced by turbulent blood flow are referred to as *murmurs*. Leaky (insufficient) valves, *stenotic* valves or vessels, and septal defects are the most frequent causes of murmurs. Murmurs are generally characterized by a swooshing sound. By correlating the swooshing sound to its timing within the cardiac cycle, murmurs will be recorded as systolic or diastolic. This information, plus the anatomic intensity of the murmur may help the cardiologist isolate a particular valve that is diseased. Appropriate stethoscope placement will focus the listener on each individual valve. On the left side of the thorax, near the costochondral junction of the third intercostal space, the pulmonic valve will be most intense. Just above the costochondral junction of the fourth intercostal space on that same side the aortic valve may be isolated. Near the costochondral junction of the left fifth intercostal space the mitral valve will be found. The right atrioventricular valve may be auscultated near the costochondral junction of the right fourth intercostal space. Valvular auscultation should be a routine part of any physical examination. Low grade murmurs will most likely be missed if this is not done. At times, the vibrations from the turbulence associated with murmurs can be so great that they can actually be palpated through the chest wall. Murmurs are generally graded on a scale of I to VI, with VI being the most severe and palpable.

One of the most common congenital cardiac defects to cause a murmur in puppies is a patent ductus arteriosus (PDA). What is it? Well, the ductus arteriosus is a vascular connection between the aorta and pulmonary artery. During fetal development, this connection is necessary to bypass the fetal lungs. At birth, the ductus arteriosus should close. If it remains open (patent), extremely turbulent blood flow is created. The murmur of a PDA is usually loud and machinery-like. Yes, it sounds very much like the "voom-voom-voom" sound of a washing machine agitating. Fortunately, a PDA is easily corrected surgically.

Electrocardiography

All of the myocardial activity of the heart is controlled by an electrical system called the cardiac conduction system (Fig. 7-15). The electrical activity acts like a battery: it discharges electrical impulses (depolarization). The end result of depolarization is myocardial contraction. After being discharged, the entire system must be recharged (repolarization) to ready itself for the next cycle of events. The *electrocardiograph* (ECG) machine is used to record this electrical activity.

The *sinoatrial node* (si"no-a'tre-al, *SA node*) is the pacemaker of the cardiac conduction system. It is located in the caudodorsal right atrium near the opening from the cranial vena cava. When it discharges, the SA node stimulates the cascade of events that occurs during the cardiac cycle. The electrical impulse quickly travels through the atrial myocardium, initiating atrial systole. The electrical activity recorded by the ECG machine during atrial depolarization

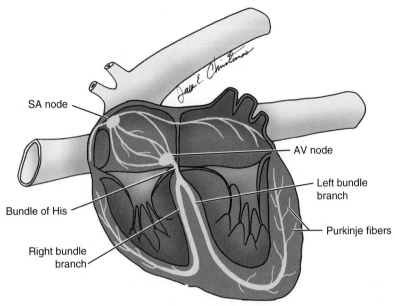

FIGURE 7-15   Cardiac conduction system anatomy.

is the *P wave* (Fig. 7-16). The impulse continues to progress through the myocardium, rapidly concentrating at a mass of specialized tissue located in the ventral right atrium, near the *interatrial* septum. This specialized mass of tissue is called the atrioventricular node *(AV node)*. As the impulse reaches this site, it is momentarily slowed. Slowing of the impulse at this time allows the atria to empty fully before the ventricles are stimulated to contract. The portion of the ECG tracing that corresponds to the AV node is referred to as the *P-R segment*. The impulse quickly continues through the rest of the cardiac conduction system. It first progresses to the bundle of His (hiss), located in the craniodorsal interventricular septum. It quickly travels through the right and left bundle branches, terminating in the Purkinje fibers (per-kin'je), and stimulates ventricular systole. Ventricular systole begins at the cardiac apex and progresses along the ventricular walls, following the impulse through the Purkinje fibers. The electrical activity from the bundle of His through ventricular depolarization is recorded on the ECG tracing as the *QRS complex*. The final electrical activity to be recorded on the ECG tracing is the *T wave,* which marks repolarization of the ventricular myocardium. The magnitude of all of the electrical activity generated through the ventricles is so great that repolarization of the atria is not detected by the ECG.

The cardiac conduction system is important for controlling the cardiac rate and rhythm. If the electrical activity is too slow, *bradycardia* will be clinically evident. When looking at an ECG tracing, bradycardia may be recognized by an excessive distance between R waves. Of course, cardiac auscultation or palpation of peripheral pulses may also be used to detect bradycardia. If the electrical activity is too fast, *tachycardia* will be clinically evident.

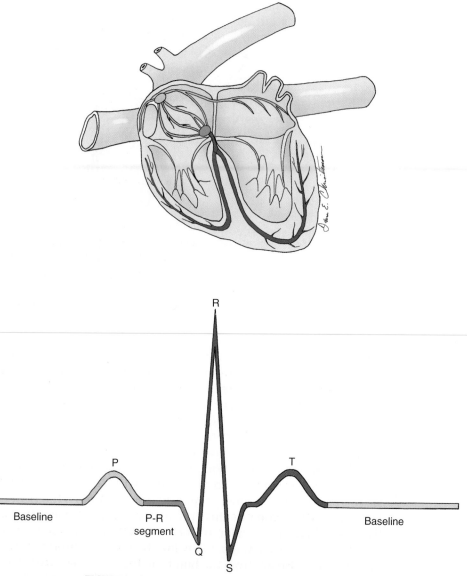

FIGURE 7-16   Electrocardiographic signal generation.

Arrhythmias develop from abnormal and uncoordinated electrical activity. The arrhythmias may be caused by a primary disease in the cardiac conduction system, whereas others may be simply the result of electrolyte imbalances in the body. One of the most common arrhythmias seen on ECG tracings is a ventricular premature complex (VPC). When this occurs, the impulse originates from the ventricles, before the SA node fires. Therefore, on ECG, it will not be preceded by a P wave. It will appear as a very large, abnormal impulse (Fig. 7-17). Because ventricular filling has been preempted, no peripheral

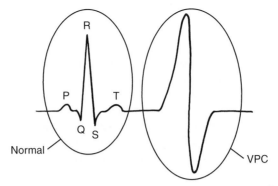

FIGURE 7-17 Ventricular premature complex (VPC).

pulse will be generated by a VPC. Rare, isolated VPCs are not a great concern. However, more frequent VPCs are an important warning sign. In an anesthetized patient, increased frequency of VPCs may be indicative of myocardial hypoxia.[6] Improving oxygenation of such a patient is imperative to prevent rapid deterioration of cardiac function. A string of three or more VPCs constitutes ventricular tachycardia (V-tach, as they frequently refer to it on emergency shows). If this is not corrected, it may rapidly progress to ventricular fibrillation[7] and then *asystole*. Any arrhythmia should always place a veterinary professional on high alert.

In addition to the electrocardiogram (ECG), the cardiologist may elect to use other diagnostic tools to evaluate cardiac patients fully. *Echocardiography* is useful in determining how well the heart can contract. In echocardiography, ultrasound (a type of sound wave, much like sonar) is used to create visual images of the heart in motion. The cardiologist may also be able to visualize abnormal chamber dilation or myocardial hypertrophy from the echocardiogram. Use of Doppler imaging with an echocardiogram can reveal location and severity of turbulence. Yes, this Doppler imaging is much like the Doppler radar shown on weather maps. Radiography is often useful for visualizing cardiomegaly. (Widening of the QRS complex may also be indicative of cardiomegaly, because it takes longer for the impulse to travel through the dilated ventricular walls.) A dorsoventral view will offer the best view of the heart with the least amount of distortion, because the heart is closest to the film. At least one lateral view should also be taken. Other special radiographic procedures, such as the *angiogram,* help outline problem areas along vessels. For this, an IV radiopaque dye is administered. On radiograph, the dye brightly outlines the vasculature. Early detection of cardiovascular problems, coupled with appropriate medical, nutritional, or surgical management, may result in happy, healthy, long-lived veterinary patients, in spite of cardiac disease.

---

[6]Hypoxia (hi-pok'se-ah [*hypo-* + *ox* (oxygen) + *-ia;* a condition of deficient oxygen].

[7]Fibrillation (fi-bri-la'shun; fibrillation of the myocardium is an uncoordinated, uncontrolled activity in which the muscle appears to simply quiver).

Pathophysiology and Disease

Heart disease, as observed in humans, is uncommon in domestic animals. Heart attacks due to myocardial infarction and the resultant myocardial ischemia are principally a human problem. Cardiac arrest in animals is more often a risk of surgery and anesthesia or the result of severe systemic disease or trauma. *Hypovolemia* that results from severe hemorrhage or dehydration may lead to cardiac arrest. Drugs used to anesthetize patients can have significant hypotensive effects. Additionally, they may also have significant negative inotropic effects, resulting in bradycardia and weak contractility. In hypotension, normal cardiac compensation should be increased heart rate and/or stronger contraction to improve cardiac output. During anesthesia, these cardiac compensatory mechanisms may be impaired. The drug-induced hypotension may result in multiple organ failure and death.

Hypertension in domestic animals does occur, although not with the frequency that it does in humans. Naturally occurring hypertension is usually a heritable condition, but may not be apparent at an early age. Congenital[8] cardiac defects, such as aortic stenosis, pulmonic stenosis, or ventricular septal defects, are usually discovered very early in life by virtue of the murmurs that they create. Many such defects may resolve with time or may be surgically corrected.

Cardiomyopathy is a very common disease. *Hypertrophic cardiomyopathy* occurs most frequently in cats. Echocardiography is used to diagnose and monitor cats with the disease. Drug therapy may be used in these cats to improve cardiac function and to prevent thrombosis. It is not uncommon for cats with hypertrophic cardiomyopathy to develop "saddle thrombus" secondarily. In saddle thrombus, a clot (most likely formed in the diseased heart) dislodges. The embolus follows circulation to the terminal end of the aorta, creating infarction of the main arterial branches that supply the hindlimbs (iliac arteries). The resultant ischemia in the affected limbs is excruciatingly painful for the cat. Owners usually find the cats crying and unable to move their rear legs. On physical examination, femoral pulses will be absent and the feet and legs will be pale and cool to the touch. Prognosis[9] is poor for these patients.

Dilatory cardiomyopathy is far more common in dogs, especially certain large breed dogs. The ventricular free walls become progressively thinner and weaker as the chamber size increases. Cardiac output becomes poor. Congestive heart failure, affecting both sides of the heart develops, resulting in retrograde backup and pooling of blood in veins, venules, and capillaries. The backup increases hydrostatic pressure in the naturally leaky capillaries and results in edematous

---

[8]Congenital (kon-jen'ï-tal [L. *congenitus*, "born together"]; a congenital defect or disease is one that an animal is born with.

[9]Prognosis (prog-no'sis [Gr. "foreknowledge"]; it is a forecast as to the probable outcome of a disease or condition).

fluids. Ascites,[10] pulmonary edema,[11] and even hydrothorax[12] may result. Dilatory cardiomyopathy is inevitably fatal.

Endocarditis can result from infectious agents (viral, bacterial, or fungal). Probably the most frequent scenario would be mobilization of bacteria from the mouth of a dog or cat with periodontal[13] disease. (See Chapter 12, "The Alimentary System," for a discussion of periodontal disease.) In this case, bacteria gain entry to the bloodstream through inflamed tissues of the mouth. Unfortunately, many such organisms have an affinity for the endocardium and valvular leaflets. If not treated promptly, complete cardiovascular collapse and death may result from endocarditis.

Heartworm disease is the most common infectious cardiac disease to affect companion animals. Originally, this disease affected only dogs. Unfortunately, the parasite that causes the disease has adapted and now frequently infects cats.

Heartworm disease is caused by the parasite *Dirofilaria immitis* (di-ro-fī-lar′e-ah im′ ĭ-tis). Adult worms live in the heart (predominantly right atrium and ventricle) and the pulmonary artery. In a patent[14] infection, reproducing adults will give birth to offspring (microfilaria). The microfilaria flow with the blood in general circulation. When a mosquito feeds on this infected dog, some of the microfilaria will be ingested. In the mosquito, the microfilaria will develop to an infective larval stage. This typically takes a few weeks. Once developed to an infective stage, the larvae will migrate to the mouth parts of the mosquito. When the mosquito feeds on another unsuspecting victim, the infective larvae will be transmitted to that animal. From the time of this infective bite, it will take an average of 6 months before this animal has fully mature, reproductively active adults in its heart. In cats and some dogs, occult infections may develop. In an occult infection, no microfilaria will be produced by the adults.

Adult heartworms living in the heart and pulmonary artery will severely impair cardiac function. Right-sided cardiomegaly will be apparent radiographically. Because the worms impede outflow from the right side of the heart, right-sided congestive heart failure will develop. This may directly affect liver and kidney function. It may also result in ascites formation. Of course, because blood is insufficiently pumped from the right ventricle to the lungs, the animal's ability to oxygenate will be impaired. The hypoxia will make the animal intolerant to activity and exercise. Additionally, circulating microfilaria, thrombosis, and pulmonary emboli may damage and diminish pulmonary function, compounding the animal's inability to exchange vital gases (oxygen and carbon dioxide). Outwardly, the animal may cough and have difficulty breathing. Progressively, the adult worms and their offspring will damage the heart, lungs, liver, and kidneys to the point that life can no

---

[10]Ascites (ah-si′tēz; abnormal abdominal fluid accumulation).

[11]Pulmonary edema: edema within the lungs, particularly the tiny air sacs where gas exchange occurs.

[12]Hydrothorax (hi″dro-tho′raks; *hydro-* "water" + *thorax;* a fluid accumulation within the chest cavity, also referred to as pleural effusion).

[13]Periodontal (per″e-o-don′tal; *peri-* + *odont(o)-* tooth + *-al;* pertaining to around teeth; periodontal disease is a syndrome that affects the teeth and all the tissues that surround them).

[14]Patent (pa′tent; open; in reference to parasitic infestations, patency means that the parasite is reproducing and able to pass its offspring to others).

longer be sustained. Death from heartworm disease is tragic because the disease is preventable.

Can animals infected with heartworms be treated? Yes, provided the damage from the parasite is not too severe. Many costly diagnostic tests must be done to determine the extent of organ damage before treatment. Even if the animal is a healthy enough candidate for treatment, the treatment itself can kill the patient. The best thing that dog and cat owners can do about heartworm disease is prevent it. Most heartworm preventives are given monthly. They are designed to kill larvae that have been transmitted to the animal over the past month. Failure to give these preventives on schedule as prescribed may permit the larvae to develop to a point that the preventive drugs can no longer kill them. Animals should be tested for heartworm disease before initiating preventive therapy. (Giving preventive therapy to an animal with a patent infection could be deadly.) Yes, heartworm preventive medication costs money. Compared with the cost of treatment, prevention is an insignificant expense. No one should ever gamble with the priceless life of a pet by not preventing this disease.

SELF-TEST

Using the previous information in this chapter, complete the following crossword puzzle using the most appropriate medical term(s). Do not use abbreviations or common names unless requested.

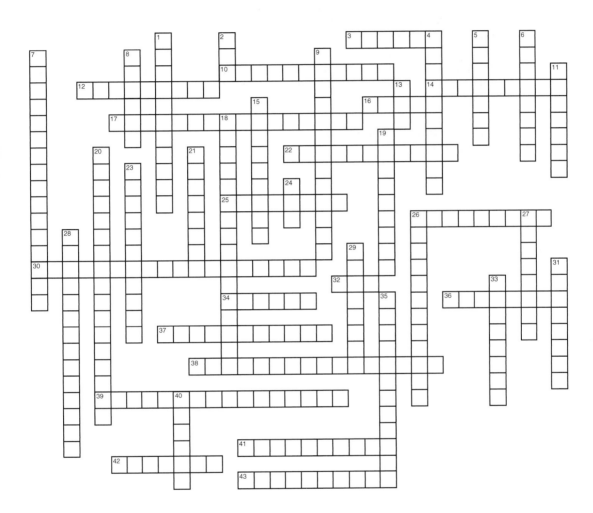

ACROSS
3	A heart chamber to which blood returns
10	A condition of a slow heart rate
12	Pertaining to an agent that influences the myocardium
14	The smallest vessel of the body
16	The large artery carrying blood from the left ventricle
17	Reduction of vessel lumen size from muscular contraction of the vessel wall
22	A condition of a fast heart rate
25	The transmitter of heartworm disease

26	An artery used as a pulse point, found on the ventral tail
30	Puncture of the sac that surrounds the heart for removal of fluid
32	Abbreviation for capillary refill time
34	An abnormal heart sound characterized by a swooshing sound from blood turbulence
36	The phase of the cardiac cycle when the heart is relaxed and filling
37	A state of abnormally low blood pressure
38	Inflammation and clotting of a vein
39	A valve found between an atrium and the next chamber
41	A condition without rhythm
42	The vein used for blood collection that is found in the ventrolateral neck
43	Blood collection from a vein; i.e., venipuncture

DOWN

1	A state of abnormally low blood volume
2	First heart sound
4	Heart muscle
5	Edematous fluid accumulating in the abdominal cavity
6	The large vein carrying blood to the right atrium (2 words)
7	A diagnostic procedure using sound waves to evaluate heart function
8	Common name for the left AV valve
9	The sum of heart rate plus stroke volume (2 words)
11	The phase of the cardiac cycle when the heart is contracting
13	The complex seen on ECG that indicates ventricular depolarization
15	A forecast for the outcome of a disease
18	An instrument used to measure blood pressure
19	The vein used for phlebotomy found on the distal rear limb
20	An ECG (i.e., the printed tracing)
21	The valve that leads to the artery that carries blood to the lungs
23	Excessive development
24	Second heart sound
26	A clinician specializing in the heart
27	Absence of cardiac activity
28	Disease of heart muscle
29	The terminal fibers of the cardiac conduction system
31	A condition of narrowing
33	Suppressed blood flow to an area
35	Heart enlargement
40	A tiny vein

Cardiovascular Challenge

1. List, in sequence, blood flow through the heart beginning with blood returning from the body.
2. Trace the blood flow of an adult animal through one complete circuit. Beginning with the systemic circulation returning to the heart, sequentially list each of the cardiac and vascular structures through which the blood passes.
3. Label each of the phlebotomy sites shown in the diagram.

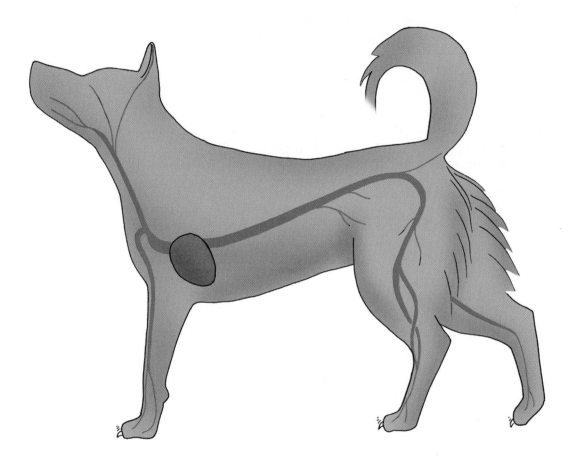

4. Label the ECG tracing.

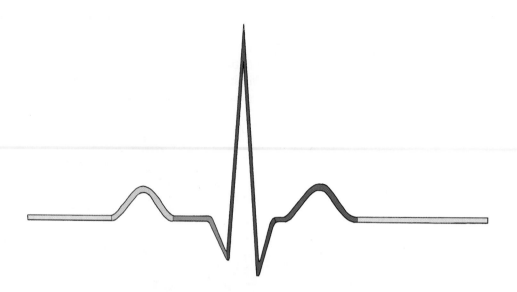

5. Label the cardiac valve locations shown on the lateral thoracic views.

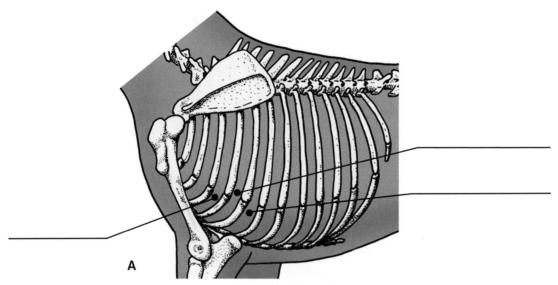

A

Left Lateral View

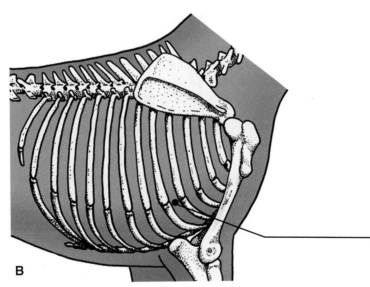

B

Right Lateral View

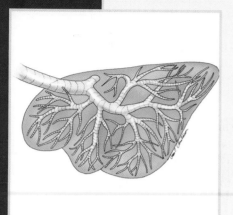

CHAPTER **8**

The Respiratory System

GOALS AND OBJECTIVES

By the conclusion of this chapter, the student will be able to:

1. Recognize common root words, prefixes, and suffixes related to the respiratory system.
2. Divide simple and compound words into their respective parts.
3. Recognize, correctly pronounce, and appropriately use common medical terms related to the respiratory system.
4. Demonstrate an understanding of respiratory and thoracic cavity anatomy.
5. Demonstrate an understanding of respiratory physiology with regard to breathing mechanisms, respiratory volumes, gas exchange, and protective mechanisms.
6. Demonstrate an understanding of the pathophysiology of common domestic animal respiratory diseases.

INTRODUCTION TO RELATED TERMS

Divide each of the following terms into its respective parts ("R" root, "P" prefix, "S" suffix, "CV," combining vowel).

1. **Pleural**   (R) _____ (S) _____
   pleural (ploor'al; pertaining to the pleura[1])

2. **Pneumonia**   (R) _____ (S) _____
   pneumonia (nu-mo'ne-ah; [Gr. *pneumonia*] a condition of the lungs; clinically refers to inflammation of the lungs with consolidation)

---

[1]Pleura (pleurae—pl., derived from [Gr. *pleura,* rib, side]) is the tissue lining the thoracic cavity and covering the thoracic viscera.

3. **Tracheobronchitis**   (R) _____ (CV) _____ (R) _____ (S) _____
   tracheobronchitis (tra"ke-o-brong-ki'tis; inflammation of the trachea and bronchi)

4. **Endotracheal**   (P) _____ (R) _____ (S) _____
   endotracheal (en"do-tra'ke-al; pertaining to within the trachea)

5. **Tracheotomy**   (R) _____ (CV) _____ (S) _____
   tracheotomy (tra"ke-ot'o-me; to incise [cut into] the trachea; clinically refers to a surgical procedure in which an incision is made into the trachea)

6. **Tracheostomy**   (R) _____ (CV) _____ (S) _____
   tracheostomy (tra"ke-os'to-me; to create a "mouth" in the trachea; clinically refers to an artificial opening created in the trachea, as well as the apparatus used to maintain patency of the opening)

7. **Rhinoplasty**   (R) _____ (CV) _____ (S) _____
   rhinoplasty (ri'no-plas"te; to form the nose; clinically this is "plastic surgery," reconstructive surgery of the nose)

8. **Rhinitis**   (R) _____ (S) _____
   rhinitis (ri-ni'tis; inflammation of the nose)

9. **Rhinopneumonitis**   (R) _____ (CV) _____ (R) _____ (S) _____
   rhinopneumonitis (ri"no-nu"mo-ni'tis; inflammation of the nose and the lungs)

10. **Pneumothorax**   (R) _____ (CV) _____ (R) _____
    pneumothorax (nu"mo-tho'raks; air of the chest; clinically refers to free air in the pleural space/chest cavity)

11. **Hemothorax**   (R) _____ (CV) _____ (R) _____
    hemothorax (he-mo-tho'raks; blood of the chest; clinically refers to blood in the pleural space/chest cavity)

12. **Pyothorax**   (P) _____ (CV) _____ (R) _____
    pyothorax (pi"o-tho'raks; pus of the chest; clinically refers to pus in the pleural space/chest cavity)

13. **Atelectasis**   (R) _____ (S) _____
    atelectasis (at"ĕ-lek'tah-sis; imperfect/incomplete expansion; clinically refers to "collapse" of the lungs)

14. **Tachypnea**   (P) _____ (R) _____
    tachypnea (tak"ip-ne'ah; rapid breathing)

15. **Bradypnea**   (P) _____ (R) _____
    bradypnea (brad"e-pne'ah, brād"ip'ne-ah; slow breathing)

16. **Hyperpnea**   (P) _____ (R) _____
    hyperpnea (hi"perp-ne'ah; excessive breathing; clinically refers to a breathing pattern characterized by increased rate and depth)

17. **Dyspnea**   (P) _____ (R) _____
    dyspnea (disp'ne-ah; difficulty breathing)

18. **Apnea**   (P) _____ (R) _____
    apnea (ap-ne'ah, ap'ne-ah; absence of breathing)

19. **Hypercapnia**   (P) _____ (R) _____ (S) _____
    hypercapnia (hi"per-kap'ne-ah; a condition of excessive carbon dioxide)

20. **Hypoxia**   (P) _____ (R) _____ (S) _____
    hypoxia (hi-pok'se-ah; a condition of deficient oxygen)

21. **Alveolar**   (R) _____ (S) _____
    alveolar (al-ve'o-lar; pertaining to an alveolus[2] or alveoli)

22. **Sinusitis**   (R) _____ (S) _____
    sinusitis (si"nŭ-si'tis; inflammation of a sinus)

23. **Intercostal**   (P) _____ (R) _____ (S) _____
    intercostal (in"ter-kos'tal; pertaining to between the ribs)

24. **Bronchiole**   (R) _____ (CV) _____ (S) _____
    bronchiole (brong'ke-ōl; a small bronchus; anatomically refers to the tiny airways that lead
    to the alveoli)

25. **Inspiration**   (P) _____ (R) _____ (S) _____
    inspiration (in"spĭ-ra'shun; the act of breathing in)

26. **Expiration**   (P) _____ (R) _____ (S) _____
    expiration (eks"pĭ-ra'shun; the act of breathing out)

27. **Aspiration**   (P) _____ (R) _____ (S) _____
    aspiration (as"pĭ-ra'shun; the act of breathing to [in]; a- is derived in this case from
    the prefix "ad-" meaning "to" or "toward"; clinically frequently refers to the inspiration
    of foreign materials into the lungs)

28. **Cyanosis**   (R) _____ (CV) _____ (S) _____
    cyanosis (si"ah-no'sis; a condition of blueness; clinically refers to blue coloration
    of the mucous membranes)

29. **Hemoptysis**   (R) _____ (CV) _____ (S) _____
    hemoptysis (he-mop'tĭ-sis; to spit blood; clinically refers to coughing up blood)

30. **Antitussive**   (P) _____ (R) _____ (S) _____
    antitussive (an"tĭ-tus'iv; pertaining to being against coughing; clinically refers to an agent
    used to suppress coughing)

31. **Epiglottis**   (P) _____ (R) _____
    epiglottis (ep"ĭ-glot'is; upon the glottis[3])

32. **Intranasal**   (P) _____ (R) _____ (S) _____
    intranasal (in"trah-na'zal; pertaining to within the nose)

---

[2]Alveolus [L. dim. of *alveus*, hollow]; alveoli are the small air sacs within the lungs.
[3]Glottis [Gr. *glottis*], the vocal apparatus; the epiglottis is the cartilaginous flap that covers the opening to the glottis (larynx).

33. **Achondral**   (P) _____ (R) _____ (S) _____
    achondral (a-kon'dral; pertaining to no cartilage)

34. **Nasopharynx**   (R) _____ (CV) _____ (R) _____
    nasopharynx (na"zo-far'inks; the nose and throat)

35. **Nasogastric**   (R) _____ (CV) _____ (R) _____ (S) _____
    nasogastric (na"zo-gas'trik; pertaining to the nose and stomach)

36. **Bronchiectasis**   (R) _____ (S) _____
    bronchiectasis (brong"ke-ek'tah-sis; dilation of bronchi)

37. **Bronchiarctia**   (R) _____ (R) _____ (S) _____
    bronchiarctia (brong"ke-ark'she-ah; a condition of bronchial constriction; cf.
    bronchostenosis)

38. **Thoracentesis**   (R) _____ (S) _____
    thoracentesis (tho"rah-sen-te'sis; puncture of the chest; cf. thoracocentesis; a clinical
    procedure in which the chest is punctured for the removal of fluid or air [i.e., using
    a syringe and needle])

39. **Hydrothorax**   (P) _____ (R) _____
    hydrothorax (hi"dro-tho'raks; a watery chest; clinically it is a condition in which fluid
    accumulates in the pleural cavity; cf. pleural effusion)

40. **Thoracotomy**   (R) _____ (CV) _____ (S) _____
    thoracotomy (tho"rah-kot'o-me; to cut the chest; clinically it is a surgical incision
    of the chest wall)

41. **Phrenic**   (R) _____ (S) _____
    phrenic (fren'ik; pertaining to the diaphragm)

42. **Oropharyx**   (R) _____ (CV) _____ (R) _____
    oropharynx (o"ro-far'inks; the mouth and throat)

43. **Lobectomy**   (R) _____(S) _____
    lobectomy (lo-bek'to-me; to cut out a lobe [as in lung lobe])

44. **Transtracheal**   (P) _____ (R) _____ (S) _____
    transtracheal (trans-tra'ke-al; pertaining to across the trachea; clinically refers to passage
    of something through/across the tracheal wall)

45. **Bronchospasm**   (R) _____ (CV) _____ (R) _____
    bronchospasm (brong'ko-spazm; bronchial contraction; clinically it is the spasmodic
    contraction of bronchial or bronchiolar muscle)

46. **Laryngoplasty**   (R) _____ (CV) _____ (S) _____
    laryngoplasty (lah-ring'go-plas"te; molding/reshaping of the larynx; reconstructive,
    "plastic surgery" of the larynx)

47. **Capnography**   (R) _____ (CV) _____ (S) _____
    capnography (kap"nah'grǎ-fe; recording of carbon dioxide; a capnograph is an instrument
    used clinically to measure CO_2 concentrations)

48. **Oxymetry** (R) _____ (S) _____

oxymetry (ok-sim'ĕ-tre; measurement of oxygen; clinically oximeters measure oxygen saturation in the blood through use of a noninvasive light source)

49. **Orthopnea** (R) _____ (CV) _____ (R) _____

orthopnea (or"thop-ne'ah; "straight breathing"; clinically this is an extreme form of dyspnea, such that the patient must remain in an upright position, usually with head and neck extended and elbows abducted)

50. **Hypoventilation** (P) _____ (R) _____

hypoventilation (hi"po-ven"ti-la'shun; a state or act of reduced fresh air supply [i.e., entering the pulmonary alveoli]; clinically it is a decreased volume of air exchanged each breathing cycle)

RESPIRATORY ANATOMY AND PHYSIOLOGY

The respiratory system, working in conjunction with the cardiovascular and hematopoietic systems, provides the body with the necessary exchange of gases (oxygen and carbon dioxide). A fully functional respiratory system is necessary for cellular respiration throughout the body to be accomplished.

Structurally, the respiratory system is a series of tubes and sacs (Fig. 8-1). Air enters the system during *inspiration* and exits during *expiration*. As air first enters through the nares,[4] it passes through numerous folds of tissue called the nasal turbinates. The nasal turbinates are covered with highly vascular mucous membranes that serve to warm, humidify, and filter the inspired air. They are covered with ciliated pseudostratified columnar epithelium. The epithelium not only produces mucus to entrap particles from the inspired air, but the cilia provide a constant caudad sweeping motion. This activity helps ensure that foreign particles and organisms are constantly being removed from the nose to the *pharynx* so that they may be swallowed. Through this protective mechanism and sneezing, veterinary patients are able to rid foreign materials from the nasal passages to protect the lower airways. Much of this protection may be lost by open-mouth breathing. Air inspired through the mouth is not warmed, humidified, or filtered as efficiently as that through the nasal turbinates. *Aspiration* of foreign materials and dehydration (drying) of lower airways are more likely to occur with open-mouth breathing. Open-mouth breathing sometimes has advantages, however. Many domestic animals (especially dogs) use a specialized form of rapid, shallow, open-mouth breathing called panting. Panting provides these animals with a means of dissipating heat from their bodies. The rapid movement of air over the moist mucous membranes of the mouth (especially the tongue) dissipates heat primarily through evaporation. Unlike the horse, dogs and cats do not have the capacity to sweat profusely for regulating body heat. Panting is by far their best natural defense against overheating.

Two major passageways are associated with the nasal turbinates, the dorsal nasal meatus[5] and ventral nasal meatus (Fig. 8-2). These two passages are merely

---

[4]Nares (na'rēz; naris, singular) denotes the nostrils of domestic animals.

[5]Meatus (me-a'tus, [L. *meatus,* a way, a path, a course]) means an opening or passage.

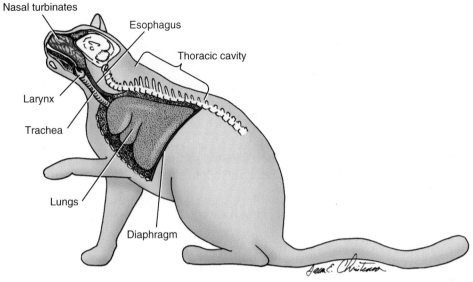

FIGURE 8-1   Feline respiratory tract.

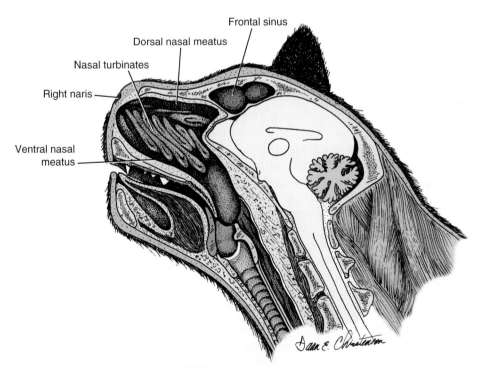

FIGURE 8-2   Nasal passages.

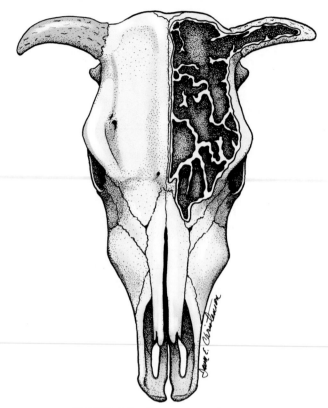

FIGURE 8-3   Bovine frontal sinus.

that, large passages. The ventral nasal meatus is clinically relevant because it is used for the *intranasal* placement of *endotracheal* tubes or *nasogastric* tubes. The dorsal nasal meatus dead-ends in the nasal turbinates. If a nasogastric tube were mistakenly passed forcefully into the dorsal nasal meatus, epistaxis[6] would likely result. Other structures associated with the nasal passages are the sinuses. The sinuses are considered dead space because air tends to stagnate in these chambers. Although sinuses do not aid in the ventilatory activity, they provide resonance during vocalization and reduce the overall weight of the head. It is important to note that in horned animals, like sheep, goats, and cattle, the frontal sinus actually communicates with the mature horn (Fig. 8-3). Therefore, it is very important to dehorn these animals before the horns develop fully, to prevent problems like *sinusitis*.

Air from the nasal passages eventually passes through the *nasopharynx*, the pharynx, and into the larynx (Fig. 8-4). To gain entry to the larynx, the *epiglottis* must be drawn ventrally and arytenoid[7] cartilages must be abducted from the opening (Fig. 8-5). The larynx is constructed of smooth muscle and chondral

---

[6]Epistaxis (ep″ĭ-stak′sis) is derived from [Gr. *epistaxis*] meaning "nosebleed."
[7]Arytenoid (ar″ĕ-tĕ′noid, ar″ĕ-te′noid; [Gr. *arytaina*, ladle + -*oid*, resembling]); refers to the pitcher-shaped cartilages associated with the larynx.

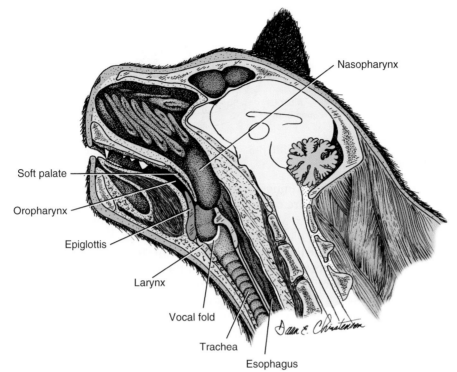

FIGURE 8-4 The pharynx and larynx.

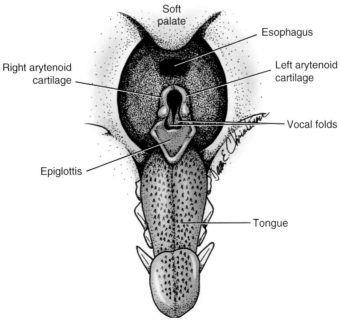

FIGURE 8-5 View of pharynx and laryngeal opening.

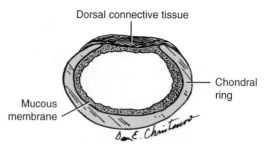

Dorsal connective tissue

Chondral ring

Mucous membrane

FIGURE 8-6   Transverse section of trachea.

plates and lined with mucous membranes. It is supported in the throat by a delicate bony structure called the hyoid (hi'oid) apparatus. The vocal folds are housed by the larynx. Vocalization occurs when muscles associated with the arytenoid cartilages place tension on the vocal folds. As air (generally expiratory air) passes over the taut vocal folds, they vibrate, creating audible sounds.

Next, the inspired air passes through the trachea. The trachea is composed of fibrous connective tissue, smooth muscle, and a series of chondral C-shaped rings (Fig. 8-6). The chondral rings provide semirigid support for the trachea, helping to maintain a patent[8] airway. The dorsal border of the trachea, which lies next to the esophagus,[9] is *achondral*. This allows for expansion of the esophagus during the passage of food. Otherwise, if the trachea was a completely rigid structure, large boluses of food would probably become lodged in the esophagus. The endotracheal mucosa is made up of ciliated pseudostratified columnar epithelium. Like the nasal turbinates, the trachea (and bronchi) have a mucociliary[10] escalator to remove mucus and debris from the caudal/lower airways. This moves mucus and debris to a point in the larger airways where it may be coughed out. (The bulk of the bronchioles, especially terminal bronchioles, do not have ciliated epithelium.) At the caudal end of the trachea is the tracheal bifurcation (bi"fur-ka'shun; a fork in the road, if you will). This marks the end of the trachea and the beginning of the bronchi.

The primary bronchi are the first branches off the trachea. From that point, the bronchi continue to branch, like a tree, becoming smaller as they progress (Fig. 8-7). The primary bronchi are quite large airways, with C-shaped chondral rings like the trachea. The secondary bronchi, the next branches from the primary bronchi, are covered with small, irregularly shaped chondral plates that provide structural support to the complete circumference of the secondary bronchi. As we progress to the tertiary[11] bronchi, the airways become even smaller and lose more cartilage. The chondral plates in the tertiary bronchi do not completely surround the airways. As we progress even further, the *bronchioles*

---

[8]Patent (pa'tent; [L. *patens*]) means "open," "unobstructed."

[9]The esophagus (e-sof'ah-gus) is the muscular passage through which food travels from the mouth to the stomach.

[10]Mucociliary (mu"ko-si'le-ar-e); pertaining to mucus and cilia; the mucociliary escalator provides a sticky surface of mucus that is moved cranially by the constant sweeping motion of the ciliated epithelium.

[11]Tertiary (ter'she-er-e) is derived from [L. *tertiarius*], meaning "third in order."

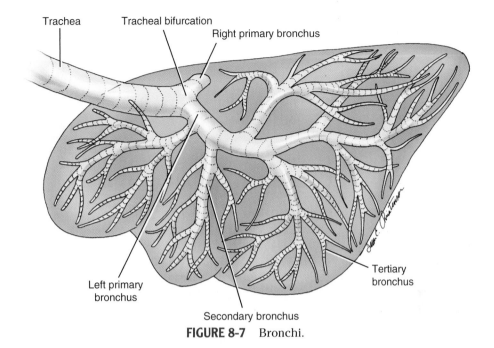

Trachea   Tracheal bifurcation

Right primary bronchus

Tertiary
bronchus

Left primary
bronchus

Secondary bronchus

FIGURE 8-7   Bronchi.

are achondral (Fig. 8-8). The bronchioles are composed entirely of smooth muscle and connective tissue, with predominantly cuboidal epithelium for their mucous membranes. The terminal bronchioles lead to the alveolar ducts, which are basically portals to the alveoli.

The alveoli are delicate clusters of sacs, composed of simple squamous epithelium. Each alveolus is surrounded by a dense network of capillaries[12] (see Fig. 8-8; and cf. Chapter 7). It is through the respiratory membrane (alveolar and capillary walls) that gas exchange takes place. The alveoli make up the bulk of the pulmonary tissue. There is species variation regarding lung lobe configuration. Most domestic animals have a configuration resembling that of the cat's lungs, with cranial, middle, and caudal lung lobes bilaterally and an accessory lung lobe dorsocaudal to the heart. The horse is the one major exception to this arrangement, because horses have only right, left, and accessory lung lobes.

The *pleural* cavity is another term for the *thoracic* cavity. It is called the pleural cavity by virtue of the tissue that lines the cavity and covers the viscera (i.e., pleura). Parietal[13] pleura lines the chest wall, and visceral pleura covers the lungs and other organs. The pleura is a continuous tissue layer. The pleural tissue actually meets in the middle of the thoracic cavity to form a thin tissue wall that envelops the thoracic viscera and serves to separate the right from the left side of the chest cavity. This centrally located tissue is called the

---

[12]Capillaries (kap-ĭ-lar'ēz) are the smallest blood vessels of the body.
[13]Parietal (pah-ri'ĕ-tal, [L. *parietalis*]) refers to the walls of a cavity.

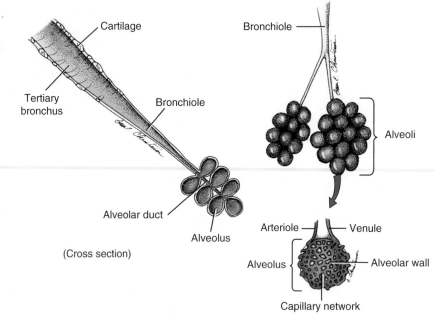

FIGURE 8-8   Terminal airways.

mediastinum.[14] All of the pleural tissue secretes small amounts of fluid into the thoracic cavity, just enough to coat the pleura with a very thin film. This fluid minimizes friction between the visceral and parietal pleurae and provides surface tension between the chest wall and the lungs. This latter attribute is discussed in the next section.

Mechanisms of Breathing

Breathing is both an involuntary and a voluntary act. The involuntary act is regulated by control centers in the brain stem. Voluntary respiratory actions involve conscious thought from higher levels in the brain. There are respiratory actions, however, both voluntary and involuntary, that do not serve to ventilate the animal (i.e., provide for gas exchange). Good examples of this type of voluntary action would be barking, meowing, whinnying, oinking, or mooing. Vocalization is a necessary form of communication, but it does not play a role in pulmonary ventilation, just as panting does not. Involuntary respiratory actions, such as sneezing and coughing, also do not contribute to *pulmonary* ventilation but are necessary protective mechanisms.

Mechanically, breathing occurs easily and relatively passively because of differences in air pressure. Air follows the path of least resistance. In fact, the entire act of breathing is analogous to the operation of a bellows used in a fireplace. When not in motion, air pressure inside and outside of the bellows is equal, at

---

[14]Mediastinum (me″de-as-ti′num, [L. a middle septum or partition]).

atmospheric pressure (760 pounds per square inch [psi] at sea level). The bellows draws air in when it is opened up. By opening up the bellows, the size of the space inside has been increased rapidly. The volume of air that filled the bellows before it was enlarged can no longer fill the new space. In essence, the air pressure inside the bellows has been lowered. Therefore, air rushes in until the air pressure inside the bellows is equal to the atmospheric pressure outside. The air will not leave the bellows until it is compressed. By reducing the size of the bellows, the new volume of air can no longer fit. The force of compression increases the air pressure inside the bellows, and therefore it rushes out into the surrounding air.

Ventilation in animals occurs similar to that of the bellows. To increase the size of the pleural cavity, muscles of respiration are used. The *intercostal* muscles (Fig. 8-9) expand the rib cage. When stimulated by the phrenic nerve, the diaphragm (di'ah-fram) contracts. The size of the pleural cavity is dramatically increased by the diaphragm contracting and moving caudally. Abdominal viscera are compressed by the contracting diaphragm. As the size of the pleural cavity and the size of the space within the lungs significantly increases, air rushes into the airways and alveoli. The lungs expand with the pleural cavity because of the surface tension between the parietal and visceral pleurae. The thin film of fluid between the pleural tissues makes them stick together, just like a wet glass sticks to a table top on a hot summer day. This surface tension can be maintained only if no extraneous substances/pressures come between the pleural tissues. For all practical purposes, the pleural cavity itself exists in a vacuum and must be maintained in such a state for pulmonary ventilation to be accomplished. Normal expiration is a purely passive motion. Most of the tissues of the lungs and the pleural cavity are elastic. Like a rubber band, these tissues spring back when stretched. Additionally, all of the abdominal viscera that were compressed by the diaphragm bounce back, pushing the diaphragm cranially. All of this reduces the available space for air in the alveoli, increasing *alveolar pressure*, and forces the air out of the lungs. This ventilatory process is repeated over and over again.

Respiratory Volumes

During every normal respiratory motion (i.e., a single breath; inspiration and expiration), a certain amount of air is moved. That volume of air that is moved during a complete respiratory motion is called the *tidal volume*. The tidal volume is adequate to meet a normal animal's needs at rest. But what if an animal is stressed? For example, what if a cat was suddenly awakened from its nap and chased by a large dog? The tidal volume is no longer enough to provide the additional oxygen needed by the cat's muscles to be able to escape. He needs pulmonary space in reserve to get him through this crisis. If normal, the cat has the ability to expand his chest farther than he routinely would at rest. To facilitate the greater expansion of his chest, the cat will put his serratus ventralis and pectoral muscles to work (see Fig. 8-9). The additional volume of air that he can now take in, over and above his normal tidal volume, is called the *inspiratory reserve volume*. If the cat is running, his muscles produce much more CO_2 than they did at rest. That

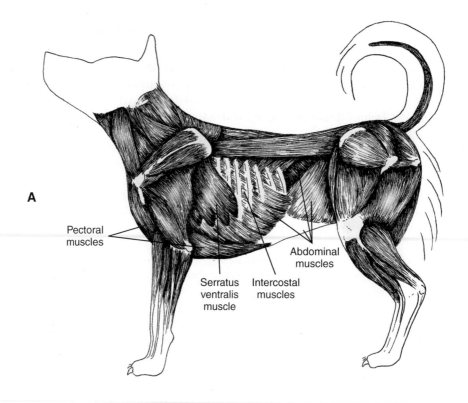

A

Pectoral
muscles

Serratus
ventralis
muscle

Intercostal
muscles

Abdominal
muscles

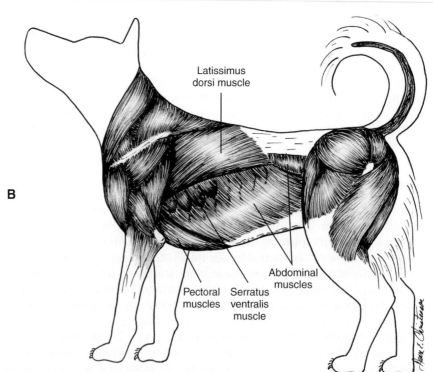

B

Latissimus
dorsi muscle

Abdominal
muscles

Pectoral
muscles

Serratus
ventralis
muscle

FIGURE 8-9 **A,** Muscles of respiration (superficial trunk muscles removed). **B,** Muscles of respiration (superficial trunk muscles intact).

CO_2 ultimately makes its way to his lungs to be diffused and blown off. He needs the ability to expire more air. Expiration will be active and forced, rather than passive. To do this, the cat will actively use his latissimus dorsi (see Fig. 8-9) and abdominal muscles. The volume of air that the cat can now expire (exhale), beyond that of his tidal volume, is called the *expiratory reserve volume*. The sum of the tidal volume, the inspiratory reserve volume, and the expiratory reserve volume is called the *vital capacity*. The vital capacity is vital to this cat, if he expects to escape the jaws of the vicious dog. If, while he was running away, he fell into a pond right after expiring a breath, there would be enough air remaining in his alveoli (the *residual volume*) to keep his tissues supplied with oxygen briefly. Hopefully, long enough to get him back to the surface. Then, by continuing to use his vital capacity, he would be able to swim to safety. The residual volume is a volume of air that cannot be expired, under any circumstances. It is there to keep gas exchange going for brief periods of time, no matter what. The residual volume also helps prevent *atelectasis* during normal respiratory activity.

Gas Exchange and Acid-Base Homeostasis

Average room air contains approximately 78% nitrogen, 21% oxygen, and 0.04% carbon dioxide. Each of these gases exerts a certain amount of weight (pressure), contributing to atmospheric pressure. Because the pressure exerted by each element is only part of what makes up the total gaseous mixture of room air, it is referred to as partial pressure. For example, if atmospheric pressure is 760 mm Hg and carbon dioxide is 0.04% of room air, then the partial pressure of carbon dioxide in room air is approximately 0.3 mm Hg ($pCO_2 = 0.3$ mm Hg). Partial pressures are exerted by gases in the body, too. In general, we are concerned with the pO_2 and the pCO_2 in the circulating blood. The net difference in the partial pressures of these gases in the bloodstream versus the alveolar spaces influences diffusion across the respiratory membrane (Fig. 8-10).

Oxygen is an essential element for life for all body tissues. Through normal cellular activities, oxygen is used and carbon dioxide is produced. The oxygen arrives at the tissues via the blood. Hemoglobin binds with the oxygen (forming oxyhemoglobin) to transport it to the tissues. Approximately 98% of O_2 is transported as oxyhemoglobin, a compound that gives the blood its red color. On arrival in the alveolar capillaries, the red blood cells are O_2 deprived. The pO_2 of blood entering the lungs is approximately 35 to 45 mm Hg in most domestic animals. The pO_2 of the alveoli is approximately 104 mm Hg. Because the pO_2 of the capillary blood is much less than the pO_2 of the alveolar lumen, diffusion across the respiratory membrane from the alveoli to the blood takes place. (The respiratory membrane is incredibly thin in normal pulmonary tissue. It consists of the alveolar wall and the capillary wall. Each of those structures is merely made up of a single, thin layer of epithelium/endothelium and a basement membrane.) Blood leaving the lungs and arriving at the tissue capillaries typically has a pO_2 of about 90 to 95 mm Hg. The body tissues have a pO_2 of approximately 40 mm Hg. So, on arrival at the body tissue capillaries, the oxygen naturally diffuses from the blood into the tissues. The opposite effect takes place concurrently with CO_2. The CO_2 diffuses from the tissues to the blood, where some

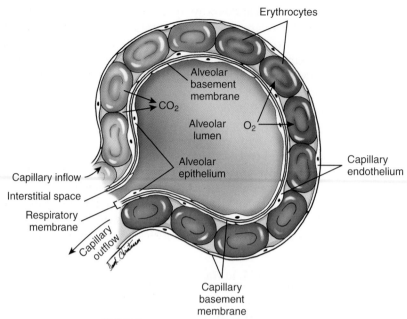

FIGURE 8-10   Respiratory membrane.

(15–25%) of it is bound to hemoglobin (forming carbaminohemoglobin, a compound that gives a blue coloration to the blood). The largest portion of CO_2 is combined with H_2O in plasma, creating the compound carbonic acid (H_2CO_3). Carbonic acid is integral to the acid-base balance of the body. The molecular structure of carbonic acid is very loose permitting rapid dissociation of CO_2 from the compound. The CO_2 carried to the lungs rapidly diffuses out of the bloodstream into the alveoli to be exhaled. The respiratory system is the single most important and most efficient body system for maintaining acid-base homeostasis. The kidneys also play a role in acid-base homeostasis, but they cannot respond and affect changes as efficiently as the lungs. (Kidney function will be discussed in Chapter 13.) Body pH must be maintained in a very narrow range of neutrality. Chemoreceptors,[15] in the brain stem, sense carbonic acid components. When too much carbonic acid is created by metabolic accumulation of CO_2, respiratory centers in the brain stem will stimulate *tachypnea* or *hyperpnea* to rapidly eliminate excess CO_2 to maintain a neutral pH. When the pH becomes too alkaline with too little carbonic acid (as it does following a meal, because of the loss of hydrogen ions into gastric juices), *bradypnea* will conserve CO_2 to permit carbonic acid to accumulate and return the pH to neutral. In anesthetized patients, using 100% O_2, *apnea* may result temporarily if we manually ventilate the patient too much and remove alveolar CO_2. In effect, we rapidly reduce pCO_2

---

[15]Chemoreceptor (ke″mo-re-sep′tor): a nerve receptor adapted for excitation by chemical substances.

and carbonic acid in the blood, causing the brain stem to react with apnea. This is a very efficient process. Fortunately with normal pulmonary function, CO_2 diffuses approximately 20 times faster than O_2, permitting efficient respiratory control over acid-base homeostasis. Gas exchange of oxygen and carbon dioxide is dynamic and must be never-ending. If gas exchange is compromised in any way, the whole body suffers.

Pathophysiology and Disease

Pulmonary gas exchange may be impaired in many ways. Certainly, changes in atmospheric concentrations of oxygen and carbon dioxide can have adverse effects on the body. Insufficient oxygen concentrations (for example, at high altitudes) may result in systemic hypoxia. Chemoreceptors located in the aorta and carotid arteries will sense significantly low blood pO_2. In response, the brain stem will stimulate compensatory tachypnea or hyperpnea. If oxygen supply still cannot keep up with metabolic demands of the body, tissue *hypoxia* will ultimately result in tissue death. It is rare for atmospheric concentrations of carbon dioxide to be so significant that alveolar diffusion is impaired. The Apollo 13 crew experienced such an event. Fortunately, most people and animals are not exposed to the extreme conditions that those astronauts were. If animals are to be exposed to high concentrations of CO_2, it will probably be during general, inhalant anesthesia. Soda lime canisters in the breathing circuit of anesthesia machines are designed to remove CO_2 from the patient's inspired air. If the soda lime becomes saturated, CO_2 will no longer be removed from the breathing circuit. Asphyxiation[16] and death would result. The use of *capnography* provides veterinary professionals with valuable monitoring of CO_2 levels of anesthetized patients so that lethal consequences can be avoided. Thankfully, carbon dioxide–related deaths are rare. More common is exposure to and death from carbon monoxide. Carbon monoxide (CO) is a by-product of combustion (e.g., burning of fossil fuels). Carbon monoxide will diffuse readily across the respiratory membrane into the bloodstream. Unlike carbon dioxide, carbon monoxide forms a very tight bond with hemoglobin (carboxyhemoglobin). This bond is very difficult to break, and it does not permit the hemoglobin molecule to carry O_2. Tissue hypoxia will develop rapidly. However, rather than the CO victim appearing pale due to hypoxia, he or she will appear to have brick-red mucous membranes. The single oxygen atom of CO provides the hemoglobin with the intense red color. Time is of the essence with CO toxicity. The longer the exposure to CO, the less likely the individual will survive. If exposure is suspected, the first course of action should be moving exposed animals and people out of the contaminated area into fresh air. Medical attention should then be sought, because oxygen therapy may be needed. Every year both people and animals die of carbon monoxide toxicity. Fortunately, the number of deaths has been reduced with the use of CO detectors in homes.

---

[16]Asphyxiation (as-fik″se-a′shun) is suffocation. The word is derived from the [Gr. *asphyxia,* "a stopping of the pulse"], because without sufficient oxygen life will cease.

Hypoxia may also occur in cases of anemia. Anemia, if severe, significantly reduces blood oxygen carrying capacity. Oxygen may be available from the atmosphere, but insufficient transportation vehicles (i.e., erythrocytes) cannot deliver sufficient quantities of oxygen to the tissues. Again, chemoreceptors will sense the low blood pO_2 and the brain stem will respond with tachypnea or hyperpnea. Tachycardia may also aid in supplying the oxygen-starved tissues of the anemic patient. Anemia may leave the body with too few oxygen transport vehicles, but if the vehicles speed up the delivery schedule, they may be able to supply just enough oxygen for the body tissues at rest. If anything increases metabolic demands for oxygen, such as activity or fever, the anemic patient will not be able to compensate for the hypoxia. As an interesting side note, pulse *oxymetry* of anemic patients may show "normal" oxygen saturation levels, in spite of significantly low pO_2. This is due to the fact that pulse oxymetry evaluates the quantity of hemoglobin that is bound (saturated) with oxygen. Hemoglobin will be well saturated in an anemic patient, giving a false normal impression of oxygenation. Arterial blood gases will more accurately determine oxygen levels, by measuring actual pO_2 present.

Structural abnormalities of the upper airways may or may not impact pulmonary gas exchange. Consider brachycephalic[17] breeds, like the English bulldog. These animals often have stenotic nares that significantly impair inspiratory movements of air. If this is the only structural abnormality in the dog, gas exchange will not be impaired. Why not? The dog will simply use the path of least resistance and breathe through its mouth. Open mouth breathing is undesirable because it bypasses the benefits of the nasal turbinates. *Rhinoplasty* can improve nasal airflow for these animals. Unfortunately, many of these brachycephalic animals also have pharyngeal and laryngeal abnormalities that also impair inspiratory air movements. Frequently they have elongated soft palates. Sometimes the palate may be so long that it actually interferes with the epiglottis and may even partially obstruct the laryngeal opening. Let's add to that excessive pharyngeal tissue with enlarged tonsils. With significant air turbulence created by these abnormalities and vibrations of tissues caused by air forces, stertorous (snoring-like) sounds will be created with every breath. Inspiratory *dyspnea* will likely be evident as well. Surgical correction is often required to remove some of the tissues interfering with inspiratory airflow. Those surgeries may include a *palatoplasty* and a tonsillectomy. During the palatoplasty, a portion of the soft palate will be removed so that it no longer interferes with the larynx and airflow. Airway patency following these procedures must be monitored closely postoperatively. If the surgical trauma results in significant pharyngeal edema, an emergency *tracheotomy* may be warranted.

Horses frequently suffer from upper airway obstruction. However, excessive pharyngeal tissues are not the problem in these animals. Instead, they suffer from a functional problem with the larynx. In laryngeal hemiplegia[18] the muscles

---

[17]Brachycephalic (brak"e-se-fal'ik; [Gr. *brachys,* short + *cephal(o)-,* head + *-ic,* pertaining to]); brachycephalic breeds have shorter than normal muzzles.

[18]Hemiplegia (hem"e-ple'je-ah; [*hemi-,* half + Gr. *plegĕ,* stroke + *-ia,* condition of]). Hemiplegia is paralysis of one side (half) of the body or a structure.

controlling abduction of one arytenoid (usually the left) will become paralyzed. At rest, this may not have a significant impact on inspired air movements. However, if the horse exerts itself and dips into its inspiratory reserve volumes, the force of inspired air will pull the paralyzed arytenoid into the laryngeal opening. Working against the partial obstruction, the horse may have inspiratory dyspnea. The partial obstruction of the larynx will create air turbulence, like blowing across a soda bottle, resulting in a loud sonorous or roaring sound. (This is why laryngeal hemiplegia is commonly called "roaring.") The sound is not problematic, but the reduced inspired air volume is. For a performance horse, this will result in hypoxia. Athletes cannot perform at peak levels if they are hypoxic. If even at rest or with minor activity, the horse is still dyspneic and hypoxic; *laryngoplasty* may be necessary. During this surgery, the paralyzed arytenoid will be tacked down in an abducted position. This will improve ventilation, but it will also leave the horse at risk of *aspiration pneumonia*. During normal swallowing, both arytenoids should be adducted to create a tight seal over the larynx with the epiglottis. That seal will be compromised once the laryngoplasty is performed. Dietary changes will be required to minimize the amount of dust and loose particles that could be aspirated.

Alterations of the respiratory membrane will have the most significant adverse effects on gas exchange. With regard to gas exchange and alveolar surface area, more is better. We need sufficient surface area to facilitate adequate diffusion of oxygen and carbon dioxide. Diseases that reduce the functional pulmonary surface area will reduce gas exchange and result in hypoxia and potentially *hypercapnia*. One such disease is pulmonary emphysema (em"fi-se'mah). This disease, commonly called "heaves," is most often seen in horses. It is much like the chronic obstructive pulmonary disease (COPD) seen in people. It usually develops from chronic inflammation of the airways, particularly the bronchioles. *Bronchiarctia* and *bronchospasm* result in air being trapped in the alveoli. Horses have tremendous inspiratory reserves. They can effectively force even more air into those already distended alveoli. This will result in *bronchiectasis* (especially of terminal bronchioles) and rupture of alveoli. Large, open, emphysematous areas will develop where numerous alveoli once were. Scar tissue will form. All of these features will profoundly reduce the functional surface area of the respiratory membrane. Too little respiratory membrane results in decreased gas exchange. Additionally, the entrapped air will not contain normal atmospheric concentrations of oxygen and carbon dioxide. The emphysematous areas will contain less oxygen and more CO_2 than normal atmosphere. This diminished diffusion gradient means less O_2 can diffuse into the bloodstream and far less CO_2 can diffuse out. Hypoxia and hypercapnia result. The hypercapnia makes the horse acidotic. Chemoreceptors sensing the blood gases and the altered acid-base state will cause the brain stem to respond with stimulation of more forced expiration. Collapse of some of the bronchiectic airways will make exhalation even more difficult. Coughing and expiratory dyspnea will likely be observed. Accessory muscles used for force expiration will become very well developed, especially along the caudal costal arch. This hypertrophic muscle is frequently referred to as a "heave line." Reduction of activity to reduce metabolic needs and by-products (i.e., O_2 needs and CO_2 produced) will be important in the management of pulmonary emphysema in horses. Also important to the management of these horses is the minimizing of environmental respiratory irritants (e.g., dust and mold). These animals are frequently pastured, because the concentration of dust and mold in a barn is usually far greater than that on pasture.

Edematous fluids can also alter the respiratory membrane. As discussed in Chapter 5, edema may result for a number of reasons including inflammation and increased hydrostatic pressure. Pulmonary edema frequently results from cardiac insufficiency. Think about it. Blood, under normal circumstances, should be oxygenated in the lungs, return to the left atrium, and then be pumped out to the body from the left ventricle (see Chapter 7). If the left atrioventricular valve is insufficient, pulmonary venous blood may become backed up. This will increase the hydrostatic pressure in pulmonary capillaries, resulting in pulmonary edema. The edematous fluid in the alveoli will make the respiratory membrane thicker, thereby interfering with diffusion of gases. Pulmonary auscultation will reveal the edematous fluid. As inspired air reaches the alveoli, it will "percolate" through the fluid creating a fine crackling sound, much like that of Rice Crispies. Fine crackles will be heard with very aqueous fluids, as in pulmonary edema. Course crackles sound more like oatmeal bubbling on the stovetop. Course crackles are indicative of thick alveolar fluids, like those found in pneumonia.

Pneumonia may develop in a number of ways. Certainly many of the infectious respiratory diseases may progress from upper respiratory symptoms to profound pulmonary disease. Fortunately, most of our common, preventable infectious respiratory diseases tend not to progress, such as feline *rhinopneumonitis* virus, canine infectious *tracheobronchitis* (kennel cough), infectious bovine *rhinotracheitis,* and equine rhinopneumonitis. Most of the upper respiratory diseases of domestic animals have very high *morbidity* and very low *mortality*. In other words, the animals appear quite clinically ill, with nasal discharges, sneezing, coughing, and depression, but most of the animals will recover, just as people do from the common cold. *Rhinitis* is uncomfortable and annoying, but it's not deadly. Certainly the dog with the nonproductive, dry, hacking cough of tracheobronchitis can be given *antitussives*. Antitussives for these dogs permit rest for the dogs and the owners. They also reduce cough-induced trauma to the upper airways that would otherwise create *hemoptysis*. Even so, with or without antitussives, most dogs with tracheobronchitis will recover. However, under the right circumstances, in an immunocompromised individual (especially the very young and geriatric patients), any of these seemingly harmless upper respiratory pathogens may open the door for secondary invaders. Bacteria are natural inhabitants of the airways. Given poor immunity and a preceding inflammatory insult by an infectious upper respiratory disease, the bacteria can flourish. The result may be a secondary bacterial bronchitis, or worse—pneumonia. Bacterial pneumonia can also develop secondary to pulmonary edema. (The pulmonary edema provides an ideal warm, moist environment for bacteria to colonize.)

In pneumonia, regardless of the etiology,[19] not only will inflammation of the alveolar walls increase the respiratory membrane thickness, but the thick

---

[19]Etiology (e"te-ol'o-je; [Gr. *aitia,* cause + *-logy*]); the study or knowledge of causes of disease (cf. pathogenesis).

purulent exudates pooling in the alveoli create a barrier and added thickness to the respiratory membrane. Gas exchange will be severely impaired in pneumonia. Life-threatening hypoxia and hypercapnia easily and rapidly develop. These patients will likely be dyspneic and *cyanotic.* Tachypnea and use of reserve volumes (seen as hyperpnea) may still be insufficient to meet their gas exchange needs. In severe pneumonia, the animal will become *orthopneic,* gasping for every breath. In an attempt to improve alveolar respiration, these patients resort to open mouth breathing. Unfortunately, open mouth breathing inspissates[20] airway secretions even further, making them so thick and sticky that they cannot be removed by the mucociliary escalator or by coughing. Inspissated secretions are more likely to completely obstruct tertiary bronchi and bronchioles. The thicker the secretions become, the more they will impair air movements and gas exchange. This is why hydration of bronchitis and pneumonia patients is so critically important. Adequate hydration keeps the secretions more fluid to facilitate easier removal. Intensive supportive care of pneumonia patients is frequently required for survival. Oxygen therapy will most likely be employed. Therapeutic oxygen (usually ~30% concentration) is most frequently delivered via intranasal catheters, allowing for natural humidification of the inspired oxygen. Intranasal oxygen should be humidified, to avoid drying of the nasal turbinates. Sometimes *transtracheal* catheters are placed for oxygen delivery. Transtracheal oxygen must be humidified so that it does not dry the mucous membranes of the airways and inspissate secretions.

Horses with pneumonia often suffer the most severe form of the disease. The structure of their lungs permits rapid, widespread involvement of the pulmonary tissues. The multilobed lungs of other domestic animals can serve to isolate pneumonic areas. (As a side note, the multilobed pulmonary structure of these animals has other advantages. For instance, with pulmonary tumors or traumatic lesions, a *lobectomy* can be easily performed with minimal impact on the animal's respiratory function.) The nonlobed pulmonary structure is why horses are more likely to develop *pleuropneumonia.* In pleuropneumonia, the inflammation progresses from the interior of the lungs and begins to involve the pleural tissues. Remember, the visceral and parietal pleurae should be very smooth and slippery in the normal state. As pleuritis develops, the pleural surfaces become roughened and sticky. Inflammatory proteins seeping into the pleural space may actually create fibrous adhesions between the lungs and chest wall. Friction between the poorly lubricated surfaces will make the inflammation worse. All of these features will make breathing extremely painful. Unlike a sprained ankle, the thorax cannot be rested to allow it to heal. Breathing is essential for life. Although they cannot stop breathing, pleuropneumonia patients will tend to *hypoventilate* to minimize pain. Yet, these patients cannot afford the reduced use of surface area from *hypoventilation,* because it will impair their gas exchange even further. If recovery from pleuropneumonia is possible, it may take months.

---

[20]Inspissate (in-spis'āt; [L. *inspissatus;* from *in-,* intensive + *spissare,* to thicken]): to thicken or dry.

Space-occupying pleural cavity disorders can also have a significant impact on gas exchange. Remember, in the normal state, there is only a thin film of fluid lubricating and, through surface tension, keeping the pulmonary and parietal pleurae "stuck" together. There should be nothing but that thin coating of fluid separating those pleural surfaces. There are times when substances may begin to fill the pleural cavity, separating the pleural surfaces. The disease syndrome will be named by virtue of the substance taking up space, such as *pneumothorax*, *hemothorax*, *hydrothorax*, and *pyothorax*. Regardless of the substance, the more pleural cavity space is occupied by a substance, the greater the separation of visceral and parietal pleurae. The end result will be *atelectasis*. Atelectatic alveoli cannot provide any gas exchange. Overall surface area for gas exchange may be so significantly reduced that the animal may not even have normal tidal volume available, let alone reserve volumes. If this is the case, treatment will be necessary. But treatment may depend on what the substance actually is. For instance, a pyothorax will require more than mere removal of the purulent[21] material, such as systemic antibiotics. A hemothorax with profound hemorrhage may require a *thoracotomy* to repair or ligate damaged *intrathoracic* vessels, in order to control the bleeding. Thoracic radiographs and/or auscultation can differentiate between free air and fluid. *Thoracentesis* may then be used to remove a portion of either the air or the fluid. Penetration of the intercostal space will be more dorsal for air and more ventral for fluids. Thoracentesis may serve as a diagnostic tool (when fluids are involved) or as a quick therapeutic tool. If further accumulation of pleural material is anticipated, a chest tube inserted and secured into the pleural cavity and connected to a sealed collection device will provide safe, continuous removal of the material. As the space-occupying material is removed, pulmonary function will gradually resume. Visibly the patient's dyspnea will be eased into a more normal breathing pattern.

Respiratory diseases are numerous and common among domestic animals. This discussion could continue until all our faces were cyanotic. But the disease details are not as important as the basic foundation of knowledge. Appropriate management of respiratory patients relies on veterinary professionals having a sound understanding of normal respiratory anatomy and physiology. Then, no matter how a particular disease interferes with airflow or gas exchange, the pathophysiologic effects of the disease can be anticipated, understood, and effectively treated.

---

[21]Purulent (pu'roo-lent; [L. *purulentus*]); pertaining to pus.

SELF-TEST

Using the previous information in this chapter, complete the following crossword puzzle using the most appropriate medical term(s). Do not use abbreviations or common names unless requested.

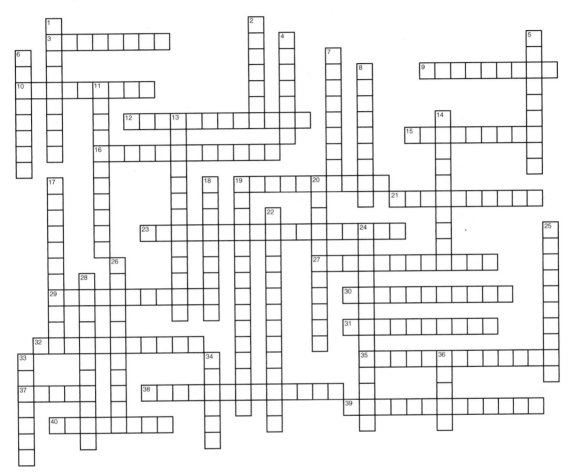

ACROSS

3   A pulmonary air sac

9   Pus in the chest

10   Cartilage bilaterally located at the laryngeal opening

12   The compound formed in plasma by combining H_2O and CO_2 (2 words)

15   Slow breathing

16   Air in the chest cavity

19   Coughing up blood

21   The chondral structure that creates a seal over the laryngeal opening during swallowing

23   Canine infectious _____, commonly called "kennel cough"

27	Within the trachea
29	A cough suppressant
30	A tube placed from the nose to the stomach
31	Blood in the chest
32	Abnormally increased pCO_2
35	Pertaining to across the trachea
37	The absence of breathing
38	The oxygen-saturated compound that gives erythrocytes their bright red color
39	The sum of tidal volume, plus inspiratory and expiratory reserve volumes (2 words)
40	Pathogenesis or the cause of disease

DOWN

1	Rapid breathing
2	Difficulty breathing
4	Oxygen deficiency
5	The major muscle of respiration that divides the chest and abdomen
6	Blueness of the mucous membranes
7	To appear quite clinically ill from a nonlethal disease
8	A nosebleed
11	The nose and throat
13	Bronchostenosis
14	An instrument used to measure CO_2 concentrations
17	Reconstructive surgery of the nose
18	Positional difficulty breathing, such that the animal probably sits or stands with its head extended and elbows abducted
19	A state of below normal tidal volume
20	An emergency incision into the trachea to provide a patent airway
22	A shorted-headed animal, like a Boston terrier or Persian cat
24	Puncture of the chest
25	A small, muscular, achondral pulmonary airway
26	Muscle found between the ribs
28	Collapse of the lungs
33	The throat
34	The tissue that lines the chest cavity and its organs
36	The volume of air moved in a normal, complete respiratory cycle

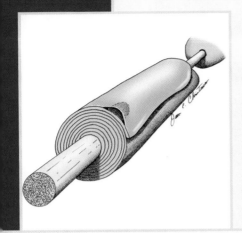

The Neurologic System

GOALS AND OBJECTIVES

By the conclusion of this chapter, the student will be able to:

1. Recognize common root words, prefixes, and suffixes related to the neurologic system.
2. Divide simple and compound words into their respective parts.
3. Recognize, correctly pronounce, and appropriately use common medical terms related to the neurologic system.
4. Demonstrate an understanding of neuroanatomy.
5. Demonstrate an understanding of neurophysiology, with regard to neurotransmission, motor and sensory pathways, autonomic pathways, and olfaction.
6. Demonstrate an understanding of the reflex arc with regard to spinal reflexes.
7. Demonstrate an understanding of and compare a pure reflex action with a response to pain.
8. Demonstrate an understanding of the blood–brain barrier.
9. Demonstrate an understanding of pathophysiology and diseases as they relate to the neurologic system.

INTRODUCTION TO RELATED TERMS

Divide each of the following terms into its respective parts ("R" root, "P" prefix, "S" suffix, "CV," combining vowel).

1. **Cerebral** (adj.)   (R) _____ (S) _____
   cerebral (ser′ĕbral, ser-e′bral; pertaining to the cerebrum [L. "brain"])

2. **Cerebellar** (adj.)   (R) _____ (S) _____
   cerebellar (ser″ĕbel′ar; pertaining to the cerebellum)

3. **Cerebrospinal** (adj.)   (R) _____ (CV) _____ (R) _____ (S) _____
cerebrospinal (ser"ĕ-bro-spi'nal, sĕ"re'-bro-spi-nal; pertaining to the cerebrum and spine [i.e., spinal cord])

4. **Hemisphere** (n.)   (P) _____ (R) _____
hemisphere (hem'ĭ-sfēr; [hemi-, half + sphere] half a ball or globe)

5. **Brachial** (adj.)   (R) _____ (S) _____
brachial (bra'ke-al; pertaining to the brachium [L. "arm"])

6. **Lumbosacral** (adj.)   (R) _____ (CV) _____ (R) _____
(S) _____
lumbosacral (lum"bo-sa'kral; pertaining to the lumbus [i.e., lumbar vertebrae] and the sacrum)

7. **Intervertebral** (adj.)   (P) _____ (R) _____ (S) _____
intervertebral (in"ter-ver'tĕ-bral, in"ter-ver-te'bral; pertaining to between vertebrae)

8. **Epidural** (adj.)   (P) _____ (R) _____ (S) _____
epidural (ep"ĭ-du'ral; pertaining to upon the dura [i.e., dura mater])

9. **Afferent** (adj.)   (P) _____ (R) _____
afferent (af'er-ent, a'fer-ent; to carry to/toward; af- derived from ad- "to")

10. **Efferent** (adj.)   (P) _____ (R) _____
efferent (ef'er-ent, e'fer-ent; to carry out; ef- derived from ex- "out")

11. **Somatic** (adj.)   (R) _____ (S) _____
somatic (so-mat'ik; [Gr. soma, somatos, body], pertaining to the body)

12. **Visceral** (adj.)   (R) _____ (S) _____
visceral (vis'er-al; pertaining to an organ or organs)

13. **Autonomic** (adj.)   (P) _____ (CV) _____ (R) _____
(S) _____
autonomic (aw"to-nom'ik; [auto-, self + Gr. nomos, law/control] pertaining to self-control; anatomically refers to the autonomic nervous system)

14. **Sympathetic** (adj.)   (R) _____ (S) _____
sympathetic (sim"pah-thet'ik; [Gr. sympathetikos] pertaining to sympathy; anatomically refers to the sympathetic portion of the autonomic nervous system)

15. **Parasympathetic** (adj.)   (P) _____ (R) _____ (S) _____
parasympathetic (par"ah-sim'pah-thet'ik; [para-, beyond] pertaining to "beyond" sympathy; anatomically refers to the parasympathetic portion of the autonomic nervous system)

16. **Cholinergic** (adj.)   (R) _____ (R) _____ (S) _____
cholinergic (ko"lin-er'jik; pertaining to choline work [Gr. ergon, work]; physiologically refers to function with the neurotransmitter acetylcholine)

17. **Sympathomimetic** (adj.)   (R) _____ (CV) _____ (R) _____
(S) _____
sympathomimetic (sim"pah-tho-mi-met'ik; pertaining to sympathy imitation [Gr. mimetikos, imitative]; clinically refers to any agent that mimics the sympathetic activity of the autonomic nervous system)

18. **Adrenergic** (adj.)   (R) _____ (R) _____ (S) _____
    adrenergic (ad"ren-er'jik; pertaining to adrenal [i.e., epinephrine] work; syn. sympathomimetic)

19. **Parasympathomimetic** (adj.)   (R) _____ (CV) _____ (R) _____
                                       (S) _____
    parasympathomimetic (par"ah-sim"pah-tho-mi-met'ik; pertaining to parasympathetic imitation; clinically refers to any agent that mimics the parasympathetic activity of the autonomic nervous system)

20. **Anticholinergic** (adj.)   (P) _____ (R) _____ (R) _____
                                       (S) _____
    anticholinergic (an"ti-ko"lin-er'jik; pertaining to against choline [acetylcholine] work; clinically refers to an agent that blocks the effects of acetylcholine; syn. parasympatholytic)

21. **Parasympatholytic** (adj.)   (R) _____ (CV) _____ (R) _____
                                       (S) _____
    parasympatholytic (par"ah-sim"pah-tho-lit'ik; pertaining to parasympathetic breakage; clinically refers to an agent that blocks parasympathetic nerve impulses; syn. anticholinergic)

22. **Neuroglial** (adj.)   (R) _____ (CV) _____ (S) _____
    neuroglial (nu-rog'le-al; pertaining to nerve "glue"; anatomically refers to the accessory, supportive structures of neural tissue)

23. **Astrocyte** (n.)   (R) _____ (CV) _____ (S) _____
    astrocyte (as'tro-sīt; a star cell)

24. **Oligodendrocyte** (n.)   (P) _____ (CV) _____ (R) _____
                                       (CV) _____ (S) _____
    oligodendrocyte (ol"ĭ-go-den'dro-sīt; a little "tree" cell; anatomically refers to a cell with few dendritic branches)

25. **Ependymal** (adj.)   (R) _____ (S) _____
    ependymal (e-pen'dĭ-mal; pertaining to the ependyma [Gr. "upper garment," "tunic"]; anatomically the ependyma lines the ventricles of the brain and the central canal of the spinal cord)

26. **Microglial** (adj.)   (P) _____ (CV) _____ (S) _____
    microglial (mi-krog'le-al, mi-kro-gle'al; pertaining to small "glue"; anatomically refers to the smallest of the neuroglial cells)

27. **Bipolar** (adj.)   (P) _____ (R) _____ (S) _____
    bipolar (bi-po'lar; pertaining to two poles)

28. **Unipolar** (adj.)   (P) _____ (R) _____ (S) _____
    unipolar (u"nĭ-po'lar; pertaining to one pole)

29. **Multipolar** (adj.)   (P) _____ (R) _____ (S) _____
    multipolar (mul"tĭ-po'lar; pertaining to many poles)

30. **Axonal** (adj.)   (R) _____ (S) _____
    axonal (ak'so-nal; pertaining to an "axle"; in neurology, refers to an axon)

31. **Dendritic** (adj.)   (R) _____ (S) _____
    dendritic (den-drit'ik; [Gr. *dendron*, tree] pertaining to a tree; in neurology dendritic fibers are branched like a tree)

32. **Synaptic** (adj.)   (R) _____ (S) _____
    synaptic (sĭ-nap'tik; pertaining to a synapse [Gr. "connection"])

33. **Neuritis** (n.)   (R) _____ (S) _____
    neuritis (nu-ri'tis; inflammation of a nerve or nerves)

34. **Meningitis** (n.)   (R) _____ (S) _____
    meningitis (men"in-ji'tis; inflammation of a meninx [Gr. membrane] or meninges)

35. **Encephalitis** (n.)   (R) _____ (S) _____
    encephalitis (en"sef-ah-li'tis; inflammation of the brain)

36. **Encephalomyelitis** (n.)   (R) _____ (CV) _____ (R) _____
                                        (S) _____
    encephalomyelitis (en-sef"ah-lomi"ĕli'tis; inflammation of the brain and spinal cord)

37. **Subdural hematoma**   (P) _____ (R) _____ (S) _____
                                   (R) _____ (S) _____
    subdural hematoma (sub-du'ral hēm"ah-to'mah; a blood accumulation under the dura)

38. **Hypoplasia** (n.)   (P) _____ (R) _____ (S) _____
    hypoplasia (hi"po-pla'ze-ah; a condition of underdevelopment)

39. **Hydrocephalus**   (R) _____ (CV) _____ (R) _____
                               (S) _____
    hydrocephalus (hi-dro-sef'ah-lus; a water head)

40. **Analgesia** (n.)   (P) _____ (R) _____ (S) _____
    analgesia (an"al-je'ze-ah; a state without pain)

41. **Nociceptor** (n.)   (R) _____ (R) _____ (S) _____
    nociceptor (no-sĕ-sep'tor; an injury [L. *nocere,* to injure] receptor [L. *capere,* to receive]; i.e., a pain receptor)

42. **Anesthesia** (n.)   (P) _____ (R) _____ (S) _____
    anesthesia (an"es-the'ze-ah; a state without sensation)

43. **Hyperesthesia** (n.)   (P) _____ (R) _____ (S) _____
    hyperesthesia (hi"per-es-the'ze-ah; a condition of excessive sensation)

44. **Paralysis** (n.)   (P) _____ (R) _____ (S) _____
    paralysis (pah-ral'ĭ-sis; a state beyond loose [Gr. *lyein,* to loosen]; i.e., immobility; loss of motor function)

45. **Paraplegia** (n.)   (P) _____ (S) _____
    paraplegia (par"ah-ple'je-ah; [Gr. *plege,* a blow, stroke] paralysis "beyond"; clinically refers to paralysis of the caudal body/limbs)

46. **Tetraplegia** (n.)   (P) _____ (S) _____
    tetraplegia (tet″răple′je-ah; paralysis of four; clinically refers to paralysis of all four limbs; cf. quadriplegia)

47. **Quadriplegic** (adj.)   (P) _____ (S) _____
    quadriplegic (kwod″rĕ-pleēj′ik; pertaining to four paralyzed; clinically refers to paralysis of all four limbs; cf. tetraplegia)

48. **Hemiplegia** (n.)   (P) _____ (S) _____
    hemiplegia (hem″e-ple′je-ah; paralysis of half; clinically refers to paralysis of one side of the body)

49. **Monoplegia** (n.)   (P) _____ (S) _____
    monoplegia (mon″o-ple′je-ah; paralysis of one; clinically refers to paralysis of one limb)

50. **Hemiparesis** (n.)   (P) _____ (R) _____
    hemiparesis (hem″e-par′e-sis; [Gr. *paresis,* relaxation] half weakness; clinically refers to weakness or partial loss of function of one side of the body)

51. **Ataxia** (n.)   (P) _____ (R) _____ (S) _____
    ataxia (ah-tak′se-ah, a-tak′se-ah; [Gr. "lack of order"] a condition without order; clinically refers to muscular incoordination/stumbling)

52. **Dysmetria** (n.)   (P) _____ (R) _____ (S) _____
    dysmetria (dis-mě′tre-ah; [Gr. *metron,* measure] a condition of difficult "measure"; clinically it refers to a difficult or improper gait)

53. **Hypermetria**   (P) _____ (R) _____ (S) _____
    hypermetria (hi″per-mě′tre-ah; a condition of excessive "measure," i.e., exaggerated gaited movements)

54. **Olfactory** (adj.)   (R) _____ (S) _____
    olfactory (ol-fak′to-re; pertaining to smell)

55. **Optic**   (R) _____ (S) _____
    optic (op′tik; [Gr. *optikos,* sight] pertaining to vision)

56. **Myelogram** (n.)   (R) _____ (CV) _____ (S) _____
    myelogram (mi′ĕlo-gram; a recording of the spinal cord)

57. **Electroencephalogram** (n.)   (R) _____ (CV) _____ (R) _____
                                       (CV) _____ (S) _____
    electroencephalogram (e-lek″tro-en-sef′ah-lo-gram; a recording of electricity of the brain)

58. **Zoonosis** (n.)   (R) _____ (R) _____ (S) _____
    zoonosis (zo″o-no′sis; [Gr. *zoon,* animal + *nosos,* disease] a disease of animals; clinically refers to disease of animals that may be transmitted to humans; pl. zoonoses)

59. **Neurotropic** (adj.)   (R) _____ (CV) _____ (R) _____ (S) _____
    neurotropic (nu-ro-tro′pik; pertaining to nerve influencing [Gr. *trepein,* to influence] cf. neurophilic)

NEUROANATOMY AND PHYSIOLOGY

The neurologic system is a complex network of interconnecting components that work together to maintain homeostasis in the body. Many body functions and actions take place because of neural stimulation. The components of the nervous system are much like the circuits of a telegraph system. Lines, transmitters, receivers, relays, and electrical current are what make a telegraph system work. For clarity, some of the following sections compare the components of the nervous system with those of the telegraph, as well as using other analogies.

Neurons

Microanatomy (Cell Types)

The nervous system has numerous types of nerve cells (neurons), each with a specific place and function within the circuit. Each cell type is described in the following list, including where it is found and what its primary function is. While we can identify individual neuron types, as well as supportive cells that surround them, it is important to remember that the "wiring" of the body is made up of millions of these cells. Collectively, they all provide a means of gathering sensory information and facilitating motor actions in response to that sensory input.

1. Unipolar neuron (Fig. 9-1)

   A *unipolar* neuron has what appears to be a single pole (axon). The cell body is eccentrically located at a midpoint along the "*axonal* fiber." Actually, one end of the fiber serves as a dendrite, to receive and relay impulses toward the cell body. The other end of the fiber serves as a true axon, carrying impulses away from the cell body. Unipolar neurons are found predominantly in sensory nerve fibers. Their dendrites make up the sensory nerve fibers of the peripheral nerves. The cell bodies of unipolar neurons are found collected in masses of neural tissue called ganglia [Gr. "knot"]. The axons of unipolar neurons continue the sensory pathway from the ganglia into the central nervous system.
2. Bipolar neuron (Fig. 9-2)

   A *bipolar* neuron has a cell body located between two poles. Actually, one end serves as a dendrite (receiver) and the other end serves as an axon (transmitter). Most bipolar neurons are associated with highly specialized sensory tissue, like that associated with vision, hearing, and *olfaction*.
3. Multipolar neuron (Fig. 9-3)

   A *multipolar* neuron has many projections (poles). The cell body of a multipolar neuron is at the receiving end of the neuron, with numerous *dendritic* processes projecting from it. Impulses are received by the dendrites, travel through the cell body, and exit by way of the axon. Multipolar neurons make up the bulk of the motor neurons of the central and peripheral nervous systems.
4. Schwann cell (Fig. 9-4)

   Schwann cells are *neuroglial* cells of the peripheral nervous system. Schwann cells wrap themselves around the axons of peripheral nerve fibers, forming a

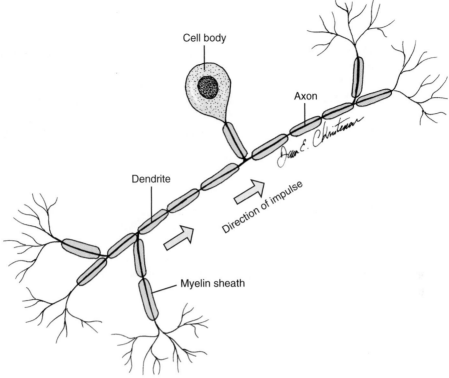

FIGURE 9-1   Unipolar neuron.

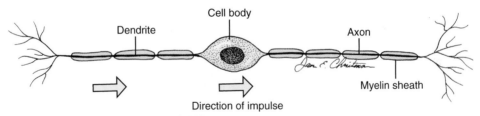

FIGURE 9-2   Bipolar neuron.

myelin sheath. The myelin sheath provides insulating characteristics for the nerve fibers, much like the rubber or plastic composites that insulate wires for electrical appliances in our homes.

5. Astrocyte (Fig. 9-5)

   Astrocytes are neuroglial cells of the central nervous system (i.e., brain and spinal cord). They have many cellular processes protruding from them, giving them a star-like appearance. They wrap their numerous appendages around neurons, as well as blood vessels, in the brain. They give structural support to the brain tissues and form scar tissue after injuries. The cellular processes that wrap around the blood vessels in the brain create the blood–brain barrier.

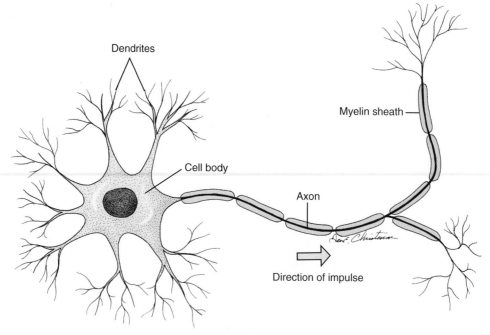

FIGURE 9-3   Multipolar neuron.

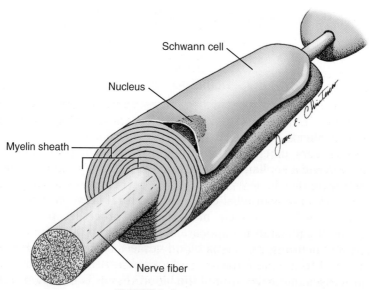

FIGURE 9-4   Schwann cell.

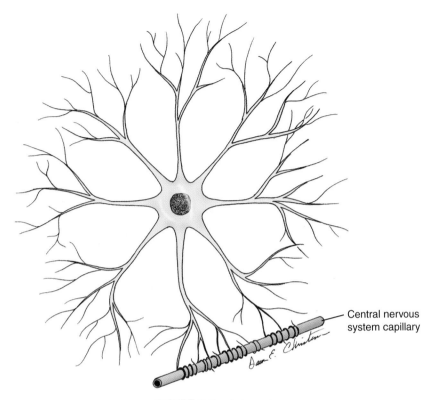

FIGURE 9-5   Astrocyte.

6. Oligodendrocyte (Fig. 9-6)
   Oligodendrocytes are also neuroglial cells of the central nervous system. They look very much like astrocytes, but with fewer processes. Oligodendroglial cells produce the myelin found in the brain and spinal cord. Unlike Schwann cells, oligodendroglial cells have numerous processes that wrap around separate axons. Therefore, a single oligodendrocyte can provide myelin for many axonal fibers.
7. Microglial cell (Fig. 9-7)
   Microglial cells are the smallest of the neuroglial cells of the central nervous system. They provide support for neurons and phagocytize organisms and debris from the tissues of the brain.
8. Ependymal cell (Fig. 9-8)
   Ependymal cells are neuroglial cells found lining the ventricles of the brain and the central canal of the spinal cord. They are actually a type of simple cuboidal epithelium.

Afferent and Efferent Neurons

Afferent neurons are those that carry impulses from the peripheral nervous system *toward* the central nervous system. They provide the sensory pathways from peripheral nerves to the spinal cord and to the brain. *Efferent* neurons are those that carry impulses *away from* the central nervous system to the

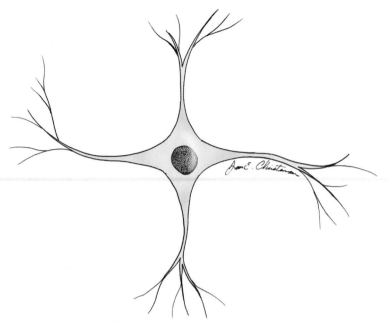

FIGURE 9-6   Oligodendrocyte.

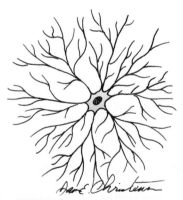

FIGURE 9-7   Microglial cell.

peripheral nervous system. They provide the motor pathways from the brain and spinal cord to the peripheral nerves and ultimately to the target organs.

Each nerve is made up of a bundle of neuronal fibers, much like electrical cords and telephone lines. Each nerve has both afferent and efferent fibers, providing pathways for sending to and receiving from the central nervous system. Nerves could be likened to expressways. They have lanes (neural fibers) set aside for strictly "northbound" traffic and other lanes designated for strictly "southbound" traffic. The afferent pathway is designed more like a toll-way, because there are very few exits. In fact, along the afferent pathway only two

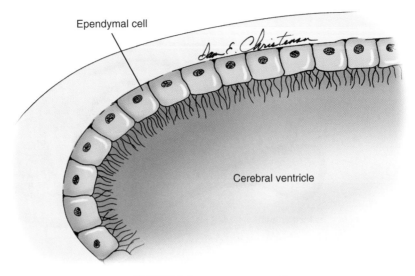

FIGURE 9-8   Ependymal cell.

exits are available for most nerves. One exit leads just to the spinal cord; this path is discussed with reflex arcs. The other exit leads to the brain. Once in the brain, there are many divided highways and side streets leading to specific destinations in the brain. Along the *efferent* pathway there are many exits, just like the interstate system throughout the United States. Ultimately, a series of exits carries the nerve impulses to a specific destination at an *effector* organ or tissue.

Upper Motor and Lower Motor Neurons

Upper motor and lower motor neurons are simply subdivisions or subclassifications of efferent neurons, based on location (see the schematic below). For the most part, those efferent pathways of the central nervous system (primarily the brain) are considered *upper motor neurons* (UMNs). Upper motor neurons ultimately control lower motor neuron activity. They have the "upper hand," if you will, controlling the subordinate lower motor neurons. The *lower motor neurons* (LMNs) are those efferent pathways of the peripheral nervous system. Disturbances of either the UMNs or the LMNs result in abnormal motor activity.

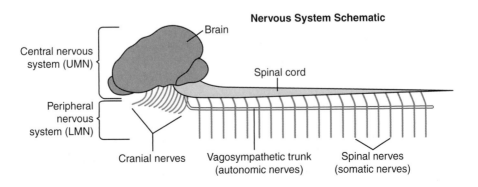

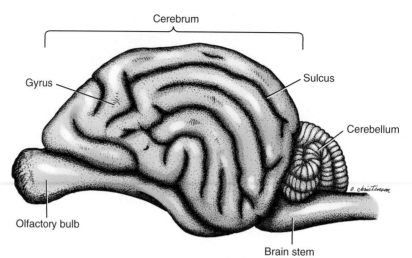

FIGURE 9-9   The brain (lateral view).

Central Nervous System Anatomy

The central nervous system (CNS) includes the brain and spinal cord. The brain serves as the central supercomputer for the body. However, unlike most computers, the brain has an almost inexhaustible amount of access and operating memory, as well as storage space. The spinal cord provides a tele-communication superhighway between the brain and the massive network of peripheral nerves. So, the spinal cord rushes important sensory information to the brain and speeds motor output from the brain to needed areas of the body. For less critical sensory input, the cord may simply reroute directly to motor output, without involving the brain. This will be discussed later with reflex arcs.

Brain

The brain, housed in the cranial vault, provides ultimate control over most activities of the body, both voluntary and involuntary. The largest portion of the brain is composed of the *cerebral hemispheres* (Fig. 9-9). The right and left cerebral hemispheres are separated by a longitudinal fissure or groove. To squeeze as much cerebral surface area into the small, confined space of the skull, the cerebral tissue is made of a series of "folds." The depressions or grooves of the cerebrum are called *sulci.*[1] The bulging ridges of the cerebrum are called *gyri.*[2] The large amount of surface area is important because all of the *gray matter* (composed of cell bodies used for data processing and storage) is spread in a thin layer over the surfaces of all the cerebral gyri and sulci. (This thin layer of gray matter is also referred to as the cerebral cortex.) The bulk of the

---

[1]Sulci (sul'ki), plural of sulcus; from [L. *sulcus,* groove, trench].
[2]Gyri (ji'ri), plural of gyrus; from [Gr. *gyrus,* ring, circle].

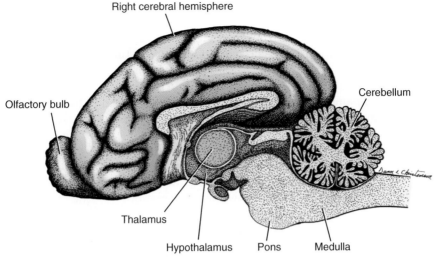

Right cerebral hemisphere

Cerebellum

Olfactory bulb

Thalamus

Hypothalamus   Pons   Medulla

FIGURE 9-10   The brain (midsagittal view).

cerebrum is composed of *white matter* (myelinated fibers). The white matter provides all of the telecommunication links for rapid transfer of information between the processing centers in the gray matter and those in the other portions of the brain and spinal cord. All conscious thought takes place in the cerebrum. The cerebrum is responsible for data processing, systems management, and data storage, much like a computer. It receives sensory information from various places in the body, analyzes the data, controls motor responses, and then commits all related information to memory. For the most part, the cerebrum exerts contralateral control over motor activity. For example, for a dog to perform the trick to "shake" with its right paw, the dog must initiate the conscious decision to do so in its left cerebral hemisphere. Motor impulses will travel to muscles of the right leg to result in the act of shaking. The coordination of those movements will be facilitated by the cerebellum.

The cerebellum is small in comparison with the cerebrum. It lies caudal to the cerebral hemispheres and dorsal to the brain stem (see Fig. 9-9). Similar to the cerebrum, the cerebellum has numerous, small convolutions and folds. A sagittal section of the cerebellum renders a dendritic appearance, somewhat like cauliflower (Fig. 9-10). The composition of the cerebellum, with regard to gray and white matter, is also much like that of the cerebrum. The bulk of the cerebellum is composed of white matter, with a thin layer of gray matter on the surface. The cerebellum is responsible for involuntary control of balance, posture, and coordination of movement. It attempts to maintain equilibrium and balance on receiving sensory information from portions of the inner ear, as well as visual and proprioceptive[3] input. Equilibrium is discussed in detail in Chapter 11, "The Ear."

---

[3]Proprioceptive (pro"pre-o-sep'tiv); a proprioceptor is a specialized sensory nerve ending designed to sense movement or position of the body.

The interbrain (diencephalon[4]) includes the thalamus and hypothalamus[5] (see Fig. 9-10). The diencephalon provides connections between the cerebral hemispheres and the brain stem. The interbrain, midbrain, and brain stem are each critical for basic life functions. The thalamus serves primarily as a relay station (like a switch-board operator or a "traffic cop"), routing all sensory information (except olfactory input) to appropriate areas of the cerebrum. As its name implies, the hypothalamus lies ventral to the thalamus. The hypothalamus provides for many of the body's basic homeostatic maintenance needs. For example, the hypothalamus controls functions such as hunger, cardiac rate, blood pressure, and body temperature.

Thermoregulation is a highly integrated system of *somatic* and *visceral* sensors and effectors. The hypothalamus acts like a thermostat, trying to maintain the core body temperature within a degree or so of the "set point." With exposure to cold, thermal sensors relay the sensory information to the hypothalamus. In response, the hypothalamus will cause vasoconstriction in the periphery to conserve heat. Fur or feathers may fluff up to increase insulation against the cold. Behaviorally, the animal may seek a warmer environment. Activity of the digestive tract, especially the liver, will increase along with hunger. This activity will act like a furnace, generating heat for the body. Finally, the animal may shiver uncontrollably, again in an attempt to generate heat. In contrast, when the animal is exposed to heat, opposite effects will occur. Peripheral vasodilation along with tachycardia will carry warm blood from the core to the surface, where heat may be dissipated. Behaviorally, the animal may seek a cooler environment. Horses may sweat profusely, to cool through evaporation. Dogs and cats will pant, to dissipate heat through evaporation and convection. Hunger will diminish, along with digestive activity, so that the "furnace" is no longer fueled. Finally, physical activity overall will slow or stop, to minimize heat generated. All of this, in a normal animal, functions like a well-oiled machine through hypothalamic and autonomic activity.

The brain stem is composed of the midbrain (mesencephalon[6]), the pons (ponz), and the medulla[7] (see Fig. 9-10). The midbrain, for the most part, simply connects the diencephalon with the rest of the brain stem. The pons is a rounded protrusion on the ventral aspect of the brain stem that forms a bridge between the midbrain and the medulla; the word *pons* in Latin literally means "bridge." The medulla forms the caudal part of the brain stem that lies ventral to the cerebellum, between the pons and the foramen magnum.[8] Both the pons and the medulla contain many control centers (cardiac, vasomotor, and respiratory centers) for functions such as heart rate, vasoconstriction and vasodilation, and respiratory rate and rhythm. Less vital, although certainly important, centers are also found in the medulla, such as those associated with coughing,

---

[4]Diencephalon (di"en-sef'ah-lon); from [*dia-*, between + *encephal(o)-*, brain]; i.e., interbrain.
[5]Hypothalamus (hi"po-thal'ah-mus); from [*hyp(o)-*, below + Gr. *thalamos,* inner chamber].
[6]Mesencephalon (mes"en-sef'ah-lon); from [*mes(o)-*, middle + *encephal(o)-*, brain]; i.e., middle brain.
[7]Medulla (me-dul'ah, me-du'lah); derived from [L. "inmost part"].
[8]Foramen magnum (for-a'men mag'num); a foramen (*foramina,* pl.) is a natural opening or passage; the foramen magnum is the hole at the base of the skull through which the spinal cord passes.

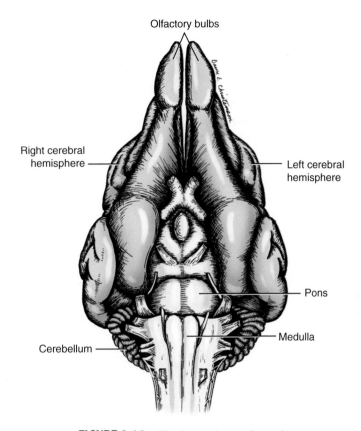

Olfactory bulbs

Right cerebral
hemisphere

Left cerebral
hemisphere

Pons

Medulla

Cerebellum

FIGURE 9-11   The brain (ventral view).

sneezing, and swallowing. In addition, 10 of the 12 pairs of cranial nerves arise
from the brain stem (Fig. 9-11). The first cranial nerve (olfactory nerve) arises
from the cerebrum, and the second cranial nerve (optic) arises from the diencephalon. The rest of the cranial nerves originate from points along the brain
stem. Structurally, the medulla oblongata is much like the spinal cord. Opposite
the arrangement of the rest of the brain, the medulla and the spinal cord are predominantly white matter, surrounding a small, centralized mass of gray matter.

Spinal Cord

The spinal cord (Fig. 9-12) begins where the brain stem leaves off, as it passes
through the foramen magnum. The spinal cord passes caudally through the
vertebral foramina to approximately the level of the caudal lumbar vertebrae.
Adipose and other connective tissues nestle around the cord, filling any space
in the vertebral canal between the spinal cord and the vertebral bone. This
prevents the cord from flopping and bumping against the boney canal during normal activity. In the lumbar/lumbosacral area, the spinal cord begins to
branch excessively, giving it a "horse's tail" appearance—hence the name cauda
equina (kaw'dah e-kwi'nah) for this portion of the cord. It is typically over this
area of the cord that *epidural analgesics* are injected.

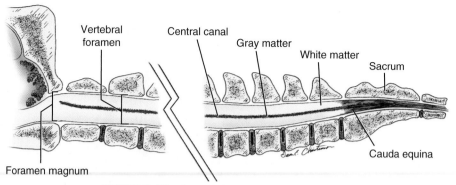

FIGURE 9-12   Spinal cord (midsagittal view).

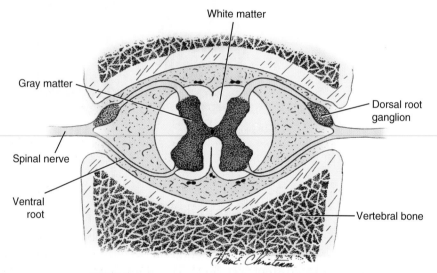

FIGURE 9-13   Spinal cord (transverse section).

As alluded to earlier, because the spinal cord serves as the telecommunication superhighway between the brain and the peripheral nerves, it is composed largely of myelinated tracts (white matter). Very specific afferent and efferent tracts transmit impulses to and from the brain and specific areas of the body. Many of these tracts are ipsilateral through the cord and into the brain. However, some tracts cross to carry impulses contralaterally. The myelinated tracts of the spinal cord give rise to the spinal nerves, which pass through the intervertebral foramina and branch into various peripheral nerves. Because of this arrangement, the white matter of the spinal cord is the most superficial and larger portion of it. The gray matter is centrally located in the spinal cord, which, in a transverse section, looks somewhat like a butterfly (Fig. 9-13). Spinal nerves branch at the cord into dorsal and ventral roots. The dorsal roots contain sensory nerve fibers and the ventral roots contain motor nerve fibers. Once again, it is evident that the northbound and southbound trafficking of neural impulses is facilitated by the physical layout of the afferent and efferent nerve fibers.

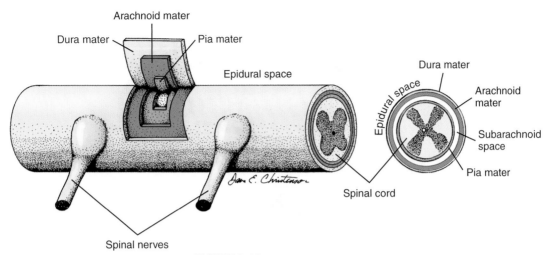

FIGURE 9-14 The meninges.

Meninges

The entire brain and spinal cord are encased in three membranes (meninges). Each meninx is somewhat different structurally and functionally. Minute spaces separate the meninges from one another.

The dura mater (du'rah ma'ter; du'rah mah'ter) literally means "tough mother." It is the most superficial of the three membranes (Fig. 9-14) and is composed of tough, protective, fibrous connective tissue. In the cranial vault, the dura mater is attached to the skull, but in the vertebral canal, there is space surrounding the dura. The space between the dura mater and the rest of the vertebral canal is called the epidural space. As mentioned earlier, this space is frequently used for regional analgesia, particularly in companion animal medicine.

The middle meninx is the arachnoid mater (ah-rak'noid; see Fig. 9-14). It is called the "arachnoid mater" because its net-like structure resembles a spider's web. Numerous strands of the arachnoid attach it to the innermost meningeal layer, the pia mater. This delicate scaffolding, if you will, creates a catacomb-like space between the two membranes, the subarachnoid space (see Fig. 9-14). This space and its importance with regard to cerebrospinal fluid will be discussed later.

The pia mater (pi'ah ma'ter; pe'ah mah'ter), meaning "soft mother," is the thinnest and most delicate of the meninges. It lies closest to the brain and spinal cord (see Fig. 9-14). It is highly vascular and closely follows the contour of the brain and spinal cord. It is therefore important for providing nutritional support by way of the bloodstream to the underlying neural tissues.

Cerebrospinal Fluid

Cerebrospinal fluid (CSF) flows in the subarachnoid space. It is produced in the ventricles of the brain by specialized clusters of capillaries from the pia mater, called choroid plexuses. The choroid plexuses are covered by epithelial-like neuroglial ependymal cells. Most of the CSF is produced by the lateral ventricles (one lateral ventricle is found per cerebral hemisphere). From there it trickles into the third ventricle, which is located in the area of the diencephalon. The

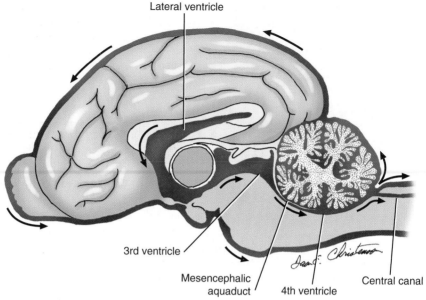

Lateral ventricle

3rd ventricle

Mesencephalic
aquaduct

4th ventricle

Central canal

FIGURE 9-15   Schematic of cerebrospinal fluid flow.

fluid must pass through the mesencephalic aqueduct[9] to reach the fourth ventricle, which is located in the brain stem, rostroventral to the cerebellum. From the fourth ventricle it flows into the central canal of the spinal cord and into the subarachnoid space around the brain and spinal cord, in essence floating these structures (Fig. 9-15). This provides a cushioning effect for everyday movement and minor trauma. Production and flow of CSF is continuous. A mechanism for reabsorption of the fluid is provided through the finger-like projections of arachnoid mater into highly vascular dural sinuses. Although the arachnoid mater is avascular, its specialized projections bring the CSF close to blood-filled dural sinuses so that it may be reabsorbed. Hundreds of milliliters of CSF are produced each day, yet in normal circumstances only a small portion of CSF is present in the subarachnoid space at any given moment in time. If something were to impair the flow of CSF (usually at the mesencephalic aqueduct), the CSF will accumulate in the "upstream" ventricles and *hydrocephalus* will result.

CSF is characteristically a transparent, colorless, acellular liquid. While it has a unique ionic composition that is high in sodium, the principle function of CSF seems to be protective. Changes in the character of the CSF generally reflect pathologic changes in the meninges, brain, and spinal cord. Disease conditions such as *meningitis, encephalitis,* and *myelitis* may be detected through microscopic, chemical, and immunologic analysis of the CSF. The fluid is collected by a CSF tap, in which a needle is inserted into the subarachnoid space and fluid withdrawn. Sites for CSF taps in domestic animals include the atlanto-occipital joint (found between the skull and first cervical vertebra), as well as the joints between the fourth and fifth and the fifth and sixth lumbar vertebrae. The skin

---

[9]Mesencephalic aqueduct (mes"en-sě-fal'ik ak'wě-dukt"); aqueduct comes from [L. "water canal"].

over the site must be carefully surgically prepped so that the spinal needle does not introduce pathogens into the subarachnoid space. These same sites are also used for *myelography*. During a *myelogram*, radiopaque dye is injected into the subarachnoid space. As the dye flows in conjunction with the CSF, structural abnormalities in the vertebral canal can be detected radiographically.

Blood–Brain Barrier

The blood–brain barrier protects the tissues of the brain and spinal cord from potentially harmful substances. It is formed, in part, by the *astroglial* cells that wrap their appendages around the capillaries in the brain. The "safety net" formed by these cells plus the unique, tightly connected endothelium of CNS capillaries selectively permits passage of only some substances into the brain and spinal cord tissues, as well as the CSF. Molecular size is probably one of the biggest factors influencing the selectivity of the blood–brain barrier. Unfortunately, this barrier is so efficient in its function that it often does not permit passage of therapeutic agents, like certain antibiotics, into the brain. This can significantly limit our ability to treat diseases of the CNS.

Peripheral Nervous System Anatomy

The peripheral nervous system (PNS) provides the body with a complex network of nerves, much like the telephone lines that stretch around the world. The PNS includes everything outside of the brain and spinal cord. This includes cranial nerves, spinal nerves, nerves of the limbs, and nerves supplying the viscera. The entire PNS is designed to receive sensory input, transmit it to the CNS, and then transmit appropriate response information from the CNS to the organs and tissues of the body.

Peripheral Nerves

The cranial nerves consist of 12 pairs of nerves originating from various regions of the brain and brain stem. The following list of cranial nerves includes a brief description of the respective nerve's function.

1. The *olfactory nerve* is the first cranial nerve. It provides for the sense of smell. Rostroventral to each cerebral hemisphere is an *olfactory* bulb (see Fig. 9-9). These bulbs (merely a portion of each olfactory nerve) lie in close proximity to the porous (ethmoid[10]) bone that separates the cranial vault from the nasal passages. The olfactory bulbs are well developed in most domestic animals. Receptors of the olfactory nerves pass through the ethmoid bone into the nasal passages. When olfactory receptors are stimulated in the nasal passages, the nerve impulses travel along the afferent fibers to the olfactory bulbs. The olfactory tracts continue to carry the impulses into the cerebrum for analysis. If you've ever witnessed a dog sniffing to track a scent, you'll notice

---

[10]Ethmoid (eth'moid); from [Gr. *ethmos,* sieve, *-oid,* resembling]; this bone has numerous holes, like that of a sieve or collander.

that the dog inspires short bursts of air into the nasal passages. This is in an attempt to concentrate the molecules of the smell for the olfactory receptors. Periodically, you'll see the dog blow from its nose in almost a mini-sneeze. This is to clear "old" scent molecules from the nasal passages to permit sniffing in fresh ones. The olfactory ability of animals far exceeds that of most humans. Dogs in particular have highly developed olfactory abilities, such that they can be trained to critically analyze specific scents for use in tracking criminals or victims of crimes, locating victims of natural disasters, discovering illicit drugs, or locating weapons or explosives. There have even been reports of dogs locating cancerous tumors in people, before the persons even knew they had a problem. Many human lives have been saved by these heros of the canine world, all by virtue of their amazing olfactory abilities.

2. The *optic nerve* is the second cranial nerve. It provides sensory fibers for vision. As you will learn in Chapter 10, each optic nerve actually carries the sensory input from each eye contralaterally into the cerebral hemispheres. Because the visual cortex is found in the caudal portions of the cerebral hemispheres, a severe injury to the caudal cerebrum may result in blindness. These individuals are said to be "cortically blind."

3. The *oculomotor nerve*[11] (cranial nerve III) provides primarily motor input for dorsal, dorsolateral, medial, dorsomedial, ventral, and ventromedial eye movements, as well as eyelid movement (opening the lids). The oculomotor nerve also provides parasympathetic fibers to the iris that reduce pupil size.

4. The *trochlear* (trok'le-ar) *nerve* (cranial nerve IV) provides primarily motor input for ventrolateral eye movement.

5. The *trigeminal* (tri-jem'ĭ-nal) *nerve* (cranial nerve V) provides large numbers of sensory fibers for parts of the face, mouth, and head. It also provides motor fibers for salivary and lacrimal (tear) glands, as well as muscles associated with chewing.

6. The *abducens* (ab-du'senz) *nerve* (cranial nerve VI) primarily provides motor input for lateral eye movement and retraction of the eye into the orbit.

7. The *facial* (fa'shal) *nerve* (cranial nerve VII) provides principal motor input to facial muscles, to provide for facial expressions and eyelid closure. Movements of facial muscles are far more important than mere expression. Many animals, such as the horse, rely on very discerning movements of the lips in order to selectively forage for food and consume it. Additional motor involvement of the facial nerve provides parasympathetic fibers to salivary as well as lacrimal glands. Sensory fibers of the facial nerves provide for much of the sensation of taste. Because of the numerous branches of the facial nerve, it is easily damaged in animals whose faces are insufficiently padded when laterally recumbent for long periods of time.

8. The *vestibulocochlear* (ves-tib"u-lo-ko'kle-ar) *nerve* (cranial nerve VIII) provides sensory fibers to areas of the inner ear associated with equilibrium and hearing. These functions will be discussed in depth in Chapter 11.

---

[11]Oculomotor (ok"u-lo-mo'tor); from [*ocul(o)-*, eye + *motor,* mover].

9. The *glossopharyngeal nerve*[12] (cranial nerve IX) provides motor input for muscles associated with the tongue and throat, as its name implies. Functionally, these fibers provide for swallowing, as well as for some salivary gland secretions. It also provides some sensory fibers for the tongue (i.e., taste) and the throat.

10. The *vagus* (va'gus) *nerve* (cranial nerve X) is a very important nerve associated largely with the parasympathetic branch of the autonomic nervous system. Its fibers are primarily motor, providing for functions such as vocalization and swallowing. Its motor input also provides autonomic control for much of the thoracic and abdominal viscera. Laryngeal hemiplegia was discussed in Chapter 8. The recurrent laryngeal nerve associated with this syndrome is one of many important branches of the vagus nerve. The influence of this nerve and its branches is far-reaching and very important with regard to the autonomic nervous system, to be discussed in more detail later. Briefly, it is important to know that stimulation of the vagus nerve slows the heart rate and accelerates gut motility. Its sensory fibers are also associated with areas of the throat and the thoracic and the abdominal viscera. It is important to note that the location of each vagus nerve as it passes through the neck is closely associated with the carotid artery and the jugular vein (see Chapter 7). This anatomy is important to remember when these vessels are used clinically.

11. The *accessory nerve* (cranial nerve XI) provides motor input for muscles of the throat, neck, and cranial back/shoulder.

12. The *hypoglossal nerve*[13] (cranial nerve XII), as its name implies, provides motor input for tongue movement.

In addition to the 12 pairs of cranial nerves, there are a multitude of peripheral nerves throughout the body. Only a few other nerves are discussed here, in keeping with those that are the most clinically relevant. The *brachial plexus*[14] is a bundle of spinal nerves that supplies all sensory and motor fibers for the forelimb (Fig. 9-16). Major blood vessels supplying the forelimb are closely associated with the brachial plexus as it enters the proximal forelimb. Severe damage to the brachial plexus results in monoplegia of the affected limb. A single nerve arising from the brachial plexus and of particular importance in the forelimb is the radial nerve. It is a large nerve that at one point passes over the lateral aspect of the humerus (see Fig. 9-16). It is easily damaged here by a severe blow to the lateral brachium or by prolonged pressure over the area (e.g., as in a recumbent animal). The radial nerve provides motor input to most of the extensor muscles of the forelimb. Damage to the radial nerve results in monoparesis, as well as significant sensory loss to the dorsal and cranial surfaces of the forelimb. Such animals tend to "knuckle-over," due to the loss of extensor muscles. Tremendous self-trauma will likely occur because the affected

---

[12]Glossopharyngeal (glos″o-fah-rin′je-al, glos″o-far-in-je′al); from [*gloss(o)-*, tongue + *pharyng(o)-*, throat + *-al*, pertaining to].
[13]Hypoglossal (hi″po-glos′al); from [*hyp(o)-*, below + *gloss(o)-*, tongue + *-al*].
[14]Plexus (plek′sus); pl. plexus or plexuses; from [L. *plexus*, braid].

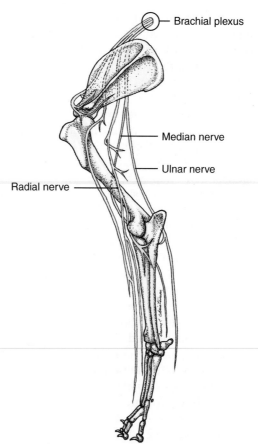

FIGURE 9-16   Brachial plexus (lateral view).

animal cannot feel the trauma. Palmar sensation will still be intact, provided the ulnar and median nerves were not damaged along with the radial nerve. Also of significance in the forelimb of horses are the digital nerves. Many of the digital nerves (front and rear limbs) are of clinical importance in equine medicine when one is trying to isolate the location and cause of lameness. By systematically blocking these sensory branches of the radial, ulnar, and median nerves with local anesthetics, the pain creating the lameness can be isolated.

The lumbosacral plexus is a bundle of spinal nerves that supply the hindlimb. Arising from the lumbosacral plexus is the *sciatic nerve* (si-at'ik; Fig. 9-17). The sciatic nerve and its branches is one of the most important nerves of the hindlimb. The sciatic nerve and its branches provide motor input to most of the flexor and some of the extensor muscles of the hindlimb, (i.e., all except those of the cranial and medial thigh). The sciatic nerve lies caudal to the femur. When using the caudal thigh muscles for intramuscular injections, particularly in companion animals, improper technique or irritating medications could damage the sciatic nerve. Varying degrees of monoparesis or monoplegia could result. All sensation to the distal limb (distal to the stifle) will also be disrupted.

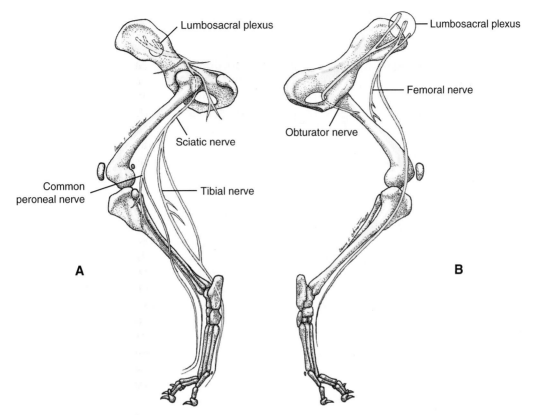

FIGURE 9-17 Lumbosacral plexus. **A,** Lateral view. **B,** Medial view.

Another nerve of the hindlimb that is of clinical importance is the *obturator nerve* (ob′tu-ra″tor; see Fig. 9-17). It provides motor input for muscles of the medial thigh (i.e., adductors). It is most frequently damaged during difficult calving (birth of a calf). This is because the nerve passes over the pelvis, in the "birth canal," before it passes through the obturator foramen and courses down the limb. With a large calf wedged in the birth canal, the obturator nerves are effectively crushed between the calf and the pelvis. Obturator nerve paralysis leaves the cow unable to support her hindquarters, because she can no longer adduct the limbs.

Autonomic Nervous System

The autonomic nervous system helps control vital functions of the body automatically. Most of the autonomic nervous system is composed of motor neurons. Functions like breathing, cardiac rate, and digestion are controlled, in part, by the autonomic nervous system. It has its own methods of checks and balances provided through its sympathetic and parasympathetic branches. Both branches are continually working, in kind of a tug-of-war arrangement. Which branch dominates at any given moment depends on the needs of the body at the time. A plethora of sensory input supplies centers in the brain with needed information to determine which type of activity is needed at a given moment.

Sympathetic System

The sympathetic branch of the autonomic nervous system provides for fight-or-flight responses. If a cat mistakenly wandered into a yard guarded by two large, fractious dogs, this portion of the autonomic nervous system would have "sympathy" for the poor cat. The sight and sounds of those frightening dogs will rapidly set the sympathetic branch of autonomics in motion. It stimulates various areas of the cat's body, making it possible for the cat to escape. Pupils will dilate to see not only the threat but any possible escape route. The cat's cardiac and respiratory rates increase. Airways will dilate to provide for ample oxygenation. Blood is redirected to vital organs (heart, lungs, and brain) while it is routed away from nonessential areas like the skin and digestive tract. If we were to look at his mucous membranes at this moment, they would be quite pale. (People in similar situations are said to "turn white as sheets.") His mouth will become dry, as salivary secretions are stopped. (This is why people frightened by public speaking develop the characteristic "dry mouth," making it difficult to speak.) While the cat might suddenly evacuate his bowels, digesting breakfast will be put on hold for a more opportune, safe, and quiet time. Blood volume is needed for more important areas, such as his major muscles, permitting him to run away or foolishly turn to fight the imposing beasts. As the rest of those sympathetic activities are stimulated, sympathetic fibers also stimulate the adrenal glands to cause them to produce larger amounts of adrenalin (epinephrine) than normal. Adrenalin has a *sympathomimetic* effect on many of these same areas of the body. The sympathetic nervous system initiates the fight-or-flight response, and the epinephrine keeps it going as long as the cat needs to fight or flee. Thankfully, the adrenal glands are only innervated by sympathetic fibers. Between the split-second response time of the sympathetic system and the "super-human strength" that epinephrine provides, survival is possible.

Parasympathetic System

The body must have a way to counter the effects of the sympathetic system. The parasympathetic branch of the autonomic nervous system provides just that. Whatever the sympathetic branch stimulates in a given organ, the parasympathetic branch has the opposite effect (except the adrenal glands, as mentioned earlier). So, as soon as that poor cat is safely inside hiding under his favorite chair, the parasympathetic system begins to overpower the sympathetic system to slow the cardiac and respiratory rates. Pupils will constrict to a normal size. Blood no longer is conserved for the vital organs, so his mucous membranes turn pink and his paws are no longer cold. The cat can relax. He may even fall asleep after his intense flurry of activity is over. That is precisely the type of activity that is stimulated by the parasympathetic system, "rest and repose" or "rest and digest." Most of the peak activity of the digestive tract is stimulated by the parasympathetic system—rightly so, because digestion is facilitated best when an animal is quietly resting. Cows and other ruminant animals demonstrate this best when they lay around for hours on end chewing their cud. See Table 9-1 for the principal responses to both the sympathetic and parasympathetic systems.

TABLE 9-1   **Principal responses to the sympathetic and parasympathetic systems**

Autonomic Nervous System Influence	
Sympathetic stimulation	**Parasympathetic stimulation**
Pupil: dilation	Pupil: constriction
Salivary secretions: decreased	Salivary secretions: increased
Heart: tachycardia	Heart: bradycardia
Airways: bronchodilation	Airways: bronchoconstriction
Digestive tract: decreased activity and secretions	Digestive tract: increased activity and secretions
Adrenal gland: increased secretion of epinephrine	Adrenal gland: no influence
Vessels: vasodilation of cardiac and major muscle vasculature; vasoconstriction of peripheral vasculature (e.g., skin)	Vessels: no influence

Neurotransmission

Neurotransmission is nothing more than a means of sending electrochemical messages throughout the body, along nerve fibers. This occurs in a way much like Morse code being transmitted over telegraph lines. A message is transmitted from a distant point and is received at another point. If a reply is needed, a message is transmitted back to the point of origin. Fortunately, as was demonstrated through the discussion of autonomics, the rate of transmission is lightening-fast. Even the methodic neurotransmission along unmyelinated nerve fibers occurs in milliseconds.

Unmyelinated Nerve Fibers

Unmyelinated nerve fibers do not have an insulating myelin sheath surrounding them. They are exposed in their entirety to interstitial fluids. Chemically, the neurons' intracellular fluids are different from the extracellular fluids. Although both fluids contain a mixture of ions, the intracellular fluid of a neuron at rest (polarized) contains large amounts of potassium ions. The extracellular fluids surrounding this resting neuron contain large amounts of sodium ions (Fig. 9-18). When the dendrites of a nerve fiber are stimulated sufficiently, through active transport, the Na^+ is taken into the neuron, while concurrently the K^+ is sent to the extracellular fluid (depolarization). The net exchanges of ions generate an electrical charge (impulse) along the neuronal membrane. The ionic exchange begins at the dendritic (receptor) end of the neuron and continues in a systematic, sequential way along the length of the neuron. Before the impulse has even reached the axonal end of the neuron, ions at the dendritic end of the cell begin reverting to their original positions (repolarization). Neurons "recharge" (repolarize) themselves, just as nickel–cadmium batteries must be recharged when they have been depleted. During depolarization and repolarization, ions are actively being exchanged across the cell membranes, via the sodium potassium pump. Therefore, the total period during which ionic exchange occurs is referred to as the *action potential* (Fig. 9-19). *Resting potential* refers to a neuron at rest, when the ions are "in the starting blocks" awaiting "firing of the starting gun" (neuronal stimulation). Neurons at resting potential are said to be "polarized."

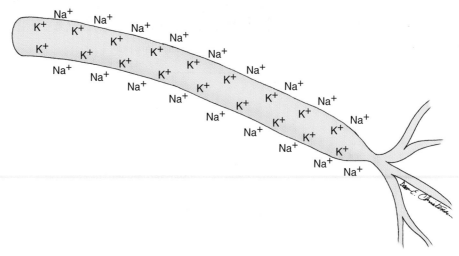

FIGURE 9-18   Polarized unmyelinated neuron.

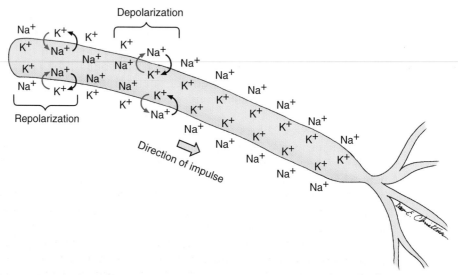

FIGURE 9-19   Action potential of an unmyelinated neuron.

Myelinated Nerve Fibers

Comparing the rate of transmission of unmyelinated nerve fibers with that of myelinated nerve fibers is like comparing the pony express with the telegraph. The pony express was fast, but the telegraph was so much faster that it put the former out of business. (Today, probably a better analogy of unmyelinated versus myelinated fibers would be to compare the speed of dial-up internet connections with that of broadband or satellite connections.) For the purpose of this discussion, the structure of the telegraph system is physically more like that of the nervous system. Of course, this is not to say that the telegraph did not have its share of problems. For instance, on long stretches of telegraph lines, especially in damp weather, much of

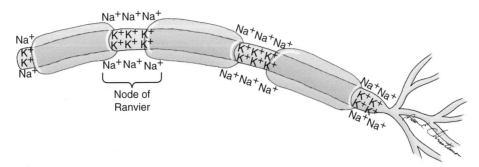

FIGURE 9-20 Polarized myelinated neuron.

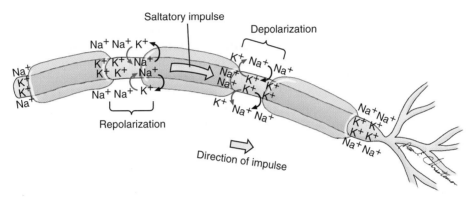

FIGURE 9-21 Action potential of a myelinated neuron.

the current traveling in the lines would "leak." Plus, some of the strength of the signal would be lost because of natural resistance in the line itself. This would result in a weak signal at its destination. To maintain the strength of the signal, the telegraph system incorporated components called relays along the lines. The relays would provide a "boost" to the telegraph signal. In addition, telegraph lines, particularly those placed underground, were insulated to minimize leakage of current. Fortunately, most of the nerve fibers in the body are myelinated. Consequently, very little of a nerve impulse "leaks" from the nerve fiber. Resistance along the nerve fiber could still weaken the impulse, however. Like the telegraph, myelinated nerve fibers are equipped with relays (nodes of Ranvier; Fig. 9-20). The bare nodes of Ranvier (rahn-ve-a′) are the only areas along a myelinated fiber at which ionic exchange takes place. The rest of the nerve fiber is insulated by myelin. The myelin prevents "leakage" of the impulse from the nerve fiber, and the nodes of Ranvier provide the impulse with a boost to maintain its strength. As a myelinated nerve fiber is stimulated, action potential occurs only at the nodes of Ranvier. The electrical charge then shoots through the myelinated portion of the fiber to the next node of Ranvier. This continues sequentially until the impulse reaches its destination, creating a saltatory[15] form of transmission (Fig. 9-21). This system provides for an extremely efficient, rapid mode of transmission of neural impulses.

---

[15]Saltatory (sal′tah-to″re); from [L. *saltatio,* to jump].

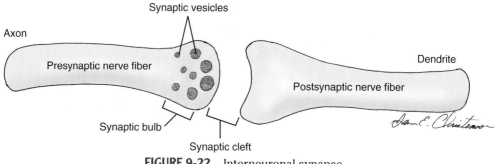

FIGURE 9-22 Interneuronal synapse.

Synapse

The synapse is another type of relay that provides a connection between two neurons or between a neuron and a target organ or tissue. Structurally, an interneuronal synapse is formed by the axon (transmitting end) of the presynaptic nerve fiber, a small space (the synaptic cleft), and the dendrites (receiving end) of the postsynaptic nerve fiber (Fig. 9-22). The end of the presynaptic nerve fiber (i.e., the presynaptic bulb) contains small vesicles filled with a chemical neurotransmitter substance. As the nerve impulse reaches the synaptic vesicles, they release the neurotransmitter substance into the synaptic cleft. As the neurotransmitter comes in contact with the receptors of the postsynaptic neuron, depolarization of that neuron is stimulated (Fig. 9-23). The most widely used neurotransmitter substance of the body is acetylcholine (as″ē-til-ko′lēn; ah-se″til-ko′lēn). The parasympathetic branch of the autonomic nervous system uses acetylcholine exclusively as its neurotransmitter substance. Consequently, parasympathetic nerve fibers are referred to as *cholinergic* nerve fibers. Many somatic nerve fibers, like those synapsing on skeletal muscle, are cholinergic nerve fibers as well. On the sympathetic side of the autonomic nervous system, acetylcholine is used only at preganglionic synapses. At most sympathetic postganglionic synapses, particularly at the organ level, norepinephrine is the neurotransmitter used. These fibers are referred to as adrenergic.

For now, let's focus on the acetylcholine. What happens to all of the acetylcholine released into the synaptic cleft? Obviously, a portion of it is used at the postsynaptic receptors. A small portion of the excess will be reabsorbed back into the presynaptic bulb and repackaged into vesicles. Most of the excess acetylcholine will be rapidly, enzymatically removed by acetylcholinesterase.[16] If it were not removed, postsynaptic receptors would continue to be stimulated until all of the acetylcholine in the synaptic cleft was used up. Curious about what happens to norepinephrine used in adrenergic synapses? Some is reabsorbed into the bulb. The rest is cleared by monoamine oxidase (MAO).

In the earlier neurotransmission discussion, the importance of sodium and potassium, along with the sodium-potassium pump, were emphasized. Calcium is another important ion with regard to neurotransmission. The threshold of

---

[16]Acetylcholinesterase (as″e-til-ko″lin-es′ter-ās; [acetylcholine + esterase]; the suffix *-ase* always indicates an enzyme).

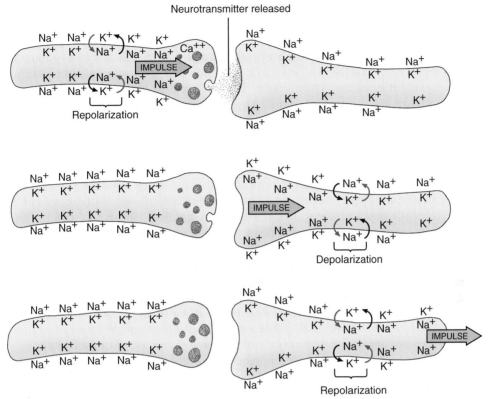

FIGURE 9-23   Synaptic neurotransmission.

stimulation required to initiate depolarization of a nerve fiber depends, in part, on the concentrations of calcium. Calcium acts as a gatekeeper for the sodium-potassium channels. With too little calcium present, depolarization may occur with very little stimulation. Too much calcium, on the other hand, could actually depress the initiation of neurotransmission. Calcium is also important for synaptic transmission. As the action potential reaches the end of the presynaptic nerve fiber, calcium must diffuse into the presynaptic bulb of the fiber to facilitate release of the neurotransmitter from its vesicle. So, with regard to synaptic transmission, hypocalcemia[17] will result in depression of neurotransmission. Homeostasis with regard to three electrolytes (i.e., sodium, potassium, and calcium) is critical for normal neurotransmission.

Neurotransmission also depends on a ready supply of energy (in the form of glucose) and sufficient oxygen for metabolism. Other cells of the body have numerous intracellular organelles for complex metabolic processes. Neurons, however, have been created for a very special electrochemical task, at which they must be efficient. Consequently, their metabolism has been simplified for aerobic glycolysis alone. Without adequate supplies of oxygen and glucose, neurons cannot function effectively, if at all.

---

[17]Hypocalcemia (hi"po-kal-se'me-ah; a condition of deficient calcium in the blood).

Reflexes and the Reflex Arc

Reflexes are protective mechanisms, reactions to stimuli, that occur independently of the will. For instance, if one were to make a menacing gesture with a finger, as if to poke a dog's eye, that dog by pure reflex action would close the eyelids and retract the eye back into the orbit. This type of action occurs independent of the conscious mind. Reflexes are designed to give rapid responses to potentially dangerous stimuli. They are intended to protect the body before the cerebrum has a chance to process sensory input about the situation. In the case of the menace reflex just described, sensory input, via the optic nerve, synapses on motor tracts of the diencephalon and "arcs" back around via the facial and abducens nerves to create the blink and eye retraction.

A reflex arc provides rapid turnaround of sensory to motor impulses. The simplest example of a reflex arc is that of the patellar reflex. With an animal in lateral recumbency and the stifle semiflexed, the patellar ligament is struck with a reflex hammer. Striking the ligament stretches it and the quadriceps tendon slightly. The stretching action stimulates receptors in the quadriceps (cranial thigh) muscles, generating a sensory nerve impulse. The impulse quickly travels along the afferent pathway through the dorsal root ganglion to the spinal cord. In the cord, the sensory nerve fibers synapse directly onto motor nerve fibers. The impulse slingshots from the spinal cord back down an efferent pathway to the cranial thigh muscles. Via the "motor end plate" (the synapse onto the muscle fibers), the quadriceps muscles are stimulated to contract, causing extension of the stifle joint. The entire process takes a split second and occurs completely independent of the brain.

A withdrawal reflex is a little more complex. The stimulus required is still minimal (perhaps tickling the toes of a dog). The afferent pathway will be stimulated from the toes all the way to the cord, as with the patellar reflex. However, the reflex motor response involves multiple muscles. Therefore, the afferent nerve fibers will synapse on multiple *interneurons* in the cord. These interneurons will provide sensory connections to many motor pathways that will result in contraction of all of the flexor muscles of the affected limb. Additionally, if the dog was standing when we tickled the toes of his left paw, interneurons will synapse on motor pathways to the contralateral limb to facilitate contraction of extensor muscles in the right leg. Again, this spinal reflex requires minimal stimulation for a rapid motor action, independent of any brain involvement.

A response to pain combines reflex actions with conscious thought. A painful stimulus is much more profound than the others we've described. In addition to those sensory fibers stimulated for a reflex, pain will result in stimulation of specialized sensory receptors *(nociceptors)* and provide for a greater number of synaptic transmissions at the level of the spinal cord. Applying a noxious (painful) stimulus, such as pinching a dog's toe, immediately initiates a reflex arc. The sensory impulse travels along an afferent pathway, through the dorsal root ganglia to the spinal cord, rapidly switches to an efferent pathway, and travels back down to the limb where the flexor muscles are stimulated to contract (as described previously for the withdrawal reflex). All the joints of the limb are flexed, and as a result the limb is withdrawn. While this protective reflex is in progress, some sensory fibers in the cord synapse on afferent pathways to the brain. On reaching the brain, the information is analyzed. The dog consciously recognizes the painful insult applied to his toe. He makes a conscious decision how to respond. That motor response is sent by efferent pathways to an appropriate target. As a result, the dog's conscious response to the pain may be vocalization, turning toward or away from the painful stimulus, biting the individual who applied the stimulus, or a combination thereof. Lower motor neurons control the withdrawal reflex and upper motor neurons control the conscious reaction. The nerve impulses initiated by the toe pinch are transmitted so rapidly that both the withdrawal reflex and the conscious response to the pain may appear to occur simultaneously. While evaluating spinal reflexes in cord injuries is very important, many times the prognosis[18] for a patient depends on the ability to stimulate the deep afferent pathways of the cord to obtain a conscious reaction to the painful stimulus. If the animal can consciously acknowledge the pain through growling or whimpering, we know that a portion of the cord is still functional, in spite of the animal currently being paralyzed. The response to deep pain gives us a glimmer of hope for the animal's recovery.

Pathophysiology and Disease

Neurotransmission can be affected in many ways. Previously, we alluded to how electrolyte imbalances could affect neurotransmission at the cellular level. Think of what the effect of hyponatremia[19] would have on the action potentials of neurons. Insufficient sodium to transport into the neurons will significantly impair depolarization. Cerebrally, this would significantly impair an animal's cognitive ability. Peripherally, hyponatremia would impair strength and mobility, by diminishing motor impulses to the skeletal muscles. Hyperkalemia[20] would have similar effects, because if neurons are surrounded by excessive potassium there is nowhere for the intracellular potassium to diffuse to. (Remember, diffusion requires movement of ions from an area of high concentration to an area of low concentration.)

What if we purposefully interfered with the active diffusion of critical ions, like sodium? What if we intentionally blocked that movement? You ask, "Why on earth would we want to do that?!" Have you ever had a minor surgical procedure performed on yourself (e.g., to suture a laceration or to remove a wart or mole)? A health care provider probably injected a solution into the skin and tissues surrounding the surgical site first, right? That solution was probably a local *anesthetic* agent like lidocaine. In a matter of moments, that area of the skin was anesthetized. How did that happen? The lidocaine blocked sodium channels, preventing depolarization of sensory neurons in the skin and surrounding tissues. But lidocaine doesn't last long, because the drug is rapidly carried away by blood flow through the area. Once again, we can interfere with normal body function, to improve the duration of the local anesthesia. How? We can cause localized vasoconstriction to slow removal of the anesthetic agent. In

---

[18]Prognosis (prog-no′sis); from [Gr. *prognosis,* foreknowledge] to forecast; clinically refers to the forecast of the probable outcome of a patient's response to a disease.

[19]Hyponatremia (hi″po-nah-tre′me-ah; a condition of deficient sodium in the blood).

[20]Hyperkalemia (hi″per-kah-le′me-ah; a condition of excessive potassium in the blood).

a fight-or-flight response, we said that the sympathetic nervous system would cause vasoconstriction in areas, like the skin, and epinephrine from the adrenal gland would sustain that response. So, what if we added a *sympathomimetic* agent, like epinephrine, to the lidocaine that we infuse? The combination of the two agents will result in local anesthesia (via the lidocaine) that is prolonged because of the *adrenergic* effects of the epinephrine. If one understands basic anatomy and physiology, one can either block or enhance normal body responses.

Let's think about a longer, much more painful procedure like a total hip replacement in a German Shepherd. Yes, the patient will be anesthetized with a general anesthetic agent, rendering her unconscious. While her conscious mind will not be aware of the pain during the procedure, nociceptors in the surgical site and in the cord will be stimulated. Repeated stimulation of these sensory neurons in the cord may result in the phenomenon called "wind-up." As its name implies, there will be a buildup of painful impulses. In this phenomenon, on awaking from anesthesia, the dog will be in profound, uncontrolled pain. To prevent this, preemptive *analgesia* may be used in conjunction with the general anesthesia. Preoperative *epidural analgesia* is a good example of this. For the epidural in our total hip replacement patient, an analgesic agent, often an opioid[21] like morphine, will be infused through the lumbosacral joint. (For animals except the cat, the lumbosacral joint lies over the cauda equina, not the cord itself. Therefore, cord injury with epidural analgesia is generally not a concern.) Because the morphine is infused into the epidural space, the drug will bathe the area including spinal nerves in the region. Because morphine binds directly to special sensory receptors, sensory input from the surgical site will be effectively blocked. The analgesia created will prevent stimulation of nociceptors in the cord and in so doing prevent wind-up. Other benefits to this regional analgesic approach include pain relief during the surgery (reducing the need for as much anesthetic agent) and postoperative pain relief. Epidural analgesia typically lasts for hours and can even be provided for days through placement of an epidural catheter for constant infusion. Analgesic therapy is very important for optimizing the recovery of surgical patients.

Synaptic neurotransmission is another area that may be diseased and/or medically controlled. Pesticides are agents that often interfere with normal neurotransmission of the pest we are trying to eradicate. Did you know that many insects and other parasites use acetylcholine as a major neurotransmitter substance? They do. Their tiny little synapses work very much like domestic animals and people, with acetylcholinesterase removing any excess acetylcholine left in the synaptic cleft. So, what would happen if we block the release of acetylcholinesterase throughout a pest's body? That's what pesticides containing organophosphates do to the pests. The tiny creatures become rigidly paralyzed from repeated depolarization of their many neurons. In the end, the parasites die from the tonic (rigid) paralysis. Naturally, care must be taken when using organophosphates for pest control on animals. If the animal is overdosed,

---

[21]Opioid (ŏp′e-oid; [Gr. *opium* + *-oid*]; opioids are synthetic narcotics that resemble opium in their actions. They are typically powerful analgesics).

similar consequences will result for the patient. Think about it. The whole parasympathetic nervous system exclusively uses acetylcholine for neurotransmission. If that branch of the nervous system is excessively stimulated by an overdose of an *anticholinesterase (parasympathomimetic)* agent, we'll see clinical evidence of parasympathetic stimulation. Such parasympathomimetic effects include constricted pupils. The animal may become critically bradycardic. The digestive tract will be extremely excited, resulting in vomiting and diarrhea. Muscle tremors and even seizures may result. To treat emergency patients like these, we again fall back to physiology. If all of these things are occurring because we cannot remove acetylcholine from the synaptic clefts, then let's block the effects of acetylcholine with an *anticholinergic (parasympatholytic)* agent like atropine. Beyond the supportive care that these animals need, this will be a principal means of managing the individual until the toxic pesticide is cleared from the body.

There are times when parasympathomimetic agents can be very beneficial for patients. Myasthenia gravis[22] is a syndrome that is most often seen in certain breeds of dogs. In this syndrome, either the animal doesn't have enough functional cholinergic postsynaptic receptors for the muscles or not enough acetylcholine is produced for those synapses. These animals will be weak and fatigue very quickly, because they deplete a limited supply of acetylcholine very rapidly. So, what if we interfere with the normal enzymatic removal of acetylcholine from the synaptic cleft? What if we give something that will selectively block the release of acetylcholinesterase at *neuromuscular* synapses? Under upper motor neuron control, postsynaptic activity like muscle contraction for walking and other movements will be stimulated until the acetylcholine is used up from the cleft. Then there is still acetylcholine to be released from other presynaptic vesicles. These animals may never be normal, but at least medication is available so that they can enjoy improved quality of life. If not medicated, these animals will spend most of their time recumbent.

Recumbency can also be created by trauma to the spinal cord. One of the most frequent disease syndromes to cause this is intervertebral disc disease (IVDD). IVDD tends to affect certain canine breeds. For many of these dogs, the intervertebral discs deteriorate at an accelerated rate. The annulus fibrosus becomes fragile and the nucleus pulposus becomes thick and mineralized (refer to Chapter 6 for intervertebral disc anatomy). The diseased discs may become compressed, with the thin, dorsal annulus actually bulging into the vertebral canal. This may create pain in the area and motor deficits caudal to the bulge. Owners may notice the *dysmetria* caused by these motor deficits as stumbling or the dog dragging its paws. During a neurologic examination, those deficits may be observed as slowed conscious proprioception. To evaluate conscious proprioception, each of the dog's feet is individually evaluated by turning the paw onto its dorsal surface. (Proprioceptors in the dorsal paw will stimulate afferent pathways to the cord, synapse on afferent pathways to the brain, and on interpretation in the brain motor impulses will descend via efferent pathways to

---

[22]Myasthenia gravis (mi″as-the′ne-ah gra′vis; [*my(o)*-, muscle + Gr. *astheneia*, weakness and L. *gravis*, heavy]).

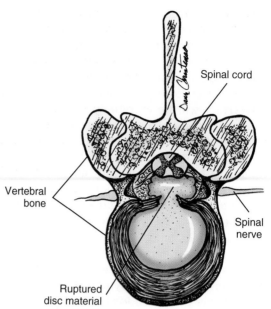

Spinal cord

Vertebral
bone

Spinal
nerve

Ruptured
disc material

FIGURE 9-24   Transverse spinal column showing ruptured intervertebral disc.

the limb for appropriate muscle contractions that will right the foot.) A normal dog should rapidly sense the inappropriate positioning and quickly reposition the paw onto its palmar or plantar surface. With proprioceptive deficits, the dog will appear slow to react. If the cord injury and inflammation is severe, the dog may not be able to right the paw at all. In mildly affected dogs, with strict rest and treatment to reduce inflammation, they may recover to lead somewhat normal existences. All too often, such a recovery is temporary.

You see unfortunately with diseased, bulging intervertebral discs, even normal movements of the spine may cause these discs to rupture. The design of the discs promotes rupture of the nucleus pulposus dorsally, directly into the vertebral canal (Fig. 9-24). Such an event most often happens in the areas of cervical, thoracolumbar, and lumbar spine. Cervical injuries result in *tetraparesis* to *tetraplegia*, depending on the severity of cord trauma. Thoracolumbar and lumbar injuries tend to result in *paraparesis* to *paraplegia*. Upper motor neuron pathways in the cord are damaged by the ventral pressure. Consequently, at the point of injury, UMN efferent impulses will be blocked. That is why the paresis and paralysis involves everything caudal to the injury. If acute paralysis resulted from the disc rupture, time is of the essence to prevent permanent loss of function. Our neurologic examination will likely be very limited, perhaps restricted to spinal reflexes and deep pain. Spinal reflexes are frequently normal or exaggerated. (The exaggeration may be due to blockage of UMN control that maintains overall muscular tone to "temper" the actual reflex.) With regard to sensation, the area near the injury may be *hyperesthetic* or anything near and caudal to the injury may appear to be anesthetic. Superficial sensations rely on intact dorsal roots of spinal nerves and superficial afferent pathways of the cord. Deep pain, however, relies on afferent pathways that are located deep within the cord, areas that will likely be the last to be lost in a traumatic injury. That is why observing a positive, conscious deep pain response is so important for the prognosis of an acutely paralyzed patient. If deep pain pathways are intact and the owners desire to do whatever is necessary for the dog, there is hope for the dog's recovery. We will need to find the exact location of injury with additional diagnostic tools, such as spinal radiographs, *myelography* CT[23] scan, and MRI.[24] If we can locate the ruptured disc, we can attempt surgical repair. Even if the disc material cannot be safely removed from the vertebral canal, we can "decompress" the area by removing a portion of the dorsal vertebral bone (i.e., dorsal laminectomy). In this way, the cord is no longer being "squished" between the disc material and the vertebral bone. The faster we can intervene with repair, the more likely the patient can recover either fully or with minimal deficits. Still, recovery may take considerable time. Remember, neurons do not have all of the intracellular organelles of other cells to be able to speed the repair of their tissues.

Of course, not all motor impairment stems from the spinal cord. Brain injury and disease can have tremendous impacts on motor function. Consider head trauma of an animal hit by a car. A significant unilateral cerebral injury may result in *hemiparesis* or *hemiplegia* contralateral to the actual injury. Closed-head injuries are often very serious. While the skull offers protection for the brain under normal circumstances, in a closed-head injury it is too confining. There is no room for the brain to swell. There is no room for a *subdural hematoma* to expand. In either case, the brain itself will be placed under extreme pressure. As the intracranial pressure increases, cerebral, cerebellar, diencephalon, and brain stem functions will decrease. *Opisthotonos*[25] is often observed near the end. Brain stem function may be diminished to the point that autonomic functions cease. Again, if we can intervene rapidly enough to minimize cerebral edema, we may be able to save the patient. Once recovered, some of these patients may experience seizure activity (*epilepsy*[26]). In these animals, the injured cerebral tissue may develop abnormal neurotransmission. At times, abnormal impulses may begin at the site of injury but then rapidly spread and involve the entire cerebrum. (An electroencephalogram may be able to detect the originating focus of the seizure activity.) The resulting seizure will typically render the animal temporarily unconscious and violently convulsing (jerking and thrashing about) from all of the abnormal, repeated upper motor neuron impulses. When the patient resumes consciousness, s/he will be exhausted. Many epileptic animals and people can "sense" an impending seizure, permitting them to seek a comfortable, safe place. (There are actually working dogs used to warn their human, epileptic owners that the person is about to have a seizure.) Seizure activity can result from many things, beyond head trauma. Sometimes it is termed *idiopathic*[27] epilepsy.

[23]CT—Computed tomography.
[24]MRI—Magnetic resonance imaging.
[25]Opisthotonos (o"pis-thot'o-nos; [Gr. *opisthen,* behind + *tonos,* tension]; an animal exhibiting opisthotonos will have extreme muscle tension along the dorsum, arching its back and extending its head and neck in extreme dorsal position as if it is trying to touch its nose to its back.
[26]Epilepsy (ep'ĭ-lep"se); from [Gr. *epilepsia,* seizure].
[27]Idiopathic (id"e-o-path'ik; [Gr. *idios,* own, peculiar + *pathos,* disease]; an idiopathic disease is one originating from one's self, often of an unknown cause.

Regardless, if seizure activity becomes frequent and severe enough, it may require *anticonvulsant* therapy.

Seizures caused by *neurotropic* pathogens may not be treatable once the animal has contracted it. Fortunately, some of these diseases are preventable through immunizations. *Equine encephalomyelitis* is such a disease. Not only does immunization protect the horse population, it also protects humans from this zoonotic threat. In both horses and humans, the encephalomyelitis that this virus causes is frequently fatal. Feline panleukopenia virus is an organism that isn't necessarily fatal and won't affect the cerebrum to cause seizures. Rather, it focuses on the cerebellum. If a queen is exposed to the disease late in pregnancy or her kittens are exposed shortly after birth, the kittens may develop *cerebellar hypoplasia*. The degree of hypoplasia will dictate the severity of motor impairment. Kittens within the litter will have varying degrees of *ataxia* and *hypermetria*. Mildly affected cats, placed in the right homes, can lead very happy lives. By the way, iatrogenic cerebellar hypoplasia may result if we immunize a pregnant queen with a modified live panleukopenia vaccine.

One of the most lethal neurotropic pathogens on the planet is the rabies virus. Immunization of our domestic animals and of veterinary professionals is very important for animal and public health. Rabies is a viral disease that is transmitted through the victim's saliva. Most people think of rabid animals being crazy, aggressive, frothing-at-the-mouth creatures that have to bite in order to transmit the deadly disease. True, it may be transmitted that way. However, veterinary professionals must be wary of a more "silent" mode of transmission to us. First, you must understand the basic progression of the disease. Let's say that an unvaccinated dog was bitten by a rabid cat on his front leg. The virus will begin to replicate in the bite wound. Then, the virus will begin retrograde movement along the motor neurons of the leg. Progressively, the dog's *neuritis* will cause *monoparesis,* perhaps even *monoplegia*. Eventually the virus will reach the spinal cord and ultimately the brain. In the brain, the virus will undergo tremendous replication and begin causing *encephalitis*. As the encephalitis develops the dog's behavior and mental ability will be altered from normal. Then the virus will travel via cranial nerves, like the trigeminal and glossopharyngeal nerves, seeking to reach the salivary glands. Viral damage will impair motor nerve fibers supplying the muscles of the jaw, tongue, and pharynx. Swallowing will be difficult (hence the classic frothing of the mouth). The clinical appearance of such a dog may be misinterpreted by the owner. The owner may bring this depressed, drooling dog to us with the complaint of a "bone caught in his throat." This should always throw up a red flag for veterinary professionals, prompting them to put on protective gloves before examining the dog's mouth and throat. If gloves are not worn, the person may become infected quietly and unexpectedly through contact of the dog's saliva with any little nick or scratch on their hands. Although the dog will not survive the disease, if a veterinary professional uses appropriate protection (including gloves and immunization), he/she will not succumb the same fate as the dog. The owners will need to undergo prophylactic immunization to be protected. The zoonotic threat in this case could have been completely avoided, had both the cat and dog owners immunized their pets against this deadly disease.

SELF-TEST

Using the previous information in this chapter, complete the following crossword puzzle using the most appropriate medical term(s). Do not use abbreviations or common names unless requested.

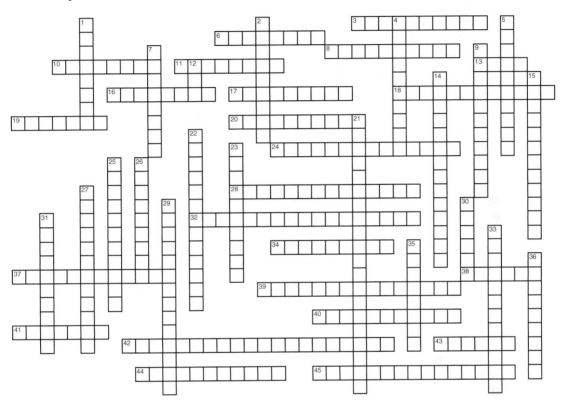

ACROSS

3	Paralysis of the hindlimbs
6	Inflammation of the spinal cord
8	The portion of the brain that coordinates motor activity
10	The portion of a neuron that receives stimulation
11	A _____ hematoma is an accumulation of blood beneath the dura mater
13	The portion of a neuron that transmits impulses away from the cell body
16	"Motor" nerve fibers
17	At resting potential of a neuron, the intracellular ion in high concentration
18	The portion of the diencephalon that controls thermoregulation
19	A "connection" providing electrochemical neurotransmission
20	Synonym for sympathomimetic
24	The phase of neurotransmission when intracellular potassium and extracellular sodium actively diffuse across the neuronal membrane
28	The discs that cushion between the spinal bones
32	Inflammation of the brain and spinal cord

34	A difficult gait
37	A condition of deficient sodium in the blood
38	The "insulation" of nerve fibers
39	The autonomic branch that provides for rest and digestion
40	The autonomic branch that provides for fight or flight
41	The major nerve of the pelvic limb that, with its branches, provides motor control for the flexor muscles of that limb
42	The enzyme that removes acetylcholine from the synaptic cleft
43	Uncoordinated stumbling
44	Nerve fibers that use the neurotransmitter acetylcholine
45	Synonym for parasympatholytic

DOWN

1	Disease transmission between animals and people
2	First cranial nerve
4	A state without sensation
5	A disease of unknown cause
7	The portion of the brain that provides for conscious thought and memory
9	Weakness, partial impairment of the hindlimbs
12	Abbreviation for upper motor neuron
14	The bare portions of myelinated nerve fibers (3 words)
15	Paralysis of all four limbs, cf. tetraplegia
21	Underdevelopment of the cerebellum caused by the feline panleukopenia virus (2 words)
22	An excessive accumulation of CSF in the cerebral ventricles
23	A pain receptor
25	An exaggerated gait
26	A diagnostic procedure in which dye is injected into the subarachnoid space
27	A condition of excessive potassium in the blood
29	The phase of neurotransmission when sodium and potassium ions return to their original locations
30	At resting potential of a neuron, the most important extracellular ion in high concentration
31	Paralysis of half (one side) of the body
33	Inflammation of the brain
35	"Sensory" nerve fibers
36	An agent that relieves pain

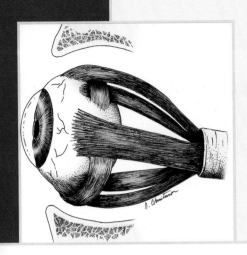

CHAPTER 10

The Eye

GOALS AND OBJECTIVES

By the conclusion of this chapter, the student will be able to:

1. Recognize common root words, prefixes, and suffixes related to ophthalmology.
2. Divide simple and compound words into their respective parts.
3. Recognize, correctly pronounce, and appropriately use common medical terms related to ophthalmology.
4. Demonstrate an understanding of ocular anatomy.
5. Demonstrate an understanding of ocular physiology with regard to aqueous production, flow, and drainage.
6. Demonstrate an understanding of the visual pathway.

Note: Chapter 9 should be completed before this chapter.

INTRODUCTION TO RELATED TERMS

Divide each of the following terms into its respective parts ("R," root; "P," prefix; "S," suffix; "CV," combining vowel).

1. **Ophthalmology** (n.) (R) _____ (CV) _____ (S) _____
   ophthalmology (of"thal-mol'o-je; study of the eye)

2. **Ophthalmologist** (n.) (R) _____ (CV) _____ (R) _____
   (S) _____
   ophthalmologist (of"thal-mol'o-jist; one who specializes in eye study; i.e., a doctor of ophthalmology)

3. **Intraocular** (adj.) (P) _____ (R) _____ (S) _____
   intraocular (in"trah-ok'u-lar; pertaining to inside the eye)

4. **Periocular** (adj.)   (P) _____ (R) _____ (S) _____
periocular (per"e-ok'u-lar; pertaining to around the eye, cf. adnexa)

5. **Extraocular** (adj.)   (P) _____ (R) _____ (S) _____
extraocular (eks"trah-ok'u-lar; pertaining to outside the eye)

6. **Optic** (adj.)   (R) _____ (S) _____
optic (op'tik; pertaining to sight/vision)

7. **Palpebral** (adj.)   (R) _____ (S) _____
palpebral (pal'pĕ-bral, pal-pe'bral; pertaining to the palpebra [L. "eyelid"])

8. **Conjunctival** (adj.)   (R) _____ (S) _____
conjunctival (kon"junk-ti'val; pertaining to the conjunctiva)

9. **Subconjunctival** (adj.)   (P) _____ (R) _____ (S) _____
subconjunctival (sub"kon-junk-ti'val; pertaining to under the conjunctiva)

10. **Corneal** (adj.)   (R) _____ (S) _____
corneal (kor'ne-al; pertaining to the cornea)

11. **Iridocorneal** (adj.)   (R) _____ (CV) _____ (R) _____
     (S) _____
iridocorneal (ir"ĭ-do-kor'ne-al; pertaining to the iris and the cornea)

12. **Scleral** (adj.)   (R) _____ (S) _____
scleral (sklĕ'ral; pertaining to the sclera [Gr. "hard"])

13. **Nasolacrimal** (adj.)   (R) _____ (CV) _____ (R) _____
     (S) _____
nasolacrimal (na"zo-lak'rĭ-mal; pertaining to the nose and lacrima [L. "tears"])

14. **Miosis** (n.)   (R) _____ (CV) _____ (S) _____
miosis (mi-o'sis; a condition of smallness; clinically refers to pupillary constriction)

15. **Mydriatic** (adj.)   (R) _____ (S) _____
mydriatic (mid"re-at'ik; pertaining to mydriasis [mid"ri'ah-sis (n.); Gr.]; clinically refers
to pupillary dilation)

16. **Heterochromia** (n.)   (R) _____ (CV) _____ (R) _____
     (S) _____
heterochromia (het"er-o-kro'me-ah; a condition of other color; in ophthalmology it refers
to the irises of an animal, each of a different color)

17. **Anisocoria** (n.)   (P) _____ (CV) _____ (R) _____
     (S) _____
anisocoria (an"ĭ-so-ko're-ah, an-e"so-ko're-ah; a condition of unequal pupils)

18. **Dyscoria** (n.)   (P) _____ (R) _____ (S) _____
dyscoria (dis-kor'e-ah; a condition of a bad pupil; typically a deformed pupil)

19. **Photophobia** (n.)   (R) _____ (CV) _____ (R) _____
     (S) _____
photophobia (fo"to-fo'be-ah; a condition of light "fear"; clinically refers to abnormal visual
intolerance of light)

20. **Uveitis** (n.)   (R) _____ (S) _____
    uveitis (u″ve-i′tis; inflammation of the uvea)

21. **Keratitis** (n.)   (R) _____ (S) _____
    keratitis (ker″ah-ti′tis; inflammation of the cornea)

22. **Keratoconjunctivitis** (n.)   (R) _____ (CV) _____ (R) _____
                                    (S) _____
    keratoconjunctivitis (ker″ah-to-kon-junk″tĭ-vi′tis; inflammation of the cornea and the
    conjunctiva)

23. **Blepharospasm** (n.)   (R) _____ (CV) _____ (S) _____
    blepharospasm (blef′ah-ro-spazm″; spasm of an eyelid; clinically refers to tonic [rigid]
    muscular spasm of the eyelids, generally in a closed position)

24. **Distichiasis** (n.)   (R) _____ (CV) _____ (S) _____
    distichiasis (dis″tĭ-ki′ah-sis; a state of a double line [Gr. *distichia,* double line]; clinically
    refers to a double row of eyelashes)

25. **Ectropion** (n.)   (P) _____ (R) _____ (CV) _____
                                    (S) _____
    ectropion (ek-tro′pe-on; an outward turning [Gr.]; clinically refers to eversion, outward
    rolling of an eyelid)

26. **Entropion** (n.)   (P) _____ (R) _____ (CV) _____
                                    (S) _____
    entropion (en-tro′pe-on; an inward turning; clinically refers to inversion, inward rolling
    of an eyelid)

27. **Retinopathy** (n.)   (R) _____ (CV) _____ (S) _____
    retinopathy (ret″ĭ-nop′ah-the; a disease of the retina)

28. **Buphthalmos** (n.)   (R) _____ (R) _____
    buphthalmos (buf-thal′mos; an ox eye; clinically refers to abnormal enlargement of the eye)

29. **Enophthalmos** (n.)   (P) _____ (R) _____
    enophthalmos (en-of-thal′mos; an in eye; clinically refers to an eye that is sunken into the orbit)

30. **Exopthalmos** (n.)   (P) _____ (R) _____
    exophthalmos (ek″sof-thal′mos; an out eye; clinically refers to an eye that protrudes from
    the orbit)

31. **Microphthalmia** (n.)   (P) _____ (R) _____ (S) _____
    microphthalmia (mi″krof-thal′me-ah; a condition of small eyes)

32. **Ophthalmoscopy** (n.)   (R) _____ (CV) _____ (S) _____
    ophthalmoscopy (of-thal-mos′ko-pe; to view the eye; i.e., the interior of the eye)

33. **Tonometry** (n.)   (R) _____ (S) _____
    tonometry (to-nom′ĕ-tre; measurement of pressure [intraocular pressure])

34. **Electroretinogram** (n.)   (R) _____ (CV) _____ (R) _____
                                    (CV) _____ (S) _____
    electroretinogram (e-lek″tro-ret′ĭ-no-gram; a recording of electricity of the retina; abbr. ERG)

OCULAR ANATOMY AND PHYSIOLOGY

Periocular Anatomy

There are many *periocular* structures, most of which serve to protect the eye itself. The orbit of most domestic animals and humans is a bony structure that surrounds the globe. The orbit of the dog and cat is incomplete along its dorso-lateral border (Fig. 10-1). This makes *proptosis*[1] of the globe much easier in the dog and the cat, particularly in *exophthalmic* breeds like Pugs and Persian cats. In other animals, the orbit would have to be fractured to facilitate proptosis. Within the orbit is much adipose and loose connective tissue to provide support and cushioning for the globe. (In dehydration those *retrobulbar*[2] tissues will shrink, giving the temporary appearance of *enophthalmos*. In some breeds, like Collies, *microphthalmia* gives the dogs an enophthalmic appearance.)

The palpebrae provide protection for the exposed surfaces of the anterior globe (Fig. 10-2). The exposed outer surface of the palpebrae of domestic animals is covered with fine hairs. Primarily, at the edges of each dorsal lid is a row of eyelashes. The remaining surfaces of the palpebrae are lined with a delicate epithelial mucous membrane called the conjunctiva. The palpebral conjunctiva is continuous with the ocular (bulbar) conjunctiva, forming a "sac" associated with each palpebra. (Bulbar conjunctiva covers the exposed portion of the sclera up to the limbus.[3] See Figure 10-9. It is the bulbar conjunctiva that is sometimes used for *subconjunctival* injections of medication. Slow absorption from the area provides a prolonged effect.) The dorsal conjunctival sac is associated with the upper eyelid and the ventral conjunctival sac is associated with the lower eyelid. The palpebral muscles permit opening and closing of the eyelids. Most domestic animals also have a "third eyelid," called the *nictitating membrane*.[4] It is most easily visualized near the medial *canthus*[5] of the eye. With gentle pressure applied to the dorsolateral palpebra and globe, the nictitating membrane elevates and covers the globe. The gland nictitans associated with this structure contributes to tear film production.

Lacrimation and the Nasolacrimal Apparatus

The lacrimal gland (Fig. 10-3), which produces most of the tear film, is associated with the dorsal palpebra near the lateral canthus. Near the medial canthus on each palpebra is a *punctum*, which is the opening to the *nasolacrimal* duct. The nasolacrimal duct is designed to drain excess tears into the nose. That is why when a person cries, his or her nose tends to run.

---

[1]Proptosis (prop-to'sis); from [Gr. *proptosis,* a fall forward]; clinically refers to displacement of the eye from the orbit.
[2]Retrobulbar (ret"ro-bul'bar) [L. *retro,* backward, behind+L. bulbur bulb, "eye"] i.e., behind the eye.
[3]Limbus (lim'bus) [L. a border]; it is the border between the sclera and the cornea.
[4]Nictitating membrane (nik"tĭ-ta'ting); from [L. *nictitare,* to wink].
[5]Canthus (kan'thus); from [Gr. *kanthos,* angle]; clinically a canthus is the angle formed by the eyelids; each eye has a medial and a lateral canthus.

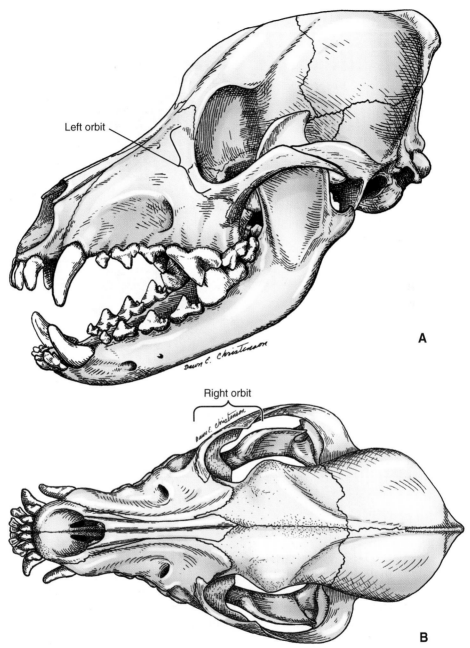

FIGURE 10-1   Canine orbit. **A,** Lateral view. **B,** Dorsal view.

Tears consist of two distinct components. The watery portion of the tears provides a constant bathing or flushing action; the oily portion of the tear film provides a longer-lasting protective coating for the eye. Collectively, tears lubricate, moisturize, and protect the delicate tissues of the cornea and conjunctiva. Blinking provides a repetitive sweeping action that continually spreads the tear film over the eye.

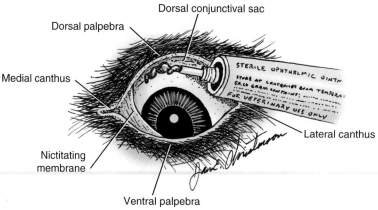

FIGURE 10-2   Palpebrae and associated structures.

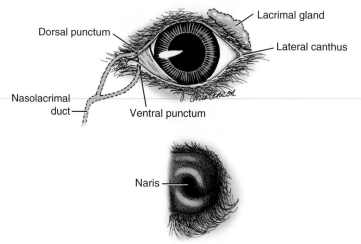

FIGURE 10-3   Nasolacrimal apparatus.

Tears, particularly the watery component, are produced predominantly by the lacrimal gland. Other periocular glands secrete more of the viscous component. The tears flow down over the eye and eventually drain out through the nasolacrimal duct. Once in the nasal passages, the tears flow with the rest of the nasal secretions, eventually to be swallowed. *Epiphora*[6] may develop with excessive production of the tears or as a result of obstruction of the puncta or of the nasolacrimal duct. Chronic (kron'ik; long-term) epiphora is easily detected in white and light-colored animals, because the tears tend to stain the periocular fur brown.

---

[6]Epiphora (e-pif'o-rah); from [Gr. *epiphora*, sudden burst]; means an overflow of tears onto the face.

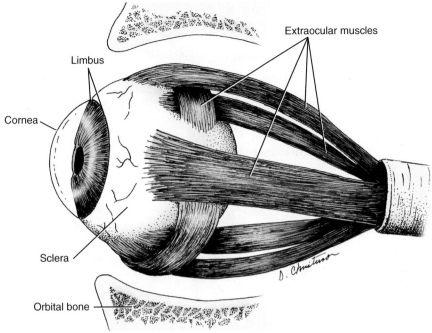

FIGURE 10-4   Extraocular muscles.

Ocular Anatomy

The globe of the eye is supported and moved by *extraocular* muscles (Fig. 10-4). They are attached to the toughest portion of the eye, the sclera. The sclera is often referred to as the "white of the eye." It is made of thick, tough, fibrous connective tissue. It actually forms and lends shape to the bulk of the globe, providing support for extraocular as well as *intraocular* structures.

The most anterior structure of the globe is the cornea (Fig. 10-5). The cornea is a dome-shaped, transparent, avascular structure, formed of layers of tissue (Fig. 10-6). The outermost layer is made of a type of stratified squamous epithelium. The thickest layer is called the stroma, which is made of a type of connective tissue. Beneath the stroma, Descemet's membrane[7] supports the innermost corneal layer of simple squamous endothelium. The cornea may be transparent and avascular, however, don't be deceived. Abundantly hidden away in the corneal matrix are numerous nociceptors, with very low thresholds for painful stimuli. (Nociceptors were discussed in Chapter 9.) Structurally, this transparent dome provides the "frontal wall" of the *anterior chamber*. Within this domed chamber is a watery, intraocular fluid called aqueous humor. (Both the cornea and the aqueous humor will refract [bend] light entering the eye.) The caudal wall of the anterior chamber is the iris. The "corner" formed by these two "walls" is the *iridocorneal angle*. (Okay, admittedly, the "corner" formed here is

[7]Descemet's membrane (des-ĕ-māz'); named after the French anatomist Jean Descemet.

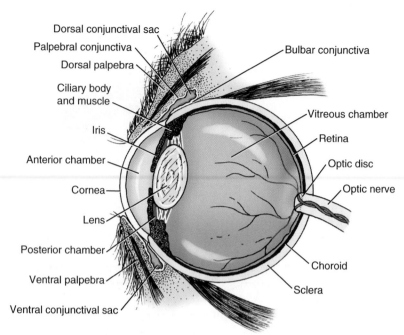

FIGURE 10-5   Sagittal section of the eye.

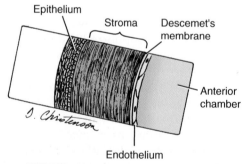

FIGURE 10-6   Corneal tissue layers.

not exactly like the perpendicular corners formed by most walls. It's actually more like taking a mixing bowl and setting it upside down on the countertop. The angle formed by the inner brim of the bowl and the counter is like that of the iridocorneal angle. We'll talk more about this later.)

The iris is an intraocular muscle that is shaped like a donut. When looking at an animal's eyes, the iris is the colored part. The color varies from animal to animal, depending on species and breed. Generally, both eyes will have the same color iris. Occasionally, *heterochromia* may be observed and is actually desired in certain breeds. The hole in the middle of the iris is the pupil (Fig. 10-7). The smooth muscle fibers of the iris are oriented in a radiating, as well as in a circular manner; each being innervated by opposite branches of the autonomic nervous system.

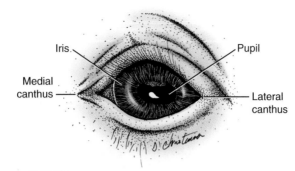

FIGURE 10-7   Anterior view of the equine eye.

This orientation permits the iris to function like the aperture of a camera or the diaphragm of a microscope. When the circular muscle fibers contract in response to parasympathetic stimulation, *miosis* results. Conversely, when the radiating muscle fibers contract in response to sympathetic stimulation, *mydriasis* results.

Directly behind the pupil and iris is the lens. The lens is a transparent, biconvex structure, like that of a magnifying glass. However, rather than rigid glass the ocular lens is formed by semifirm layers of material, much like an onion. All of this marginally flexible material is contained within the lens capsule (like an onion shrink-wrapped in plastic). The tough lens capsule is attached to the muscles of accommodation, the ciliary (sil′e-er″e) muscles, by tough strands of connective tissue fibers (zonular[8] fibers). As the ciliary muscles contract and relax, they change the shape of the lens. This changes the way light passing through the lens is focused within the eye. Closely associated with the ciliary muscles is the ciliary body. The ciliary body is responsible for aqueous humor production (to be discussed in a later section). The small space formed by iris, lens, and the ciliary tissues is called the posterior chamber (see Fig. 10-5). It is a very small space immediately behind the iris that cannot be seen with routine examination of the eye.

The largest, most posterior intraocular cavity, behind all of the previously mentioned structures, is filled with vitreous[9] (vit′re-us). The vitreous is a transparent, gelatinous substance that is also called the vitreous humor or the vitreous body. The vitreous helps maintain the shape of the globe. The walls of this vitreous-filled cavity are lined by a series of tissue layers. The innermost of these layers is the retina. There is actually a fine matrix of transparent fibers within the vitreous that attach to the retina. With age-related shrinkage of the vitreous, some of these fibers may detach from the retina. In people, this event may create "shadows" in the visual field referred to as "floaters." Vitreous detachment generally does not seriously affect vision. Infrequently, if the vitreous shifts with movement and one of its firmly attached fibers pulls on the retina, rather than detaching from it, retinal detachment or a retinal tear may occur.

---

[8]Zonular (zon′u-lar); derived from [L. dim. *zona*, "a girdle"].
[9]Vitreous (vit′re-us); derived from [L. *vitreus*, "glassy"].

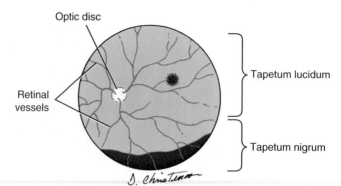

FIGURE 10-8   Normal canine fundus.

The retina is a thin, transparent structure composed of specialized neural tissue. The specialized sensory receptor cells (rods and cones) of the retina are embedded in the pigmented tissue layer of the choroid. The function of the retina is pure and simple: collect visual, sensory input to be sent to the brain. Detachment of the retina from the underlying choroid will result in visual loss in the detached area. The importance of this connection between the pigmented tissue layer and the rods and the cones is discussed further in the section on the visual pathway. All of the sensory neurons of the retina converge at the optic disc.

The brightly colored pigmented epithelial tissue of the choroid found in the eyes of domestic animals is unique. The choroidal epithelium actually contains two distinctly different pigments. The black pigment is called the tapetum nigrum,[10] and the unique, brightly colored, iridescent pigment is called the tapetum lucidum.[11] The tapetum lucidum is found predominantly in the dorsal and central region of the fundus[12] near the optic disc (Fig. 10-8), whereas the tapetum nigrum covers the remaining area up to the ciliary process. The tapetum lucidum is found in abundance in predatory animals, such as dogs and cats. It is designed to "amplify" or enhance incoming light in low-light situations. Think about the effects of snow cover on a winter night, compared with grass cover on a summer night. In the same location, with the same dim lighting of the street light, it is far easier to see with winter snow cover. The reflection of the snow enhances the same minimal light source. Like the snow, the tapetum lucidum's reflective characteristics plus an abundance of rods in the retina give animals night vision that is far superior to humans. The more tapetum lucidum an animal has (like cats), the better their night vision. That is why cats make such superb night predators. Have you ever driven down a dark, winding, country road at night, only to see a pair of bright green, glowing eyes from the side of the road looking back at you? That was no demon. It was probably a cat or a raccoon.

---

[10]Tapetum nigrum (tah-pe'tum ni'grum); derived from [L. "black carpet"].
[11]Tapetum lucidum (tah-pe'tum lu'sid-um) [L. lucidus "luminous carpet"].
[12]Fundus (fun'dus); in ophthalmology the fundus refers to the interior surface of the eye behind the lens. Structures usually associated with the fundus are the optic disc, intraocular blood vessels, the macula, and the retina.

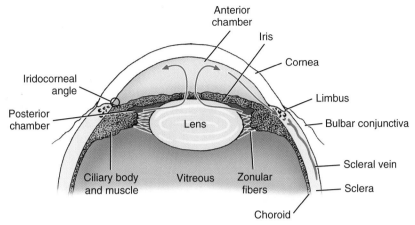

FIGURE 10-9   Schematic of aqueous flow.

The tapetum lucidum vividly reflected the headlights of your oncoming car, giving a bright green glowing appearance to the eyes. (Human eyes reflect only red ["red eye" as seen in photos], because we have no pigmented epithelium like that of the tapetum lucidum, only the vascular tissue of the choroid and light-absorbing pigments.) The whole choroid is sandwiched between the retina and the sclera. The choroid is the largest part of the uvea (the vascular "tunic" or vascular layer of the eye). The choroid provides vascular, nutritive support to the retina, as well as vascular supply to the rest of the uvea. The other two parts of the uvea include the ciliary tissues (body and muscle) and the iris.

Aqueous Production, Flow, and Drainage

The production, flow, and drainage of aqueous humor can be likened to the workings of a kitchen sink. Water flows out of the faucet into the sink and flows out through the drain of the sink. Instead of having a drain in the center of the sink, let's increase the efficiency of drainage and decrease the chance of completely plugging the drain by placing a series of drain holes all the way around the bottom margin of the sink. So, how does this actually work in the eye? Our faucet (the ciliary body) produces the intraocular fluid called aqueous. As it is produced, it flows into the tiny posterior chamber. This would be like having our faucet directed into a bottle or small bowl in the sink. Eventually, it will be full and overflow. The overflow will follow the path of least resistance. Within the eye, this path of aqueous will flow from the posterior chamber through the pupil into the anterior chamber (the sink in our analogy). Once the anterior chamber is full, the aqueous eventually drains through small portals found around the entire circumference of the iridocorneal angle (Fig. 10-9). From there it is picked up by scleral blood vessels and eventually joins the rest of the venous return. The goal here is to have a constant turnover of fresh fluid, while keeping the sink just full. Aqueous humor is constantly being produced and drained within the eye and plays an important role in providing nutrients to avascular structures like the cornea. Aqueous humor also helps maintain the domed shape of the cornea, by having just the right volume of fluid exerting enough pressure to hold the cornea up. That is the biggest difference between the eye and the kitchen sink. While the water of our kitchen sink could evaporate or overflow onto the floor, the aqueous humor of the eye is contained within a closed system. This creates a pressurized situation within the eye (intraocular pressure). So, with changes in production or drainage of aqueous humor, the pressure within the eye can change. Even a simple thing like occluding the jugular veins can increase intraocular pressure. Just the right amount of intraocular pressure keeps the anterior chamber (covered by the cornea) "inflated" (like those big holiday lawn ornaments). If excessive, especially with chronic increases, intraocular pressure can damage critical parts of the eye. This will be discussed later with glaucoma (glaw-ko′mah).

Visual Pathway

Light entering the eye first passes through the cornea and anterior chamber (Fig. 10-10). Both the cornea and the aqueous humor refract or bend the light, concentrating it at the pupil. The pupil will control the volume of light permitted through the lens. As the light passes through the pupil and the lens, the lens, by virtue of the ciliary muscles, focuses the light on the fundus. Because the lens is biconvex, the actual image focused on the fundus is upside down. (Look at a distant object at arm's length through a magnifying glass to observe this effect.) The light passes through the transparent retina and strikes the pigmented tissue layer (Fig. 10-11). At the interface of the retinal sensory neurons (rods and cones) and the choroid epithelium, a photochemical reaction takes place. That photochemical reaction stimulates the rods and cones, initiating the cascade of neural impulses. The stimulated rods and cones synapse on retinal sensory nerve fibers that transmit the impulses toward the optic disc (i.e., the initial portion of the optic nerve; Fig. 10-12). Once at the optic disc, the neural impulses will be carried by the optic nerves, with most crossing contralaterally at the optic chiasm, and following the optic tracts into the brain. Ultimately, the sensory input will arrive at the visual cortex of the cerebrum for perception of the visual image. In the visual cortex, the image is "righted" and perceived in the correct position.

It should be noted that any light focused directly on the optic disc will not generate sensory impulses. The optic disc is a blind spot. Remember, a photochemical reaction is necessary to initiate the sensory impulse from the rods and cones. There are no rods or cones over the optic disc, nor is there any pigmented epithelium to facilitate the photochemical reaction. The optic disc is merely a portal or connection for the optic nerve.

Binocular versus monocular vision makes all the difference in the world for depth of field and being able to judge distances. The placement of the eyes in the head will determine whether an animal has a predominance of binocular or monocular vision, as well as how large the actual visual field is. If you think about predators, they need very good depth perception in order to accurately attack their prey. Binocular vision provides such visual precision. Cats, dogs,

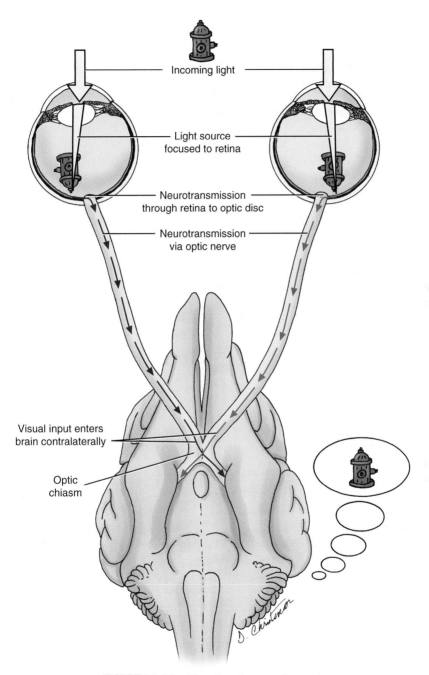

FIGURE 10-10 Visual pathway schematic.

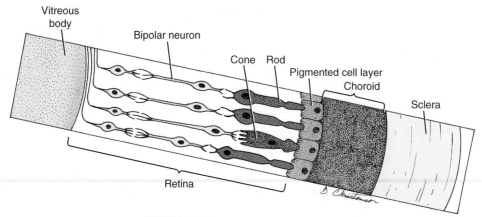

FIGURE 10-11   Retinal cross section.

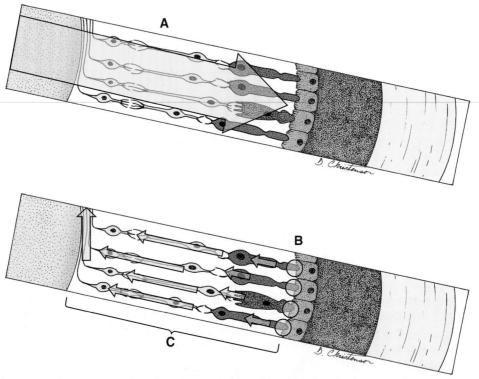

FIGURE 10-12   Sequential retinal activity. **A,** Light passes through retina and strikes pigmented cell layer. **B,** Photochemical reaction stimulated at sensory cell–pigmented epithelium interface. **C,** Neurotransmission to optic disc.

and owls provide us with wonderful examples of animals that have a large binocular area to their visual field. The close frontal placement of the eyes permits the triangulation of vision on a focal object. This allows for better interpretation visually of the distance between prey and predator to optimize the attack. On the flip side, monocular peripheral vision is limited in these animals. Now think of our prey animals (like sheep, cattle, horses, rabbits, and many birds). Their eye placement is more lateral. This does not provide for a very large binocular portion of the visual field (if at all). However, the monocular visual fields provide for tremendous peripheral vision. With a large range of peripheral vision, the prey animal may be able to see the predator coming, before it is too late. The visual field of animals must be considered for veterinary professionals to appropriately and safely handle them. The horse, for instance, has somewhat lateral eye placement and a very long muzzle. For someone to be squatting directly in front of the horse could be very dangerous for the person. The horse may not even be able to see the individual because of the natural blind spot in its visual field. That is why horses are typically handled from the side near the shoulder. The horse can see the handler in that location.

It has been stated by many that animals see only in black and white. If this were true, then animals would not be equipped with both types of sensory receptor cells in the retina. Rods transmit black and white images, whereas cones transmit images of color. Rods require less light to be stimulated than do cones. Although the retinas of most domestic animals contain more rods than cones, they do contain both. Therefore, in appropriately lighted situations, animals can perceive some color. The distribution of numbers of rods versus cones varies tremendously among the different species of the animal world. Many species of birds have particularly abundant cones in their retinas. It only stands to reason that this should be so. Why else would so many birds have such brilliantly colored plumage? If they were unable to perceive it visually, it would not be very helpful for identifying potential mates or enemies.

Pathophysiology and Disease

Visual impairment can develop many different ways. Of course, human optometry has made tremendous strides in compensating for visual impairment of conditions like nearsightedness, farsightedness, and the like. Animals can experience similar visual problems. However, unlike their human counterparts, most domestic animals do not have the need for corrective lenses. Most of the time, they have no need for visual acuity. It is only in special circumstances, like canine agility or equestrian events, that we may notice a problem. In such a circumstance, the dog or the horse may miss a gate, turn, or jump because it lacks precise vision. Most of the time, we don't notice optic problems until there is loss of vision.

Blindness (loss of vision) can be created many ways. Think about the visual pathway alone. There are so many ways and locations either to block light from reaching the sensory receptors or to block the sensory neurotransmission itself. Let's look at this (no pun intended) in a systematic way. Let's begin by interfering with light entering the eye. The first structure that could block light is the cornea. Remember the cornea is a transparent, avascular dome. If it is injured or becomes inflamed for any reason, its transparency will be lost. *Keratitis* responds like any other inflamed tissue, with pain and edema. The ocular pain will stimulate parasympathetic fibers to the iris, causing *miosis*. (If unilateral, this may be viewed and noted as *anisocoria*.) The miosis alone will limit the amount of light entering the eye. With corneal edema, edematous fluid in the stroma makes the tissue opaque (bluish-gray). Additionally, in an attempt to heal the area, *neovascularization* will infiltrate the cornea. All of these factors will impede light entering the eye and thereby impair vision. Once the keratitis resolves, transparency should be restored (provided there is no significant scarring). *Entropion* and *distichiasis* are two common palpebral disorders that may lead to keratitis and corneal ulceration. Both of these conditions chronically abrade and irritate the cornea. Both can be surgically corrected. *Ectropion* may contribute to *keratopathies* as well. In ectropion, foreign material is easily caught in the ventral conjunctival sac and may lead to corneal damage. As with the other palpebral problems, ectropion can be surgically corrected. Of course, even with normal anatomy, if insufficient lubrication is available, even the palpebral conjunctiva may cause similar abrasive corneal damage. That is the case with *keratoconjunctivitis sicca*[13] (KCS). With this syndrome the lacrimal glands no longer produce sufficient quantities of the watery portion of the tear film. Compensation will be attempted, by producing more of the oily, more viscous portion of the tear film. All this tends to do is produce a buildup of thick, stringy ocular discharge. Without sufficient lubrication, keratitis will appear as described earlier, along with appearing dull due to the dryness. Plus, because of the chronic nature of the irritation, the epithelium of the cornea will become hyperpigmented. The bulbar conjunctiva will appear hyperemic and dull. KCS may not be curable, but it is manageable with application of ophthalmic lubricants and/or medications to stimulate better lacrimation. If controlled, corneal integrity can be preserved.

The lens is the next most common structure to interfere with light entering the eye. *Cataract* formation is nothing more than development of lens opacity. If one looks at an animal with mature cataracts, the animal's pupils will appear whitish. This is quite contrary to the typical "black hole" impression that the pupil usually offers. Often, cataracts develop over such a long period of time that the animal adjusts to the gradual loss of vision. These animals begin to rely more on olfaction and hearing to help them navigate through the home. Many dogs with cataracts compensate so well for the gradual visual loss that the owners never notice. A common complaint with such a dog may be acute (sudden) blindness. The only reason the dog appeared to go suddenly blind is because the owners suddenly changed the furniture around. Consequently, the dog began bumping into the furniture. As in human ophthalmology, cataract surgery is a reality in veterinary medicine today. Most often the dense core of the lens is the portion that becomes opaque. That portion can be removed. Whether or not an artificial lens is replaced into the remaining lens capsule is irrelevant. The animal will become visual again, simply from removing the opaque lens material. Of course, before cataract surgery is performed, retinal integrity should be assessed. Intraocular ultrasound will permit the ophthalmologist to detect intraocular defects, such as retinal detachment. *Electroretinograms* (ERGs) will evaluate the retinal function

---

[13]Sicca (sik'ah); from [L. *siccus,* dry].

and the visual pathway. If these diagnostics indicate that the animal will be blind regardless of the cataracts, there is no point in removing the cataracts.

How might the retina be damaged? Some breeds of dogs are prone to progressive retinal atrophy (PRA). With this inherited *retinopathy,* the retina progressively deteriorates. Night vision for these animals will be the first to go. As the disease progresses, the tapetum will become hyperreflective. Owners may notice the brightly reflecting eyes and become frustrated by the dog's reluctance to venture out after dark. *Ophthalmoscopy* will typically reveal shrinking retinal vessels that eventually disappear. The optic disc becomes small and pale. Ultimately, dogs with PRA will go blind, often at a young age. Even so, these dogs can lead very happy, long lives. With dogs' keen senses of olfaction and hearing, they can compensate extremely well for the complete visual loss.

Retinopathies can also be secondary to other disorders, such as *uveitis.* Equine recurrent uveitis (commonly called moon blindness) is a syndrome that will cause progressive visual loss. Uveitis is a painful event. These horses typically demonstrate that pain with classic symptoms of *epiphora, photophobia, miosis,* and *blepharospasm.* The actual inflammatory intraocular event goes far beyond pain, however. Inflammation of the choroid may cause retinal detachment and intraocular hemorrhage. If the inflammation begins to involve the retina itself, it may develop direct permanent damage. The proteins and cellular infiltrates seeping from the inflamed anterior uveal tissues may cause a hazy appearance to the aqueous humor (aqueous flare). The proteins themselves may cause the iris to adhere to the lens, referred to as *synechia* (sin-ĕk′e-ah). How does this happen? Remember the discussion of plasma proteins, like fibrinogen, in Chapter 4? Fibrinogen is a principal protein associated with inflammation. It can do only one thing, and that is convert to fibrin. In this situation, the miosis plus the proteins provide the perfect environment for synechia to develop. (This may lead to *dyscoria.*) The iris itself may even bleed into the anterior chamber. This is referred to as *hyphema* (hi-fe′mah). Obviously, aggressive antiinflammatory therapy will be needed for a horse with uveitis. Analgesics may be administered as well. Plus, *mydriatics* will be administered. The mydriatics will actually serve two purposes. First, by using an anticholinergic agent, iris and ciliary muscles will be paralyzed so that the muscular spasm will not be contributing to the intraocular pain. (Think of how painful a muscle cramp is in your lower leg. Stopping the spasm relieves much of the pain.) Second, mydriasis will minimize synechia development by reducing physical contact between the iris and the lens. Each acute episode of uveitis can be treated. However, the damage done, particularly to the retina, will ultimately result in visual loss. Repeated episodes of uveitis may also lead to glaucoma.

Glaucoma can be a primary or a secondary disease syndrome. What is it? Glaucoma is an ophthalmic disease in which intraocular damage results from prolonged increased intraocular pressure. Not all intraocular pressure increases will result in damage. Every time a jugular vein is occluded, intraocular pressure increases. As soon as the vein is released, pressures return to normal. No damage is done. In glaucoma, intraocular pressure is chronically increased. "How?" you ask. Let's think about our normal physiology for a moment. Earlier, we said that aqueous humor was constantly produced and drained, with just the right amount always present to keep the anterior chamber "inflated." Considering the faucet and drain analogy, there are really only two ways for excesses of aqueous to create increased pressure. Either aqueous humor is produced in too great a volume or the iridocorneal angle drainage is impaired. The latter is more common. Regardless of the actual cause, glaucoma will ultimately damage the retina and optic disc, resulting in permanent visual loss. Patients with glaucoma may be medically managed. Monitoring of pressures with *tonometry* will be very important, to ensure that medical therapy is working as intended. Medical therapy may include agents to reduce production of aqueous humor, improve outflow of aqueous through the iridocorneal angle, or a combination thereof. In cases of severe acute glaucoma, pressures may become so great that they actually stretch the globe, resulting in *buphthalmos*. A *buphthalmic* eye likely has irreparable visual damage. Better to be blind without the diseased eye than to be blind with the chronic discomfort of the diseased eye. Therefore, enucleation[14] is often performed in such cases.

Veterinary ophthalmology has an arsenal of diagnostics and therapeutics to manage a wide range of ocular diseases. Our goal is preservation of vision for our patients, if at all possible. In order to accomplish that goal, early detection of problems along with cooperation and compliance of owners are critical to a successful outcome.

---

[14]Enucleation (e-nu"kle-a'shun): removal of the eye.

SELF-TEST

Using the previous information in this chapter, complete the following crossword puzzle using the most appropriate medical term(s). Do not use abbreviations or common names unless requested.

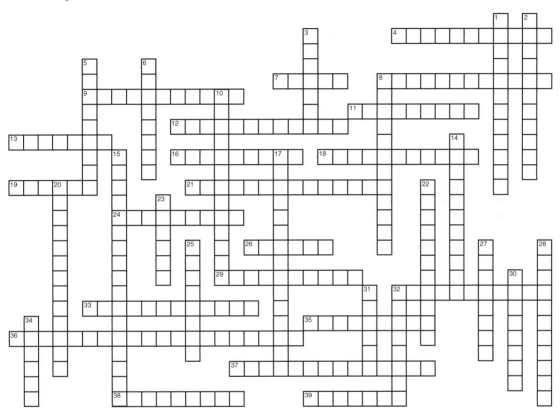

ACROSS

4   A disease of the cornea
7   Pertaining to vision
8   An eye that bulges from the orbit, as in brachycephalic breeds
9   A disease of the retina
11 Complete displacement of the eye from the orbit
12 A double row of lashes
13 Inflammation of the vascular layer of the eye, including the choroid, ciliary tissues, and iris
16 Inward rolling of an eyelid
18 Excessive, abnormal eye enlargement
19 The anatomic border between the cornea and the sclera
21 A condition of small eyes
24 Measurement of intraocular pressure
26 The tough, white fibrous connective tissue of the globe

29   A condition of unequal pupils
32   Muscles outside the globe that move the eye in various directions
33   The drainage angle formed by the iris and cornea
35   Outward rolling of an eyelid
36   Inflammation of the cornea and conjunctiva
37   Use of an instrument to view the fundus and other intraocular structures
38   Pupillary dilation
39   Bleeding into the anterior chamber

DOWN
1   The duct that naturally drains tears from the puncta to the nose
2   Aversion to light
3   An angle or corner formed by the eyelids
5   Inflammation of the cornea
6   Adherence of the iris to the lens
8   Sunken eyes, as in dehydration
10   A condition of differently colored irises
14   The delicate mucous membrane lining of the eyelids and globe
15   A recording of neural impulses of the retina
17   A doctor who specializes in the eye
20   Muscular spasm of an eyelid
22   The third eyelid or _____ membrane
23   The transparent, dome-shaped anterior structure of the eye
25   A lens opacity
27   A bad (deformed) pupil
28   Pertaining to within the eye
30   An ocular disease caused by prolonged increased intraocular pressure
31   Pupillary constriction
32   Overflow of tears onto the face
34   The intraocular neural tissue layer containing rods and cones

CHAPTER 11

The Ear

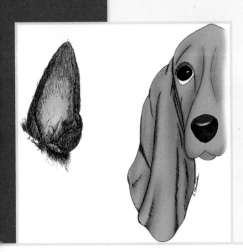

GOALS AND OBJECTIVES

By the conclusion of this chapter, the student will be able to:

1. Recognize common root words, prefixes, and suffixes related to the ear.
2. Divide simple and compound words into their respective parts.
3. Recognize, correctly pronounce, and appropriately use common medical terms related to the ear.
4. Demonstrate an understanding of otic anatomy.
5. Demonstrate an understanding of otic physiology with regard to the auditory pathway and equilibrium.
6. Demonstrate an understanding of common otic pathophysiology and disease.

Note: Chapters 9 and 10 should be completed before this chapter.

INTRODUCTION TO RELATED TERMS

Divide each of the following terms into its respective parts ("R," root; "P," prefix; "S," suffix; "CV," combining vowel).

1. **Otic** (adj.) (R) _____ (S) _____
   otic (o'tik; pertaining to the ear; cf. aural)

2. **Acoustic** (adj.) (R) _____ (S) _____
   acoustic (ah-koos'tik; pertaining to sound)

3. **Audiology** (n.) (R) _____ (CV) _____ (S) _____
   audiology (aw"de-ol'o-je; the study of hearing)

4. **Vestibular** (adj.) (R) _____ (S) _____
   vestibular (ves-tib'u-lar; pertaining to a vestibule [L. "chamber"])

5. **Semicircular** (adj.)   (P) _____ (R) _____ (S) _____
   semicircular (sem"ĭ-ser'ku-lar; pertaining to a partial circle)

6. **Cochlear** (adj.)   (R) _____ (S) _____
   cochlear (kok'le-ar; pertaining to the cochlea [L. "snail shell"])

7. **Vestibulocochlear** (adj.)   (R) _____ (CV) _____ (R) _____ (S) _____
   vestibulocochlear (ves-tib"u-lo-kok'le-ar; pertaining to the vestibule and cochlea)

8. **Tympanic** (adj.)   (R) _____ (S) _____
   tympanic (tim-pan'ik; pertaining to the tympanum [Gr. "drum"])

9. **Aural** (adj.)   (R) _____ (S) _____
   aural (aw'ral; pertaining to the ear; cf. otic)

10. **Otoscope** (n.)   (R) _____ (CV) _____ (S) _____
    otoscope (o'to-skōp; to examine the ear; clinically refers to an instrument used to examine the external ear)

11. **Ototoxic** (adj.)   (R) _____ (CV) _____ (R) _____ (S) _____
    ototoxic (o"to-tok'sik; pertaining to ear poison; clinically refers to any agent that may be toxic to components of the inner ear or auditory nerve)

12. **Ceruminal** (adj.)   (R) _____ (S) _____
    ceruminal (sĕ-roo'mĭ-nal; pertaining to cerumen [L. cera, wax]; i.e., earwax)

13. **Retrograde** (adj., adv., v.)   (R) _____ (CV) _____ (S) _____
    retrograde (ret'ro-grād; going backward)

14. **Otolith** (n.)   (R) _____ (CV) _____ (R) _____
    otolith (o'to-lith; an ear stone)

15. **Dynamic** (adj.)   (R) _____ (S) _____
    dynamic (di-nam'ik) from [Gr. dynamis, power]; pertaining to power or motion)

16. **Otitis** (n.)   (R) _____ (S) _____
    otitis (o-ti'tis; inflammation of the ear; clinically otitis is subdivided into otitis externa [inflammation of the external ear], otitis media [inflammation of the middle ear], and otitis interna [inflammation of the inner ear])

17. **Otalgia** (n.)   (R) _____ (R) _____ (S) _____
    otalgia (o-tal'je-ah; a condition of ear pain)

18. **Otorrhea** (n.)   (R) _____ (CV) _____ (S) _____
    otorrhea (o"to-re'ah; a discharge of the ear)

19. **Otopyorrhea** (n.)   (R) _____ (CV) _____ (R) _____
                                   (CV) _____ (S) _____
    otopyorrhea (o"to-pi"o-re'ah; a discharge of ear pus)

20. **Otoplasty** (n.)   (R) _____ (CV) _____ (S) _____
    otoplasty (o'to-plas"te; to reform/reshape the ear; i.e., surgery to reshape the ear)

21. **Otodectes** (n.) (R) _____ (CV) _____ (R) _____

otodectes (o"to-dek'tez; an ear biter; [Gr. *dēktēs*, a biter] *Otodectes* is the genus name of the ear mite of dogs and cats)

22. **Otoacariasis** (n.) (R) _____ (CV) _____ (R) _____
(CV) _____ (S) _____

otoacariasis (o"to-ak"ah-ri'ah-sis; a condition of ear mites; actually any infestation of the ears with mites [Gr. *akari*, a mite]; a parasitic otitis)

OTIC ANATOMY AND PHYSIOLOGY

Otic Anatomy

The *external ear* (Figs. 11-1 and 11-2) is composed of the pinna (ear flap), external acoustic meatus,[1] and tympanic membrane (eardrum). Ear pinnae come in a variety of shapes and sizes, depending on the species and breed of animal (see Fig. 11-1). Those animals with large, erect pinnae have very sharp hearing. The external acoustic meatus in most domestic animals is relatively long, with a slight L shape. The shape of the ear canal helps prevent perforation of the tympanic membrane by foreign objects. However, the L shape also tends to contribute to accumulations of cerumen and other secretions near the tympanic membrane.

The *middle ear* is housed by the tympanic bulla[2] (Fig. 11-3). Contained within the tympanic bullae are the otic ossicles[3]: the malleus,[4] the incus,[5] and the stapes[6] (see Fig. 11-2; Fig. 11-4). These are the smallest bones found in the body. The malleus is attached to the inner surface of the tympanic membrane. So, when the tympanic membrane moves, the malleus moves with it. All of the otic ossicles are interconnected, like other bones, by ligaments (tiny ligaments, but ligaments nonetheless). Does that mean that if the malleus moves, the incus and stapes will move as well? That's right! However, they don't have full freedom of movement at all times. When subjected to abrupt, high decibel sounds, tiny muscles within the middle ear will (via a reflex arc) contract to minimize the movement of the ossicles. (Those muscles are strategically attached to the malleus and the stapes.) This tympanic reflex helps prevent damage to the auditory portion of the inner ear. (Damage to that portion of the inner ear would result in hearing loss.) The tympanic bullae are connected to the pharynx (throat) by the eustachian tubes.[7] Each eustachian tube equalizes pressure and drains the

---

[1]Meatus (me-a'tus); from [L. *meatus*, a way, a path, a course]; meaning an opening or passage; the external acoustic meatus is also referred to as the "ear canal."
[2]Bulla (bul'ah); bullae—pl.; from [L. *bulla*, a large vesicle]; the tympanic bullae are osseous chambers found at the base of the skull; they house the middle ear.
[3]Ossicle (os'sĭ-kl); from [L. *ossiculum*, a small bone].
[4]Malleus (mal'e-us); from [L. *malleus*, hammer].
[5]Incus (ing'kus); from [L. *incus*, anvil].
[6]Stapes (sta'pēz); from [L. *stapes*, stirrup].
[7]Eustachian (u-sta'ke-an); the eustachian tubes are named after an Italian anatomist, Bartolommeo Eustachio.

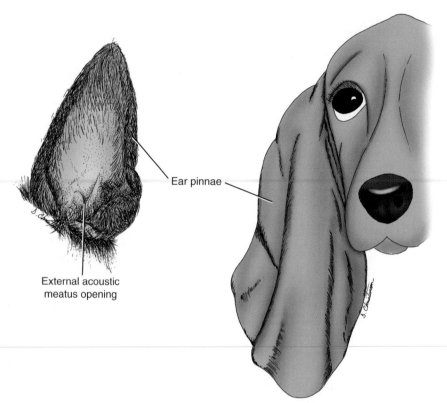

Ear pinnae

External acoustic
meatus opening

FIGURE 11-1 Pinnae.

middle ear. The drainage is important to keep the middle ear free of fluid accumulations. Fluid will develop in the middle ear only in the presence of disease, such as a retrograde bacterial otitis media. (This will be discussed later.) Under normal circumstances, only air should be found in the middle ear/tympanic bullae. Have you ever driven to a high altitude or flown in an aircraft? During the ascent and descent you probably found it difficult to hear. Some folks even find such events painful. The reason for the difficulty hearing was due to the difference in atmospheric pressure compared with that within your middle ear. That difference in pressure is exerted on the tympanic membrane, stretching it out. When stretched, the tympanic membrane cannot move as freely; therefore, hearing is temporarily diminished. By yawning, swallowing, or chewing gum, you probably found that the hearing issue was resolved. Why? Those actions physically help open the eustachian tubes, allowing for equalization of the air pressure within the middle ear. This is the principal purpose of the eustachian tubes. Without them, we could not prevent damage (even rupture) of the tympanic membrane. Horses have very unique eustachian tubes. Two out-pouchings are found along each eustachian tube, called guttural pouches (Fig. 11-5). What the true purpose of each guttural pouch is may continue to be a mystery. Do they help with vocal resonance? Do they cool blood going to the brain during exercise? Horses aren't divulging their secret. Regardless of what nature

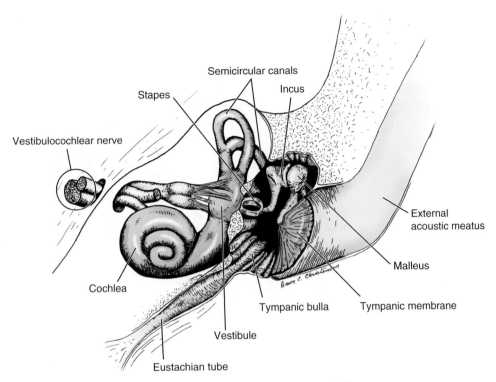

FIGURE 11-2 Schematic cross section of the ear.

intended for guttural pouches, they can serve as a focus of disease. Regarding guttural pouch disease, you might think, "Big deal!" However, when you consider the numerous critical structures that guttural pouches are near, like the carotid arteries; the cervical sympathetic trunk; and the vagus, accessory, glossopharyngeal, and hypoglossal nerves, guttural pouch disease may be worthy of our attention. That is why it will be discussed later. For now, let's continue to focus on the ear.

The inner ear (see Fig. 11-2; Fig. 11-6) is composed of the cochlea and the vestibular apparatus (i.e., the vestibule and semicircular canals). The components of the inner ear are actually encased in the temporal bone of the skull. (Liken it to pouring concrete around an object. That's the way the bone of the skull envelopes the parts of the inner ear.) If that's the case, how do we access those parts? Well, from the middle ear, a small, membrane-covered opening exists called the oval window. (The stapes is held in place at this window. We'll talk about its purpose there later.) On the other side of the temporal bone, a small opening provides passage of the vestibulocochlear nerve from the brain in the cranial vault. What is the nerve connected to? Why the cochlea and vestibule, of course. Let's take a closer look at these structures, starting with the cochlea. The cochlea is so named because it resembles a snail shell. Spiraled within the hard outer shell of the cochlea are fluid-filled tubular ducts. The ducts are divided into three distinct compartments: upper (scala vestibuli), middle

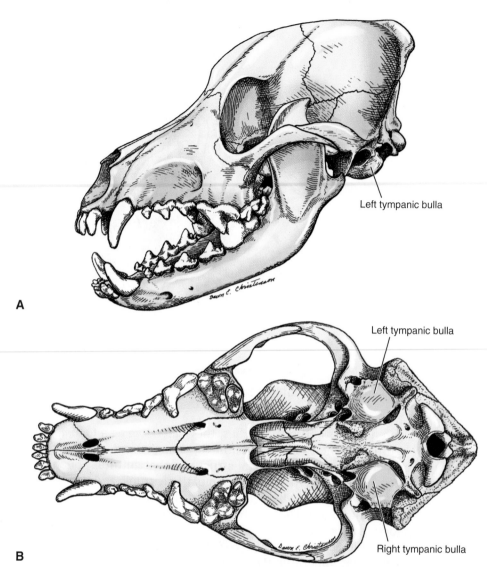

FIGURE 11-3   Tympanic bullae. **A,** Lateral view. **B,** Ventral view.

(cochlear duct), and lower (scala tympani). All of these compartments are separated by flexible membranes. Remember the oval window mentioned earlier? Well, that flexible window communicates with the scala vestibuli. Move the flexible oval window and fluid waves are created in the scala vestibuli. Those fluid movements will be transmitted progressively through the flexible membranous walls separating the three compartments. Those fluid movements will stimulate auditory receptors in the cochlear duct. Eventually, fluid movements progress to the scala tympani, at the base of which is another membranous window, the round window. The membrane of this window also separates the tympanic bulla

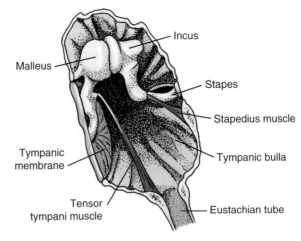

FIGURE 11-4   Middle ear.

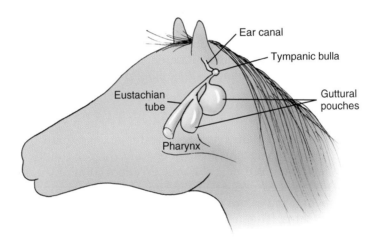

FIGURE 11-5   Equine guttural pouches.

from the inner ear. Ultimately, any fluid waves initiated at the oval window will be dissipated at the round window. We'll talk more about this later, when we discuss the auditory pathway.

The vestibule is also fluid filled and contains two smaller chambers within it. The chambers within the vestibule are important for static[8] equilibrium. The semicircular canals are rigid tubes that connect to and openly communicate with the vestibule. They are also fluid filled. Each semicircular canal (there are three with each inner ear) is oriented so that it is associated with a major body plane. This orientation will focus sensory stimulation of dynamic equilibrium,

---

[8]Static (stat'ik); from [L. *staticus*]; meaning at rest or not in motion.

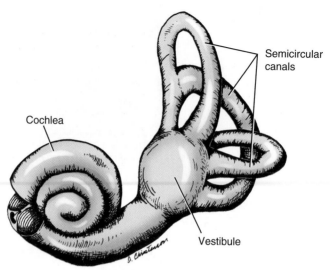

FIGURE 11-6 Inner ear.

according to the directional movements of the head. No, these brief descriptions regarding equilibrium are insufficient for understanding. This is merely a preview of the balance and equilibrium discussion yet to come.

Audiology

The auditory pathway is a delicate, intricate path by which sound waves are converted to mechanical energy and then to fluid waves, ultimately resulting in stimulation of neural impulses. Disruption of the pathway anywhere in the sequence of events results in some form of hearing loss.

Sound waves are collected by the pinna and directed to the external acoustic meatus. The sound waves, on reaching the tympanic membrane, cause it to vibrate. Because the malleus is attached to the tympanic membrane, it and the other otic ossicles begin to move. Earlier we said that the stapes was attached at the oval window. When the stapes moves, the oval window moves, creating a fluid wave within the scala vestibuli. That wave will progress into the cochlear duct. Within the cochlear duct, the wave will cause movement of auditory receptor cells against a tectorial[9] membrane. It is intense movement of these receptors against the roof of the tectorial membrane that ultimately results in stimulation of a neural impulse. That neural impulse is rushed to the brain, via the cochlear branch of the vestibulocochlear nerve, for interpretation of the sound. The fluid wave that progresses into the scala tympani will be dissipated (like a shock absorber) at the round window. Interestingly, the frequency or pitch of the original sound wave corresponds to the size of the fluid waves created in the cochlea. The waves of low-frequency sounds could be likened to

[9]Tectorial (tek-tor′e-al); [L. *tectum,* roof].

the ring of large waves created by throwing a large rock into a pond, whereas a little pebble, like high-frequency sounds, creates tiny, close-set waves in the pond. Each different pitch moves specific sensory receptor cells. Now, think about listening to an orchestra playing a musical arrangement. Think about all of the various sound waves from all of the various instruments impacting your tympanic membrane. Think about the chain of events that must take place from there for you to actually perceive and hear each and every note and tone. Amazing isn't it? Take care of that great hearing apparatus, because any sensory receptor cells destroyed by trauma or disease are not replaced. Attrition of these cells will create hearing loss, per the frequency of receptors lost.

Equilibrium

There are two types of equilibrium associated with the inner ear: static equilibrium and dynamic equilibrium, as mentioned earlier. Each uses a different portion of the vestibular apparatus, and both send their sensory input to the brain. Although the vestibular apparatus is vital to balance and equilibrium, it is not an exclusive component. A tremendous amount of sensory input is required from the inner ear, vision, and proprioception. With all of the collective input, the brain will respond with motor output, coordinated by the cerebellum, to effectively maintain balance and an upright posture. Proprioceptive input was discussed in Chapter 9 and visual input in Chapter 10. Let's focus on the components of the inner ear and then put the whole sensory package together, shall we?

Static equilibrium relies on the two chambers within the vestibule of the inner ear (Fig. 11-7). Each fluid-filled chamber is lined with specialized sensory receptor cells. On top of the sensory cells is a layer of gelatinous material, and stuck to the surface of the gelatinous material are tiny otoliths. The function of this portion of the vestibular apparatus is based entirely on gravity: however the head is positioned, gravity causes the otoliths to slide along the gelatinous material to the lowest point within the chamber. Wherever the otoliths fall to rest, the pressure exerted by their weight stimulates the associated sensory receptors. This initiates a neural impulse that is sent to the brain for interpretation of head and body position. Gravitational forces (g-forces) exerted by acceleration and deceleration will also stimulate receptors within the vestibular chambers. Imagine sitting in an automobile at a stoplight. While sitting there waiting for the light to turn green, otoliths are resting at the bottom of your vestibular chambers. The sensory stimulation from the vestibule, in part, indicates to your brain that you are in an upright posture and motionless. As the light turns green and you step on the accelerator, your posture hasn't changed. Yet, your brain perceives, from vestibular input, that you are moving forward. How? The forces of acceleration have suddenly shoved, if you will, the otoliths across the bottom toward more caudal portions of the vestibular chambers. The perception? Forward movement. Once you reach highway speed and maintain it, g-forces are no longer causing the change in otolith movement and position. The otoliths slide back down to the bottom of the chambers. Without visual input at this point, you'd have no concept of movement. This is particularly true when

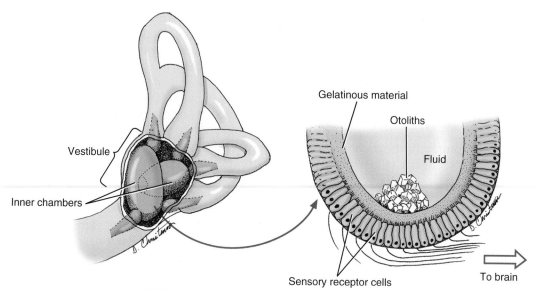

FIGURE 11-7   Vestibule and associated structures.

flying in commercial airliners. Once the cruising altitude is reached, passengers have no clue that they are actually moving at hundreds of miles per hour. Until the vehicle in which we are traveling begins to slow, our brains will perceive from the vestibule that we are simply sitting quietly, statically still.

Dynamic equilibrium uses the semicircular canals of the inner ear (Fig. 11-8). It is dynamic, meaning it is based on actual movements of the head (e.g., turning to the right or left, looking up or down). In the ampulla of each semicircular canal is a specialized sensory receptor cell. Each canal is fluid-filled and openly communicates with the greater vestibule. Whenever the head is turned, the semicircular canal associated with the plane of movement moves around the fluid contained within it. What? Did I just say that the canals moved AROUND the fluid? Yes, I did. To demonstrate this (e.g., a solid object moving around its liquid contents), fill a bowl with water and place a few ice cubes in the center of the water. Make sure that everything is sitting perfectly still before proceeding. Then, spin the bowl on the table top. Notice that initially the bowl moves but the ice cubes remain stationary; they have remained stationary because the bowl, not the water, has moved. Now, if the semicircular canals move around the fluid within them, what effect does this have on the sensory receptor cells attached to the walls of the ampullae? The receptor cells are dragged through the fluid. Because the fluid creates resistance against the receptor cells, they are forced to bend. Going back to the fluid-filled bowl experiment, try sticking flexible objects of tape or plastic to the inner wall of the bowl. When the bowl is still, the strips of plastic simply stick straight into the water, pointing to the center of the bowl. Ah, but when the bowl is spun, those plastic strips bend as they are dragged through the water. Notice that the plastic strips point counterclockwise when the bowl is spun clockwise and visa versa. The same effect occurs when an arm and hand are moving through the water while swimming. The

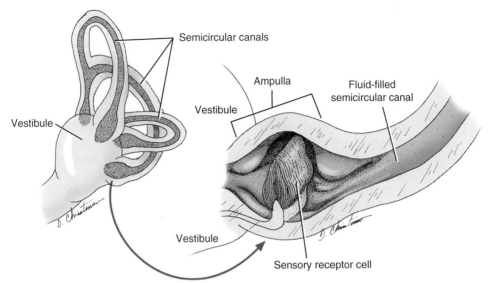

Semicircular canals

Ampulla

Fluid-filled
semicircular canal

Vestibule

Vestibule

Vestibule

Sensory receptor cell

FIGURE 11-8   Semicircular canals.

hand bends pointing in a direction opposite the direction of movement of the arm through the water. The same is true for the sensory receptor cells. As they are bent, they are stimulated and initiate neurotransmission to the brain, via the vestibular branch of the vestibulocochlear nerve. That neural input from each receptor is different, depending on the direction of its bend. Remember, there are two inner ears, one on each side of the head. Because they are on opposite sides, the effect of the rotational head movement will be opposite the other side. This reciprocal activity within each inner ear will be valuable as the brain tries to interpret direction of movement. The brain ultimately interprets the direction of movement and stimulates appropriate motor responses elsewhere in the body to maintain balance.

As stated earlier, neither static nor dynamic equilibrium alone or collectively are enough to maintain balance and equilibrium. Sensory input from vision and proprioception must also be used for the brain to accurately determine body position, direction of movement, and how to make appropriate corrections for maintenance of balance. All of that sensory input must be congruent. If incongruities are present, overreaction to the input will result. Let's think about some of those childhood games we used to play. Remember taking someone and making him or her spin in one spot with her/his eyes closed? What happened when the person stopped spinning? Ataxia, right? Why did the ataxia develop? Let's see, proprioceptive input indicated standing still. Vestibular input indicated standing still. Even visual input indicated standing still. Alas, the semicircular canals indicated spinning. Why? When we initiated the spin, the receptors in the ampullae were bent by dragging them through the fluid, initiating the dynamic input of the spin. However, with continued spinning, inertia eventually caused the fluid to move. When the individual stopped spinning, the fluid kept moving. This secondary fluid movement bent the receptors, indicating (incorrectly) that the person was still spinning. Based on that incorrect input, the brain (particularly the cerebellum) responded with exaggerated corrective movements (ataxia). If you were to look at the person's eyes immediately after stopping the spin, you'd observe nystagmus.[10] That temporary horizontal "bouncing" of the eyes is simply an exaggerated oculomotor response to the inaccurate input.

How does motion sickness fit into the scheme of things? Motion sickness is nothing more than a profound overreaction to incongruent sensory input. Many people and animals suffer from motion sickness. These individuals are highly sensitive to incongruities in sensory input associated with equilibrium. Here's a common scenario. Place the individual in the back seat of the car, unable to see out of the window. What does her brain perceive? Visually, "I'm sitting still in the back seat." Proprioceptors indicate a seated, upright, motionless posture. Ah, but the inner ear indicates otherwise. Acceleration, deceleration, and g-forces exerted by going over hills stimulate receptors in the chambers of the vestibule, indicating movement. Turning the vehicle moves those semicircular canals around their fluid contents. Again, sensory input indicates movement. To the brain, this makes no sense. Unfortunately, the end result is central stimulation of the CTZ (chemoreceptor trigger zone). When the CTZ is stimulated, nausea develops. Fortunately, for our motion sickness–prone friends, centrally acting drugs can depress this reaction. Of course, they often depress the rest of the CNS too, inducing a somnolent (sleepy) state. From the perspective of the motion sickness–prone individual, sleep is far, far better than nausea. (Of course, veterinary patients don't operate heavy machinery or motor vehicles. So, becoming sleepy doesn't really matter.)

Otic Pathophysiology and Disease

Deafness and partial hearing losses can be caused by many different disruptions of the auditory pathway. When trying to determine the cause of hearing loss, a systematic approach that evaluates external, middle, and internal ear components is required. An otoscopic examination may reveal a very quick answer. Excessive ceruminal accumulations in the external acoustic meatus impair sound waves from reaching the tympanic membrane. Block the sound waves and hearing loss results. *Otoacariasis* is a frequent contributor to such a scenario, especially in kittens. *Otodectes cynotis* living and breeding in the kitten's ear canals are irritating. The irritation causes *otorrhea*. Plus, all of the little mites add to accumulations of material in the ear canal with their excrement. With severe cases, the entire canal can become plugged. Imagine being able to hear only the chewing and scampering movements of those tiny creatures in your ears. Feeling this activity must be incredibly annoying. That's why animals infested with *Otodectes* dig furiously at their ears and shake their heads violently. Often the head shaking will flap the pinnae around so hard that vessels within the pinnae

---

[10]Nystagmus (nis-tag′mus) from [Gr. *nystazein*, to nod]; an ocular involuntary, rapid, rhythmic movement of the globe that may be horizontal, rotary, or vertical. Vertical nystagmus generally indicates central disease (i.e., CNS) rather than peripheral disease.

break, resulting in an *aural hematoma*.[11] *Otodectes* can be eradicated. Once the little creatures are gone and all cerumen and debris are cleaned from the canals, the kitten's hearing will be restored.

Of course, otitis externa doesn't simply result from parasites. Bacterial otitis is very common resulting in *otopyorrhea*. Exposure to moisture (e.g., swimming) and big, heavy pinnae (like Spaniels and Basset Hounds) will promote bacterial growth. However, many cases of recurrent otitis externa involve underlying health issues, like allergies. During the actual otitis event, inflammation and the pus accumulations can significantly diminish hearing. With chronic,[12] recurrent otitis externa the walls of the ear canal will actually begin to *hypertrophy*.[13] Even when there is no active bacterial otitis, the hypertrophic canal will impair hearing. In severe cases of hypertrophy, the ear canals may be completely obstructed. These patients must endure chronic *otalgia*. Hypertrophy makes medical management of the ears nearly impossible. *Otoplasty* may be required to not only restore some hearing but to make management of the diseased ears possible, for the welfare of the patient. The surgery may involve merely removing the lateral wall of the vertical canal or the entire vertical canal. Chronic, recurrent otitis externa often leads to otitis media. Think of how fluid and pus accumulations in the tympanic bulla would impair movement of the eardrum and the tiny ossicles. It may even lead to arthritic changes to the ossicles, again impairing their movement. It is very difficult to treat disease within the tympanic bulla. If it cannot be treated effectively, for the sake of the patient, the otoplasty may also involve removal of the entire ear canal and creation of an opening into the bulla (total ear canal ablation[14] and bulla osteotomy[15]). Unfortunately, this will remove the tympanic membrane and ossicles, rendering the affected ear completely deaf. This is an extreme circumstance that may have been prevented by managing an underlying allergic condition.

Earlier when we discussed otic anatomy, we mentioned that the eustachian tubes could provide a mechanism for retrograde otitis media. Certainly, with an upper respiratory disease and associated pharyngitis, micro-organisms could traverse the eustachian tubes to inflame and infect the middle ear. In horses, the scenario, more often than not, will affect the guttural pouches first, resulting in guttural pouch *empyema*.[16] It may progress no further. Whether we look at inflammation and infection of the guttural pouches of the horse or the otitis media of a dog, either way surrounding structures can be significantly affected. The cervical branch of the sympathetic trunk passes very near both of these structures. Disease of the middle ear or the guttural pouches could adversely affect the sympathetic trunk, perhaps even permanently. How would you know that this happened? By looking at the eyes of the animal, you'd readily see effects of

---

[11]Hematoma (he-mah-to'mah); from [*hemat(o)-*, blood + -*oma,* swelling]; a hematoma is an accumulation of blood under the skin.
[12]Chronic (kron'ik); from [Gr. *chronos,* time]; means to persist over a long period of time.
[13]Hypertrophy (hi-per'tro-fe); overgrowth or above normal/excessive development.
[14]Ablation (ab-la'shun); from [L. *ablatio,* detachment, removal].
[15]Osteotomy (os"te-ot'ŏ-me); to cut bone; i.e., surgical cutting of a bone.
[16]Empyema (em"pi-e'mah); [Gr. *empyema*] an abscess; containing pus.

unilateral damage to the sympathetic trunk. Grossly, you'd observe anisocoria. On closer observation, the pupil of the affected side is miotic and highly sensitive to light. Isn't it amazing how parts of the body that seem so distinctly separate physically and functionally can affect other parts?

Affecting other parts of the body is very apparent when considering the inner ear. Yes, otitis interna locally can certainly result in hearing loss. Believe it or not, some of the drugs used to treat otitis externa can actually be *ototoxic* and create some level of hearing loss (by damaging the receptor cells in the cochlea). Let's not forget, however, that the inner ear also includes the vestibular apparatus. Peripheral vestibular disease is quite common and most definitely affects more than just the inner ear. What causes vestibular disease? Ototoxicity and viral organisms are possible *etiologies*.[17] Why, even meningoencephalitis could progress easily to the inner ear, as could otitis media. Many times vestibular disease is *idiopathic*.[18] What happens in the disease? Let's think back to our discussion of motion sickness. Like motion sickness, a portion of the sensory input is indicating to the brain a stationary individual, while the vestibular apparatus (due to inflammation this time) is indicating otherwise. The brain's perception of these disparities leads to marked physical overcompensation and nausea (yes, due to stimulation of the CTZ). Imagine feeling like the room is spinning out of control, the floor is moving, and you have the need to vomit. Your cerebellar overcompensation would make it incredibly difficult to navigate to an appropriate place to vomit, let alone the act of vomiting itself. It is not a pleasant experience, as any person who has had vertigo would tell you. On physically examining a vestibular disease patient, you will typically find a very ataxic, nauseated individual, perhaps with a head tilt. If he/she can walk, the animal may walk in circles. Finally, when you look at the eyes of the animal, nystagmus will be present. The nystagmus is the brain's way of ocular compensation for the "spinning" room. No, it's not really spinning, but the brain perceives that it is. Any normal individual, when turning his head, will "spot" on objects visually as they pass by. That's what the brain thinks it is doing with this vestibular disturbance. None of this is pleasant for the affected individual. Fortunately, most people and animals with peripheral vestibular disease do recover. Often in a few weeks, they are back to normal. Until full recovery, medication can be given to control some of the symptoms.

As you can see, the ear does far more than simply provide hearing. Certainly, otic pathology can result in much more than simply hearing loss. That is why veterinary professionals must be thorough in their history taking and physical examinations. Who knows, the answer for a significant neurologic problem could lie in a simple *otoscopic* examination. We owe it to our patients to leave no stone unturned.

---

[17]Etiology (e″te-ol′ŏ-je); [Gr. *aitia,* cause + *-logy*] the causes or origin of a disease or disorder; cf. pathogenesis.

[18]Idiopathic (id″e-o-path′ik); disease of unknown origin.

SELF-TEST

Using the previous information in this chapter, complete the following crossword puzzle using the most appropriate medical term(s). Do not use abbreviations or common names unless requested.

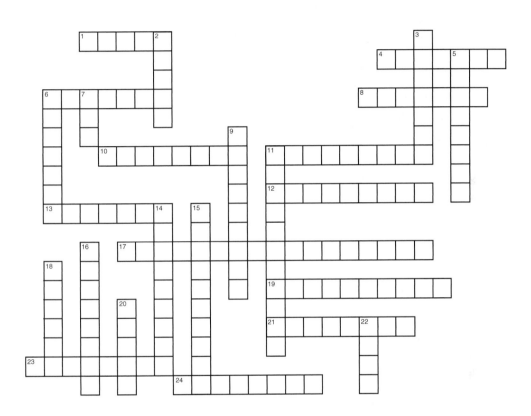

ACROSS

1	An ear flap
4	Ear pain
6	The portion of the inner ear associated with hearing
8	An ear stone
10	An instrument used to examine the external ear
11	Genus name of the canine and feline ear mite
12	Surgical restructuring of the ear
13	Ear wax
17	Cranial nerve VIII
19	To move backward
21	The cause of a disease
23	Tiny bones
24	Pertaining to sound

DOWN

2	Pertaining to the ear
3	The bone of the middle ear attached to the eardrum
5	The pouches along a horse's eustachian tubes
6	Persisting for a long time
7	Abbreviation for the vomiting center in the brain
9	That portion of the inner ear whose chambers provide for static equilibrium
11	Discharge of ear pus
14	The "bouncing" of the eyes that often accompanies vestibular disease
15	Pertaining to a disease of unknown origin
16	Pertaining to a drum
18	Inflammation of the ear
20	The tympanic _____ houses the middle ear
22	The window that the stapes impacts for sound wave transmission

CHAPTER 12

The Alimentary System

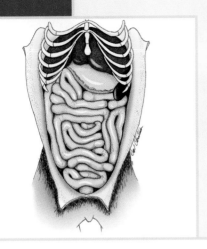

GOALS AND OBJECTIVES

By the conclusion of this chapter, the student will be able to:

1. Recognize common root words, prefixes, and suffixes related to the alimentary system.
2. Divide simple and compound words into their respective parts.
3. Recognize, correctly pronounce, and appropriately use common medical terms related to the alimentary system.
4. Demonstrate an understanding of alimentary anatomy of simple monogastric animals, hindgut fermentors, and ruminants.
5. Demonstrate an understanding of comparative dentition and dental formulas.
6. Demonstrate an understanding of digestive physiology with regard to simple monogastric animals, hindgut fermentors, and ruminants.
7. Demonstrate an understanding of basic nutrients and nutrition.
8. Demonstrate an understanding of common pathophysiology and disease conditions of domestic animal digestive tracts.

Note: It is strongly advised that all previous chapters be completed before this chapter. Familiarity, particularly with hematologic, respiratory, cardiovascular, and neurologic terminology and information, is recommended.

INTRODUCTION TO RELATED TERMS

Divide each of the following terms into its respective parts ("R," root; "P," prefix; "S," suffix; "CV," combining vowel).

1. **Glossal** (adj.)   (R) _____ (S) _____
   glossal (glos'al; pertaining to the tongue; cf. lingual)

2. **Lingual** (adj.)   (R) _____ (S) _____
   lingual (ling'gwal; pertaining to the tongue, cf. glossal)

3. **Buccal** (adj.)   (R) _____ (S) _____
   buccal (buk′al; pertaining to the cheek)

4. **Labial** (adj.)   (R) _____ (S) _____
   labial (la′be-al; pertaining to the lip)

5. **Palatal** (adj.)   (R) _____ (S) _____
   palatal (pal′ă-tal; pertaining to the palate)

6. **Periodontal** (adj.)   (P) _____ (CV) _____ (R) _____ (S) _____
   periodontal (per″e-o-don′tal; pertaining to around the teeth)

7. **Gingival** (adj.)   (R) _____ (S) _____
   gingival (jin′jĭ-val, jin-ji′val; pertaining to the gingiva ["gums"])

8. **Oropharynx** (n.)   (R) _____ (CV) _____ (R) _____
   oropharynx (o″ro-far′inks; the mouth and the throat)

9. **Esophageal** (adj.)   (R) _____ (CV) _____ (S) _____
   esophageal (e-sof″ah-je′al, e-so-fa′je-al; pertaining to the esophagus)

10. **Gastric** (adj.)   (R) _____ (S) _____
    gastric (gas′trik; pertaining to the stomach)

11. **Pyloric** (adj.)   (R) _____ (S) _____
    pyloric (pi-lor′ik; pertaining to the pylorus; from [Gr. *pyle,* gate])

12. **Enteric** (adj.)   (R) _____ (S) _____
    enteric (en-ter′ik; pertaining to the intestines)

13. **Duodenal** (adj.)   (R) _____ (S) _____
    duodenal (du″o-de′nal, du″od′en-al; pertaining to the duodenum)

14. **Jejunal** (adj.)   (R) _____ (S) _____
    jejunal (jĕ-joo′nal, je-joo′nal; pertaining to the jejunum)

15. **Ileocecal** (adj.)   (R) _____ (CV) _____ (R) _____ (S) _____
    ileocecal (il″e-o-se′kal; pertaining to the ileum and the cecum)

16. **Hepatic** (adj.)   (R) _____ (S) _____
    hepatic (hĕ-pat′ik; pertaining to the liver)

17. **Biliary** (adj.)   (R) _____ (S) _____
    biliary (bil′e-a-re; pertaining to bile)

18. **Pancreatic** (adj.)   (R) _____ (S) _____
    pancreatic (pan″kre-at′ik; pertaining to the pancreas)

19. **Peritoneal** (adj.)   (R) _____ (S) _____
    peritoneal (per″ĭ-to-ne′al; pertaining to the peritoneum)

20. **Peristalsis** (n.)   (P) _____ (R) _____
    peristalsis (per″ĭ-stal′sis; around contraction; from [Gr. *stalsis,* contraction])

21. **Haustration** (n.)   (R) _____ (S) _____
    haustration (hos-tra'shun; pertaining to a haustra; from [L. *hustor,* drawer]; haustrations are small pouches or sacculations found in the colon and rectum)

22. **Deglutition** (n.)   (R) _____ (S) _____
    deglutition (deg"loo-tish'un; the act of swallowing)

23. **Defecation** (n.)   (R) _____ (S) _____
    defecation (def"ĕ-ka'shun; the act of defecating [evacuation of the bowels; a bowel movement])

24. **Postprandial** (adj.)   (P) _____ (R) _____ (S) _____
    postprandial (post-pran'de-al; pertaining to after a meal)

25. **Mucus** (n.)   (R) _____ (S) _____
    mucus (mu'kus; the presence of slime)

26. **Mucous** (adj.)   (R) _____ (S) _____
    mucous (mu'kus; pertaining to mucus)

27. **Mucosal** (adj.)   (R) _____ (CV) _____ (S) _____
    mucosal (mu-ko'sal; pertaining to mucus)

28. **Mucoid** (adj.)   (R) _____ (S) _____
    mucoid (mu'koid; resembling mucus)

29. **Submucosal** (adj.)   (P) _____ (R) _____ (CV) _____ (S) _____
    submucosal (sub"mu-ko'sal; pertaining to beneath mucus)

30. **Lacteal** (adj. or n.)   (R)_____ (CV) _____ (S) _____
    lacteal (lak'te-al; [L. *lacteus,* milky] pertaining to milky)

31. **Lipase** (n.)   (R) _____ (S) _____
    lipase (li'pās; an enzyme of fat)

32. **Amylase** (n.)   (R) _____ (S) _____
    amylase (am-ah-lās; [Gr. *amylon*, starch] an enzyme of starch)

33. **Coprophagia** (n.)   (R) _____ (CV) _____ (R) _____(S) _____
    coprophagia (kop"ro-fa'jah; the process of feces/dung eating)

34. **Hematochezia** (n.)   (R) _____ (CV) _____ (R) _____ (S) _____
    hematochezia (hĕm"ă-to-ke'ze-ah; a condition of bloody feces [Gr. *chezein,* to defecate])

35. **Melenic** (adj.)   (R) _____ (S) _____
    melenic (mĕ-le'nik; [Gr. *melas,* black] pertaining to black; clinically refers to the passage of black feces)

36. **Steatorrheic** (adj.)   (R) _____ (CV) _____ (R) _____ (S) _____
    steatorrheic (ste"at-o-re'ik; pertaining to fatty flow; clinically refers to passage of loose, fatty feces; [Gr. *steatos,* fat; *rhoia,* flow])

37. **Lipemia** (n.)   (R) _____ (R) _____ (S) _____
    lipemia (li-pe'me-ah; a condition of fatty blood; [Gr. *lipos,* fat])

38. **Hypersialosis** (n.)   (P) _____ (R) _____ (CV) _____ (S) _____
    hypersialosis (hi"per-si"ah-lo'sis; a condition of excessive saliva)

39. **Gastroenteritis** (n.)   (R) _____ (CV) _____ (R) _____ (S) _____
    gastroenteritis (gas"tro-en-ter-i'tis; inflammation of the stomach and intestines)

40. **Colitis** (n.)   (R) _____ (S) _____
    colitis (ko-li'tis; inflammation of the colon)

41. **Peritonitis** (n.)   (R) _____ (S) _____
    peritonitis (per"ĭ-to-ni'tis; inflammation of the peritoneum)

42. **Icteric** (adj.)   (R) _____ (S) _____
    icteric (ik'ter-ik; pertaining to icterus [Gr. *ikteros,* jaundice])

43. **Bilirubinemia** (n.)   (R) _____ (R) _____ (S) _____
    bilirubinemia (bil"ĭ-roo"bĭ-ne'me-ah; a condition of bilirubin in the blood [bilirubin
    is a yellow-pigmented by-product of hemoglobin breakdown])

44. **Dysphagia** (n.)   (P) _____ (R) _____ (S) _____
    dysphagia (dis-fa'je-ah; a state of difficult eating)

45. **Stomatitis** (n.)   (R) _____ (S) _____
    stomatitis (sto-mah-ti'tis; inflammation of the mouth [Gr. *stoma,* mouth])

46. **Anorexia** (n.)   (P) _____ (R) _____ (S) _____
    anorexia (an"o-rek'se-ah; a state without appetite)

47. **Intussusception** (n.)   (P) _____ (R) _____ (S) _____
    intussusception (in"tus-sus-sep'shun; the act of receiving within; from [L. *intus,* within
    + *suscipere,* to receive]; clinically refers to telescoping of part of the intestine into an
    adjoining part)

48. **Necrotic** (adj.)   (R) _____ (CV) _____ (S) _____
    necrotic (ne-krot'ik; pertaining to necrosis; from [Gr. *nekros,* dead])

49. **Chylothorax** (n.)   (R) _____ (CV) _____ (R) _____
    chylothorax (ki"lo-tho'raks; [L. *chylus,* juice] juice in the chest; chyle is a milky, fat-laden
    fluid)

50. **Orogastric** (adj.)   (R) _____ (CV) _____ (R) _____ (S) _____
    orogastric (o"ro-gas'trik; pertaining to the mouth and stomach; clinically refers
    to the administration of food or medication by the passage of a tube from the mouth to the
    stomach)

51. **Antiemetic** (adj.)   (P) _____ (R) _____ (S) _____
    antiemetic (an"tĭ-e-met'ik; pertaining to being against vomiting [Gr. *emein,* to vomit])

52. **Antidiarrheal** (adj.)   (P) _____ (R) _____ (S) _____
    antidiarrheal (an"ti-di"ah-re'al; pertaining to being against diarrhea)

53. **Laparotomy** (n.)   (R) _____ (CV) _____ (S) _____
    laparotomy (lap"ah-rot'o-me; to cut the flank/abdomen [Gr. *lapara,* flank]; i.e., surgical
    cutting through the abdominal wall; an abdominal surgery)

54. **Enterotomy** (n.)   (R) _____ (CV) _____ (S) _____
   enterotomy (en"ter-ot'o-me; to cut the intestine; clinically refers to a surgical procedure
   in which the intestine is incised/cut into)

55. **Colectomy** (n.)   (R) _____ (S) _____
   colectomy (ko-lek'to-me; to cut out the colon; i.e., to surgically remove part or all
   of the colon)

56. **Gastrostomy** (n.)   (R) _____ (CV) _____ (S) _____
   gastrostomy (gas-tros'to-me; creation of a stomach "mouth"/opening; i.e., surgical
   creation of an artificial opening into the stomach)

57. **Omentopexy** (n.)   (R) _____ (CV) _____ (S) _____
   omentopexy (o-men'-to-pek"se; [Gr. *pĕxis*, fixation] fixation of the omentum; i.e., surgical
   fixation/suturing of the omentum, often to the abdominal wall)

58. **Gastropexy** (n.)   (R) _____ (CV) _____ (S) _____
   gastropexy (gas'tro-pek"se; fixation of the stomach; i.e., surgical fixation/suturing
   of the stomach usually to the abdominal wall)

59. **Gastroscopy**   (R) _____ (CV) _____ (S) _____
   gastroscopy (gas-tros'ko-pe; viewing of the stomach; i.e., inspection of the stomach
   using an endoscope)

60. **Palatoschisis** (n.)   (R) _____ (CV) _____ (S) _____
   palatoschisis (pal"ah-to-ske'sis; a cleft palate [Gr. *schisis*, cleft])

ALIMENTARY ANATOMY AND PHYSIOLOGY

Comparative Oral Cavities and Dentition

Have you ever really inspected the oral cavity of animals? The mouth is an
essential part of the anatomy that most people simply take for granted. Let's
look closely at the remarkable structures it contains. The tongue is probably one
of the most remarkable of all (Fig. 12-1). Okay, so you've seen it lying along the
ventral part of the mouth or hanging out of an animal's mouth. Ah, but have you
looked closely at it and how it is used? Think about it. Dogs especially can use
that saliva-soaked tongue hanging from their happy mouths to help them cool
when they pant. As a muscular instrument, the tongue is absolutely amazing!
Animals use its muscular prowess to consume food and drink. Did you know
that animals like dogs and cats actually form a little ladle with the tips of their
tongues (curling the tip caudoventrally) to drink liquids? That's why after drinking they always have little dribbles on their chins. (Most of our other domestic
animals use suction to drink.) What about taking care of an itch or grooming or
showing affection or even taking care of that runny nose? The glossal ability of
animals far exceeds that of people. The dorsal surface of the tongue is covered
with numerous small projections (papillae[1]). These projections contain taste

---

[1]Papillae (pah-pil'e); plural of papilla (pah-pil'ah); from [L. *papilla*, a small, nipple-shaped
projection].

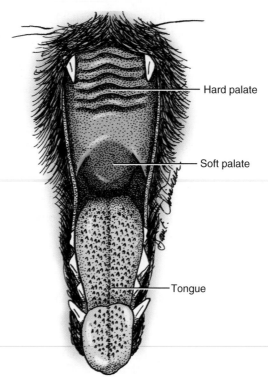

FIGURE 12-1   Feline oral cavity (frontal view).

receptors. In cats, the projections are pronounced and sharp, aiding with normal feline grooming practices. (Being licked by a cat feels like having sandpaper dragged across your skin.) The base (caudal-most portion and attachment) of the tongue is located in the ventrocaudal oropharynx. A sublingual band of connective tissue on the ventromidline of the tongue connects the remainder of the tongue to the floor of the oral cavity. This band of connective tissue is called the *frenulum*[2] (Fig. 12-2). It is very important in small animal medicine to take care to not traumatize the frenulum during intubation for anesthesia. If traumatized, salivary ducts in the area may become inflamed or even obstructed, resulting in *ranula* or *sialocele*[3] formation. This sublingual area is also a very important area to inspect for foreign bodies, such as string; this is particularly important in cats. The dorsal border of the oral cavity is formed by the hard palate. The hard palate provides a bony separation between the oral and nasal cavities. It is covered by connective tissues and mucous membranes, formed in ridges. For dogs who chew on things like sticks or bones, such objects may traumatize the tissues of the hard palate or even become wedged against the palate. Always examine the hard and soft palates for foreign bodies and trauma. Caudal to the

[2]Frenulum (fren'u-lum); from [L. dim. of *fraenum*, a small bridle].
[3]Ranula (rahn'u-lah)/sialocele (si-al-o-sēl; [*sial(o)-* saliva + *-cele,* cyst]); a salivary cyst.

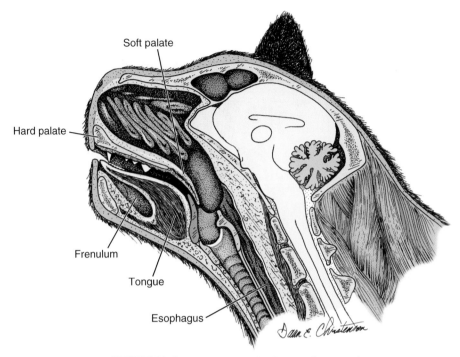

Soft palate

Hard palate

Frenulum

Tongue

Esophagus

FIGURE 12-2 Oral cavity (midsagittal section).

hard palate, in the oropharynx, is the soft palate. The soft palate separates the nasopharynx from the oropharynx, providing protection for the nasal passages during *deglutition.* Particularly in newborn animals, it is important to evaluate the mouth for *palatoschisis.* Even a small cleft can significantly impact a newborn's ability to nurse and certainly its ability to thrive or survive.

The *gingiva* (or "gums") is the periodontal mucous membrane that covers the bone of the upper and lower jaws. The *gingival sulcus* is the tiny groove formed between the neck of the tooth and the free edge of the gingiva (Fig. 12-3, *A*). The gingiva is the most common tissue to be used for evaluation of mucous membrane color and capillary refill time. This tissue, in a quick glance, can tell us much about the animal's health status. The *neck* of the tooth is found at the gingival margin, where the *crown* and the *root* meet. When looking at teeth of carnivores (e.g., those of dogs, cats, and ferrets), the crown of each tooth is covered in *enamel,* the hardest substance found in the body. Each root is covered in a mineralized substance called *cementum.* Directly beneath the enamel and cementum is a porous, bony substance called *dentin;* dentin makes up the bulk of each tooth. At the center of the dentin of each tooth is a canal, filled with soft tissue, blood vessels, and nerves (i.e., pulp). This is the *pulp cavity.* Nerves and vessels enter and exit the pulp cavity through the *apical delta,*[4] found at the apex of the root.

---

[4]Apical delta; apical, pertaining to an apex; delta, as in a delta found at the mouth of a river, with numerous small divisions leading to the destination.

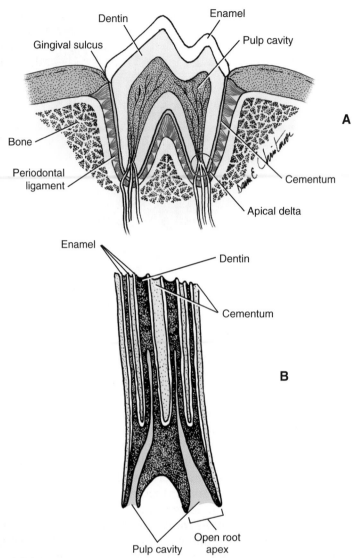

FIGURE 12-3   Comparative tooth anatomy. **A,** Carnivorous tooth (premolar). **B,** Herbivorous tooth (premolar).

The tooth is held in the bone of the jaw by the *periodontal ligaments.* A carnivore's teeth are designed for ripping and tearing tissue from a carcass. They are not designed for chronic wear. Comparatively, a herbivore's teeth must account for all of the constant, chronic grinding of forages. So, instead of a single layer of hard material covering the crown, herbivores maximize hardness and minimize wear by "scrolling" cementum, enamel, and dentin throughout the vertical length of the root and crown (Fig. 12-3, *B*). By having many folds of harder material always present at the exposed, *occlusal* (o-kloo'zal) surface, the tooth will wear away more slowly. Additionally, the root apices for most herbivores remain open for years (in rabbits, for their lifetime). This means that even though the crowns are slowly wearing away, the teeth are slowly and chronically erupting (growing) to replace what was lost. This is not true for carnivores and omnivores. In these animals, once adult teeth have fully erupted, the root apices will close and no longer provide for growth. Therefore, carnivores and omnivores who wear through the enamel covering the crown can rapidly wear the tooth all the way down to the neck of the tooth, and it will never be replaced. When this happens, the pulp will recede and the pulp cavity will be filled with darker, reparative dentin.

In veterinary dentistry, it is important to be able to report/chart dental abnormalities. Noting the specific location of those abnormalities is essential for follow-through of appropriate treatment and management. To that end, specific surfaces of teeth and the individual teeth themselves must be identified. Regarding surfaces, some dental surfaces are designated as either *labial, buccal, palatal,* or *lingual,* by virtue of the mucosal tissue with which the tooth surface comes in contact. The terms *distal* and *mesial* correspond to caudal and rostral, respectively (Fig. 12-4, *A*), when looking at any teeth, particularly those along the lateral teeth of the dental arcade. (The arcade will be discussed in a moment.) For incisors, mesial and medial could be used interchangeably, where distal or lateral would distinguish the opposite surface. (Please note that in veterinary dentistry, mesial and distal are the most appropriate terms to be used.) The *occlusal* surface of a tooth is that which comes in contact with another tooth by design. Carnivores have very little, if any, occlusal surface on their teeth. Herbivores, on the other hand, have occlusal surfaces on most, if not all, of their teeth. Teeth are arranged in what is referred to as a *dental arcade,* because their orientation in the mouth forms an "arch." The arrangement of teeth in the arcade is the same, regardless of animal. Incisors are always the most rostral teeth in the mouth, while molars are always the most caudal. How many of each type of tooth (incisors, canines, premolars, and molars) are present will vary widely among domestic animals. Adult dental arcades may be found in Figure 12-4 for dogs, cats, ruminants, pigs, and horses. Adult dental formulas may be found in the table on page 244. Regardless of the animal, dental abnormalities must be recorded for the specific tooth involved. To simply say that dental caries (i.e., cavities) are present on a molar is insufficient. Which molar? Upper or lower? On what surface? Where?! No one providing follow-up care for that animal should have to search for or question where the abnormality is located. If charted appropriately, the follow-up caregiver should be able to go directly to the affected location. So, individual teeth are named according to right or left, maxillary (upper) or mandibular (lower), and the sequence number within the tooth type. A sequence number does not apply to the canine teeth because there is only one right and one left canine tooth on each jaw. For sequentially numbering other teeth of the mouth, they should be counted beginning mesial to distal. Dental formulas provide veterinary professionals with a guide as to the types and numbers of teeth that should be found in an animal's mouth (Figs. 12-5 and 12-6). To interpret a dental formula, one must consider that the

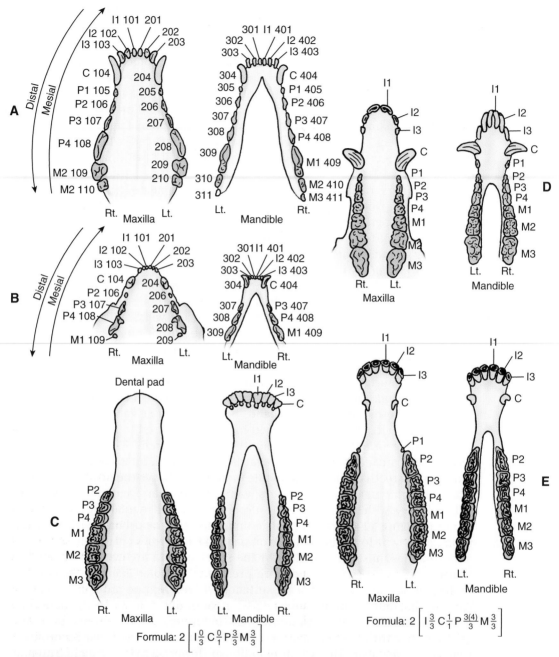

FIGURE 12-4　Comparative dental arcades. **A,** Canine. **B,** Feline. **C,** Bovine, ovine, and caprine. **D,** Porcine. **E,** Equine.

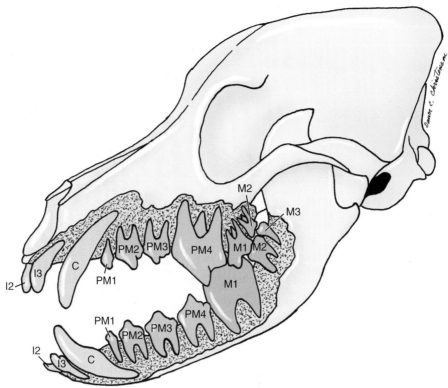

FIGURE 12-5 Canine dentition schematic. *I,* incisor; *C,* canine; *PM,* premolar; *M,* molar.

"fractions" included are actually numbers of maxillary teeth over mandibular teeth. Notice that these "fractions" are contained within brackets and multiplied by a factor of 2. This is because the numbers within the "fractions" account for only half of the dental arcades of the mouth. One side of the mouth is a mirror image of the other. Because we can look at only one side of the mouth at a time, it makes sense to know how many of each tooth we should be seeing as we look at one side. Within the dental formulas, each type of tooth is abbreviated as follows: "I" (incisors), "C" (canines), "P" (premolars), and "M" (molars). Notice, comparatively, that ruminants have no maxillary incisors or canines. Instead of these maxillary teeth, ruminants have a tough, leathery, dental pad. This unique dental structure is true for all domestic ruminants, including sheep, goats, and cattle. Note also the variability in the horse's dental formula. Not all horses have canines, and the maxillary first premolar may or may not be present. The maxillary first premolar is often referred to as the "wolf tooth." In dogs and cats, a modified Triadan numbering system has been developed, giving each tooth its own individual number. Both means of identifying canine and feline teeth have been included in Figure 12-4. The Triadan system may seem confusing at first. However, once you're familiar with it, it is quite easy and efficient to use. Just remember to always begin counting on the upper right for the 100-series, then

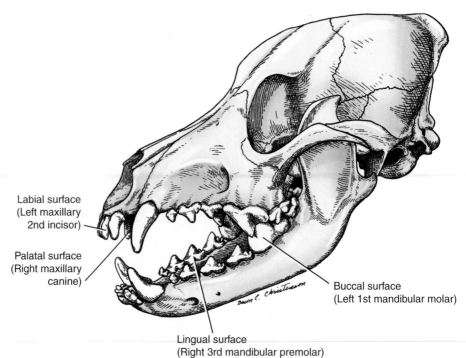

Labial surface
(Left maxillary
2nd incisor)

Palatal surface
(Right maxillary
canine)

Buccal surface
(Left 1st mandibular molar)

Lingual surface
(Right 3rd mandibular premolar)

FIGURE 12-6   Canine dentition.

Comparative Dental Formulas

Cats	$2\left[I\frac{3}{3}C\frac{1}{1}P\frac{3}{2}M\frac{1}{1}\right]$
Dogs	$2\left[I\frac{3}{3}C\frac{1}{1}P\frac{4}{4}M\frac{2}{3}\right]$
Ferrets	$2\left[I\frac{3}{5}C\frac{1}{1}P\frac{3}{2}M\frac{1}{2}\right]$
Horses	$2\left[I\frac{3}{3}C\frac{1(0)}{1(0)}P\frac{3(4)}{3}M\frac{3}{3}\right]$
Pigs	$2\left[I\frac{3}{3}C\frac{1}{1}P\frac{4}{4}M\frac{3}{3}\right]$
Rabbits	$2\left[I\frac{2}{1}C\frac{0}{0}P\frac{3}{3}M\frac{3}{3}\right]$
Ruminants	$2\left[I\frac{0}{3}C\frac{0}{1}P\frac{3}{3}M\frac{3}{3}\right]$

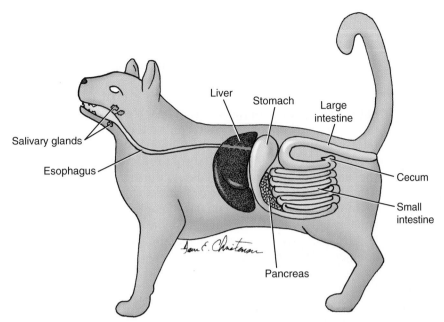

FIGURE 12-7   Schematic of the feline gastrointestinal tract.

progress to the upper left for the 200-series, then to the lower left for the 300-series and finally to the lower right for the 400-series. Then, using the rule of 4 and 9 is very helpful for orienting yourself in the mouth, especially when the animal is missing a few teeth. What is the rule of 4 and 9? The canine teeth numbers always end in 4 (104, 204, 304, and 404). The first molar numbers always end in 9. Just in case you run across a retained deciduous (baby) tooth, you can determine its Triadan number by simply adding 400 to the respective adult tooth that should have fully replaced it. (For example, if 104 is erupting but the deciduous tooth is retained, the actual number of the retained tooth is 504.)

Simple Monogastric Digestive Anatomy

Animals with a simple monogastric digestive system include the dog, cat, pig, and ferret (and even humans). Let's look at the magnificent simplicity of the digestive tract of these creatures first. Then we'll take a comparative look at hindgut fermentors like horses, rabbits, and guinea pigs. Finally, we'll look at ruminants. Thus far, we've looked at the oral cavity. Alas, that is only the beginning. Most of the digestive tract is simply a series of tubes. Let's look at each segment of those tubular structures, shall we?

Stemming from the pharynx, the esophagus is a muscular tube that serves as a passage from the pharynx to the stomach (Fig. 12-7). It lies dorsal to the trachea as it traverses the neck and thoracic cavity, slipping just a little to the left of the trachea about mid-neck. (Can you imagine how long the esophagus of a giraffe is?! No, giraffes are not simple monogastric animals, but it sure is fun to think about them compared with dogs and cats.) Peristalsis moves food through the esophagus to the stomach. (Boy, that's a good thing or it might take forever for food to reach that giraffe's stomach!) We'll discuss peristalsis more when we get to the small intestine. For now, let's move on to the stomach. The stomach is a pouch-like structure that lies in the left craniolateral quadrant of the peritoneal cavity. When empty, it lies very close to the diaphragm, liver, and spleen, partially protected by the caudal ribs. The fundus is the billowing, curved portion of the stomach near the gastroesophageal opening. Muscles of the distal esophagus, while contracted, help prevent reflux of gastric contents and juices into the esophagus, (this is often referred to as the "cardiac sphincter"[5]) (Fig. 12-8). The body of the stomach is the portion that lies between the fundus and the pylorus. The pylorus is the narrow segment of the stomach, near the duodenum. (It more or less acts like a funnel to move pulverized stomach contents into the intestinal tract. Actually, it's a little more like a pastry bag, squeezing things out through a tiny opening.) Unlike a pastry bag, the opening from the pylorus has an active, powerful muscular sphincter—the pyloric sphincter. This sphincter is generally tightly closed, except during active gastric emptying. Only small volumes of liquid, like water, can trickle through the pyloric sphincter when it is closed. The wall of the stomach is muscular and has numerous folds called rugae (roo'gay). These folds provide tremendous expansive ability for the stomach and help pulverize food. The gastric mucosa is covered with a thick layer of protective mucus. Without the protective mucus, the stomach wall would be in direct contact with the hydrochloric acid and other gastric juices. (Ouch!)

The small intestine is composed of the duodenum, jejunum, and ileum. The duodenum is the proximal portion of the small intestine (see Fig. 12-8). It lies in the right lateral peritoneal cavity, from the pyloric sphincter to the jejunum. Its Latin origin, [*duodeni*, twelve at a time], was derived because, in humans, it is approximately 12 fingerbreadths long (~12 inches). Obviously, with the size variances in domestic animals, the name cannot be used to estimate the length of this section of bowel. The duodenum is a critical section of small intestine where much of the bile and enzymes used for digestion will enter the enteric lumen. The jejunum is the middle portion of the small intestine, which actually makes up the longest segment of bowel (Fig. 12-9). It occupies the greater portion of the peritoneal cavity in simple monogastric animals. In any animal, the jejunum is a principle region for digestion and absorption of nutrients. The distal portion of the small intestine is the ileum, which lies between the jejunum and the cecum (Fig. 12-10). Note that this ileum is spelled differently from that of the pelvis. This ileum contains an "e" for enteric.

As alluded to earlier, the entire small intestine is simply a tube-like structure. So, just exactly how do you move squishy contents through a long, flexible tube? Think about it, if we randomly squeeze that tube, we might empty that small portion of the tube, but we won't really make any progress in effectively moving things along in one direction (i.e., to ultimately move things into the colon to reach the "back door" for emptying the "trash," so to speak). The wall

---

[5]Sphincter (sfingk'ter); from [Gr. *sphingkter*, that which binds tight]; a sphincter is a ring-like band of muscle fibers that constricts a natural opening.

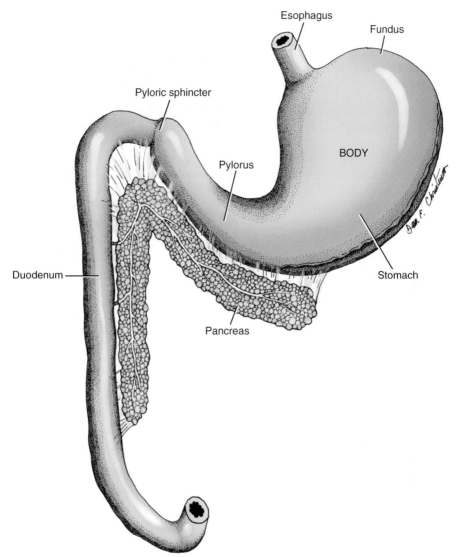

FIGURE 12-8   Canine stomach, duodenum, and pancreas.

of the small intestine is very muscular, with the muscle fibers oriented in both a longitudinal and a circular fashion. Coordinated muscular contractions create the worm-like, propulsive action called peristalsis. Peristalsis will rhythmically move enteric contents along at a steady pace—not too fast and not too slow—to allow for digestion and absorption of nutrients. To maximize that digestion and absorption, the enteric mucosa is composed of billions of finger-like projections called villi[6] (Fig. 12-11). The villi increase the surface area of the small intestine for maximal absorption of nutrients. Each villus is covered by simple columnar

---

[6]Villi (vil'ī), plural of villus (vil'us); from [L. *villus*, a tuft of hair].

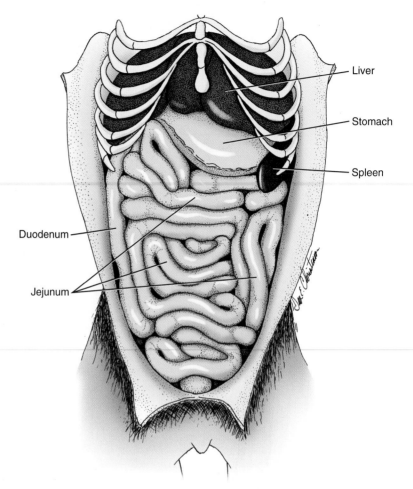

FIGURE 12-9   Canine abdominal viscera (omentum removed).

epithelium. Even the epithelial cells have their own finger-like projections, called microvilli, which increase the absorptive surface area even further. Near the bases of the villi are small crypts, also lined with simple columnar epithelium. The epithelium of the crypts produces protective mucus that coats the surface of the enteric lumen (hence, enteric mucosa). In the center of each villus are a lymphatic vessel and capillaries. The lymphatic vessel found at the center of each villus is called a lacteal (lak′te-al). These vessels will transport absorbed nutrients to their destinations. These digestive and absorptive processes will be discussed later in this chapter.

Moving right along, the cecum is a vestigial structure in most simple monogastric animals, like the dog, cat, and ferret. In the pig, it is a modest-sized structure, perhaps up to a foot long. The cecum in any of these animals marks the end of the small intestine and the beginning of the large intestine or colon (see Fig. 12-10). It is a small, blind sac in dogs, cats, and ferrets, through which very

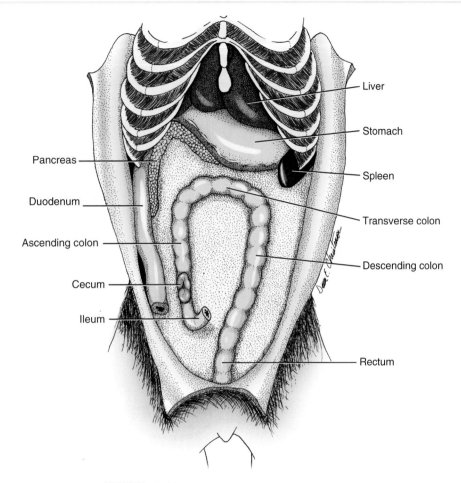

FIGURE 12-10   Canine ileum, cecum, and colon.

little intestinal contents flow. In the pig, ileal contents enter directly into the cecum before passing into the colon.

The colon or large intestine is composed of several segments (see Fig. 12-10). In carnivores, like the cat and dog, the ascending colon lies along the right side of the peritoneal cavity. It courses cranially from the cecum to the transverse colon. The transverse colon crosses the peritoneal cavity from right to left, between the ascending and descending portions of the colon. The descending colon lies on the left side of the peritoneal cavity and runs caudally, between the transverse colon and the rectum. The colon of omnivores, like the pig, has more bends and turns before it reaches the rectum and anus. The rectum is the terminal portion of the colon, associated with the anal opening. An internal and an external anal sphincter are found at the anus. The internal sphincter is under autonomic control, while the external sphincter is under conscious control. Young animals must be taught to control that external sphincter, hence "potty training" for dogs and cats. But that's a story to be discussed at another time.

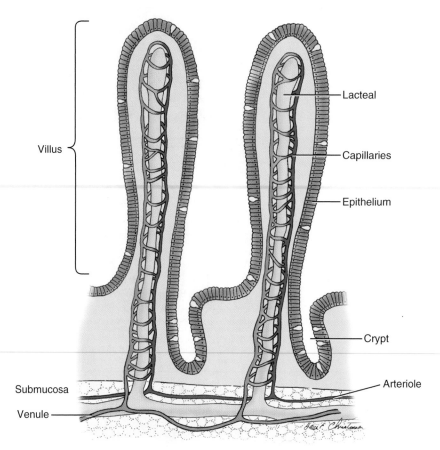

FIGURE 12-11　Enteric villi.

The muscular arrangement and activity of the colon is different from that of the small intestine. Of course, this is because the purpose of the colon is different. Rather than playing a pivotal role in digestion and absorption of nutrients, the colon's job is to slowly and methodically reclaim water from its contents. To that end, it is designed to squeeze and turn fecal material for optimal surface area contact. The entire colon contains numerous large haustrations. These sac-like haustrations, coupled with musculature that focuses on segmentation (squeezing and turning its contents) rather that peristalsis, effectively turn the fecal matter like anyone would use a spade or shovel to turn soil. The mucosal surface of the colon also differs from that of the small intestine, in that it does not have villi. Absorption of water doesn't require such an intricate mucosal surface. Weak peristaltic waves will eventually move the semidried fecal material toward the anus and eventually out the "back door." If you've ever seen some cats' feces, you know that the colon can be a powerful drying "machine." Rocks come to mind as I think of that.

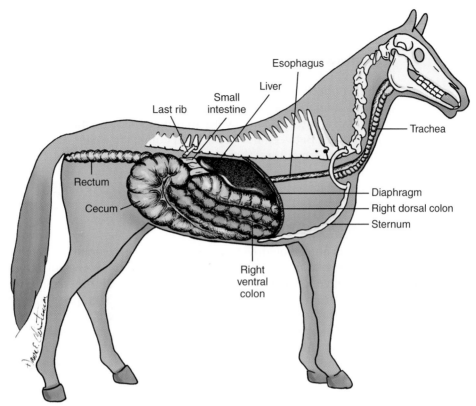

FIGURE 12-12   Equine abdominal viscera.

Hindgut-Fermentor Digestive Anatomy

How are hindgut-fermenting animals (i.e., horses, rabbits, and guinea pigs) different from our simple monogastric animals? Well, aside from external appearances being quite different, they are actually quite similar to our other monogastric friends. The esophagus, stomach, duodenum, jejunum, and ileum are very much the same. It is the cecum that is incredibly different. They even have a well-developed ileocecal valve. The cecum itself in these animals is big. Aw, let's face it, it's HUGE! Look at Figure 12-12. Just look at the size of the cecum in that horse. It takes up a great deal of space along the entire floor of the ventral abdomen. Why is it so big, you ask? Up until now, when talking about monogastric animals, we've been discussing carnivores and omnivores. Now, we are talking about monogastric herbivores. The mainstay of horse, rabbit, and guinea pig diets are roughages and forages like grasses and hay. A simple monogastric digestive tract cannot adequately break these rough-ages down to usable, absorbable nutrients. Herbivores need a team of happy micro-organisms to help with the digestion of these materials, through a process called microbial fermentation. The "happy home" in which most of this fermentation takes place is the cecum. It's a big job. So, those microbes need a big place to do it. Okay, now you're probably asking, "Why are they called hindgut fermentors?" Well, the cecum is located kind of at the tail end of the digestive tract. After all, the only thing we have to traverse from here is the colon. After that, hello world here we come! Of course, the colon in these herbivores is a bit different from the other monogastric animals too. It is way longer, because it's going to help contribute to the fermentative process and absorb a portion of the wonderful by-products (like volatile fatty acids). Structurally, the colon in these animals is a plumber's nightmare. The colon is very long with numerous twists and turns, along with stenotic areas and many more well-developed haustrations. Between the cecum and colon, it's easier to plug up the plumbing in hindgut fermentors than in other monogastrics. By the way, it's those well-developed haustrations in the terminal colon and rectum that give the fecal material passed by these animals its distinctive shape.

Ruminant Digestive Anatomy

Ruminants are herbivores too. What makes these animals, including our sheep, goats, and cattle, so different is the fact that they are not monogastric. They actually have a multichambered forestomach before reaching what is called a "true" stomach. The esophagus of these animals empties into the rumen, the largest of the chambers (Fig. 12-13). You thought just the cecum of a horse was big. The rumen is enormous! The rumen is the reason these animals are called ruminants (go figure). The rumen is a veritable microbial party-heaven. The microbes in that rumen can party 'til the cows come home. (Yes, the pun was intentional.) The huge, fermentative vat of the rumen is very muscular. One to three times a minute the rumen will churn its contents through powerful muscular contractions, called (what else?) ruminations. Periodically too, ruminants will eructate (more or less belch) some of the rumen contents back up into the oral cavity for further chewing of the forages. Cattle chew their "cud" for many, many, many *(many)* hours during the course of the day. This makes the microbes' job easier, because chewing pulverizes the food to create more surface area for the microbes to work on. What a win-win situation this is. The microbial fermentation creates gaseous by-products, like CO_2 and methane, that make the eructation easier, and the eructation and cud-chewing makes the microbial fermentation more efficient. Cranial to the rumen is the second, smaller chamber called the reticulum. The walls of the reticulum are very unique, with a net-like or honeycomb appearance. It is that appearance that led to the name of this chamber. Contents may freely slosh between the rumen and the reticulum. If anything heavy was consumed (like metal objects) they will frequently accumulate in the reticulum. The consequences of this will be discussed later. The third chamber in the series is the omasum. The omasum has many layers of muscular "leaves" or folds of tissue within it. These serve to further pulverize the ingesta. Finally, we arrive at the abomasum, frequently referred to as the "true stomach" of ruminants. Structurally and functionally, the abomasum is similar to the monogastric stomach. Note the normal location of the abomasum (see Fig. 12-13). It lies along the ventral abdomen, ever so slightly to the right of midline. (The importance of that positioning will be discussed later, when we talk about

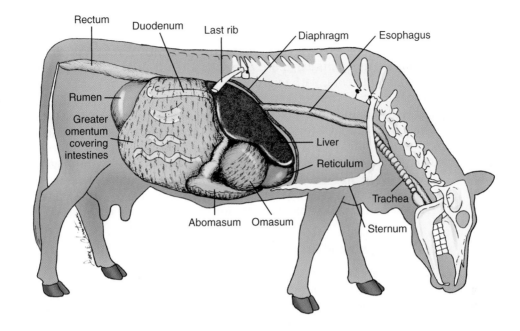

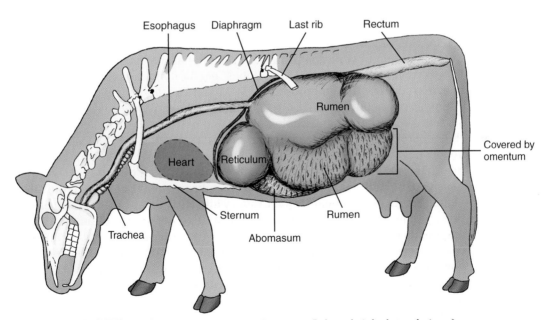

FIGURE 12-13   Bovine abdominal viscera (left and right lateral views).

displaced abomasums; i.e., DAs.) From this point, the digestive tract of ruminants is sequentially the same as our monogastrics. Obviously, ruminants don't require a large cecum, because all of the fermentative work was done up front. This makes ruminants far more effective when it comes to digestion and absorption of nutrients. With microbial fermentation occurring prior to the small intestine, most of the nutrients produced by the fermentative process can be easily digested and absorbed by the small intestine. Fecal matter produced by a ruminant is pure waste. Hindgut fermentors, comparatively, will actually lose some of the valuable fermentative by-products like B vitamins and volatile fatty acids in their fecal matter. Actually, that's why rabbits are coprophagic. Yes, rabbits will eat the initial soft fecal pellets that they produce each day, to recoup those valuable nutrients. By the way, the fermentative by-products lost by the horse makes its manure much better for the garden than cow manure.

Accessory Organs and Tissues

Liver and Biliary Tree

It's not much to look at, but the liver is an amazing organ. It occupies approximately the cranial third of the peritoneal cavity in most domestic animals (see Fig. 12-9). In cattle, it's relatively small, comparatively, and occupies only the right cranial third of the abdomen. The liver lies immediately caudal to the diaphragm and is well protected by the caudal ribs. In a dog or cat, during abdominal palpation, you will probably have to slip your fingers just under the caudal ribs to feel the margins of the liver lobes. If you feel the margins of the liver extending beyond the protective ribs, hepatomegaly probably exists. The liver is composed of several large lobes, each of which is highly vascular and is constructed with numerous sinuses, channels, and canals lined with simple cuboidal epithelium (Fig. 12-14). The hepatic cells lining these biliary canals secrete bile and bile salts. Cholesterol is one of the precursor elements used by the hepatocytes to produce bile and bile salts. (So, not all cholesterol is bad.) Yellow bile pigments come from bilirubin, which is a by-product of hemoglobin degradation. Backup of these pigments into the blood, due to hepatic disease, may result in icteric-appearing mucous membranes and skin, due to the bilirubinemia. Fortunately, a healthy liver is very efficient at transforming bilirubin into bile and bile salts, which are excreted into the biliary tree. All of the many biliary canals converge into larger bile ducts. The common bile duct connects all of the hepatic bile ducts with the duodenum (Fig. 12-15). The gallbladder is also connected to the common bile duct. The gallbladder merely serves as a storage area for bile. Bile is concentrated while it is stored in the gallbladder. Smooth muscle in the walls of the gallbladder contracts during a meal to express the concentrated bile into the common bile duct. This is especially important when meals high in fat are consumed. (By the way, horses do not have a gallbladder. I guess it's a good thing horses don't eat pizza, eh?)

The liver has many other functions, in addition to bile and bile salt production. All of the blood from the mesentery (mes"en-ter'e) must pass through the liver before entering general circulation. This ensures that blood in general circulation is detoxified and is free of microbes from the gut. In addition, the

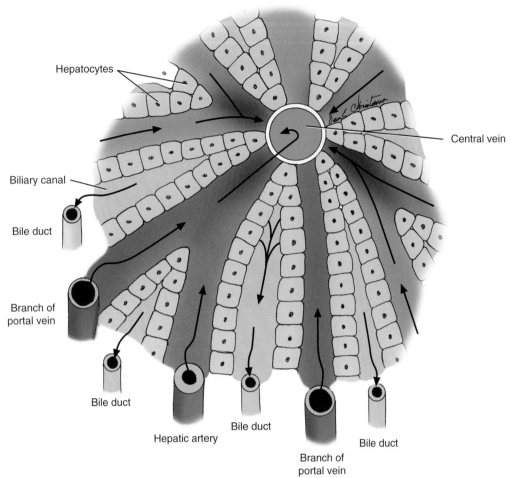

Hepatocytes

Biliary canal

Bile duct

Branch of
portal vein

Bile duct

Hepatic artery

Bile duct

Branch of
portal vein

Central vein

Bile duct

FIGURE 12-14   Hepatic anatomy.

liver is responsible for producing most of the plasma proteins, particularly
many of the clotting factors. The liver can metabolize or, if necessary, it can
store many nutrients in its tissues, like lipid-soluble vitamins, as well as sources
of energy. It can also create, from "scratch," simple sugars to be used for energy
(gluconeogenesis[7]). How cool is that?! The liver is important for metabolism
and biotransformation of many of the drugs administered to animals. The list of
hepatic functions goes on and on. Animals cannot survive without the liver. Fortunately, the liver is not easily destroyed and has a tremendous ability to repair
and regenerate its tissues when damaged. Just how important is the liver? Suffice it to say, when thinking about important physiologic concepts and body
health, think either liver or water.

---

[7]Gluconeogenesis (gloo″ko-ne″o-jen′ĕ-sis); *gluc(o)-,* sugar + *ne(o)-,* new + *gen-,* produce + *-sis,*
the process of.

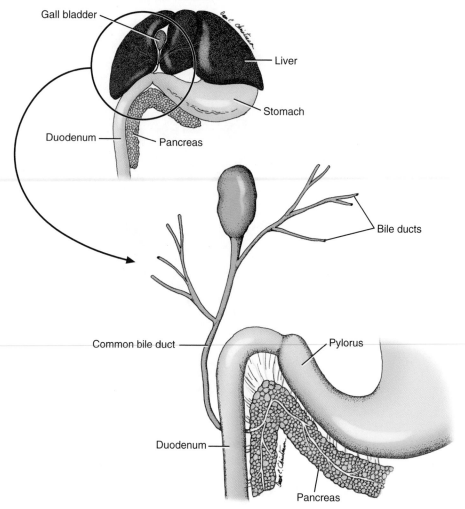

FIGURE 12-15   Biliary tree and gallbladder.

Pancreas

Ah, the pancreas is another organ that plays dual roles. The pancreas is a glandular organ that lies along side the duodenum and pylorus (see Fig. 12-15). Ducts from the pancreas enter the duodenum, providing passage for pancreatic enzymes. So, what about those dual roles I mentioned? Well, this complex organ provides both exocrine (digestive) functions as well as endocrine functions. Endocrine functions of the pancreas are discussed in Chapter 15. No, we won't discuss pancreatic exocrine function yet either. If we did it now, you'd have no reason to read the rest of the chapter.

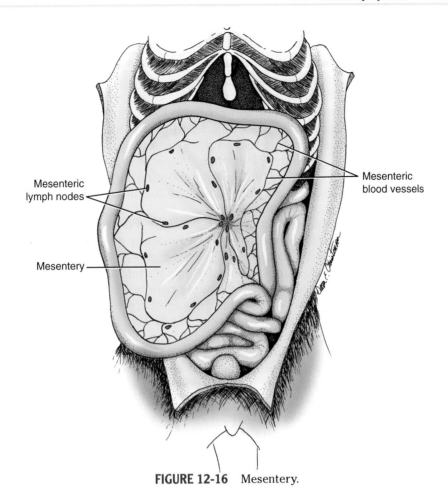

Mesenteric lymph nodes

Mesenteric blood vessels

Mesentery

FIGURE 12-16 Mesentery.

Peritoneum, Omentum, and Mesentery

Lest we forget, there are very important tissues that hold all of the marvelous peritoneal organs and structures together in an organized fashion. The peritoneum is the tissue that lines the walls of the abdominal cavity and covers the abdominal viscera. Parietal peritoneum[8] is that which lines the walls of the abdominal cavity, and visceral peritoneum is that which covers the organs. The parietal and visceral peritoneum are, for all practical purposes, continuous with one another. (Think of it as one sheet of plastic wrap that starts on one side of the abdominal wall, envelopes each loop of bowel and organ, and then continues on to cover the rest of the abdominal wall.) The large portion of peritoneal tissue that connects visceral and parietal portions is the mesentery (Fig. 12-16). The main attachment for the mesentery is found along the dorsum of the abdominal cavity. Okay, admittedly this is a difficult thing to visualize if you've never seen it. So, take a big sheet of plastic wrap and begin placing it in a large bowl or pan.

---

[8]Parietal (pah-ri′ĕ-tal, [L. *parietalis*]) refers to the walls of a cavity.

(The bowl or pan represents the abdominal walls.) Start by sticking one edge of the plastic wrap at one edge of the bowl and run it down the side of the bowl to the bottom. Now, begin creating a pouch of the plastic wrap billowing up from the bottom of the bowl, carefully sticking under and within that pouch objects to represent intestines and organs. Once you've covered those objects, continue with the sheet of plastic wrap back down to the bottom of the bowl and bunch it up at the base to hold those objects within it securely. Finally, you may finish by extending the sheet of plastic wrap up over the other inside wall of the bowl. Whew! That was a lengthy description, but what does it really represent? The plastic wrap on the sides of the bowl represent the parietal peritoneum. The plastic wrap that is directly stuck to the objects in the middle is the visceral peritoneum. But there is a lot of seemingly extra or wasted plastic wrap in between all of those objects contained within that pouch we secured to the bottom of the bowl. That, my friends, is the mesentery. In a real body, the mesentery is more of a fan-like membrane that supports all of the mesenteric blood vessels, lymph nodes, lymphatic vessels, and nerves that supply the intestines and other abdominal organs. The mesentery provides the supportive attachments for most of the intestinal tract. The omentum[9] is a much more delicate tissue, made of loose connective tissue and adipose (see Fig. 12-13; Fig. 12-17). It looks rather lacy. Attachments for the omentum are found from the fundus to the pylorus of the stomach (in ruminants it attaches to the abomasum and rumen). The rest of the omentum drapes loosely over the intestines of monogastric animals and lies freely on the floor of the ventral abdomen. In ruminants, it more or less drapes from the dorsal right abdomen down and around to the lower left abdomen attaching to the abomasum and rumen. (Place a kitchen towel over the bowl that we just plastic wrapped and tuck it in around the edges. That's the omentum.) Omentum helps hold the intestines, stomach/abomasum, and spleen in place. The truly unique characteristic of the omentum is that it can seal off or wall off small damaged areas along the intestinal tract. This could minimize or even prevent peritonitis in the case of a small defect. Plus, the omentum can come in handy for surgically repositioning and securing a displaced abomasum. We'll tell the rest of that story later.

Digestive Physiology

The digestive process actually begins preprandially. Come now, we have all watched TV commercials or the Food Channel and begun salivating and had to listen to our stomachs growl as a result. Almost any stimulus could initiate this—seeing the food, smelling the food, or even just hearing the clanking of pans or a food bowl. Once one learns what the sight, smell, or sound truly means (yummo!), it will stimulate a parasympathetic response whenever presented with it. (Remember, the parasympathetic branch of the autonomic nervous system is responsible for digestive activities.) Pavlov proved this by training a group of dogs to respond to the sound of a bell in anticipation of a meal. Once trained, the dogs would exhibit hypersialosis whenever the bell was rung. Not only is saliva produced excessively, in anticipation of a meal, but gastric and

---

[9]Omentum (o-men'tum); from [L. *omentum*, fat skin].

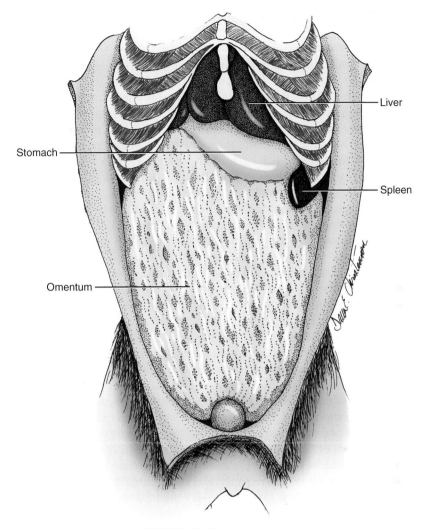

FIGURE 12-17   Omentum.

other digestive juices begin to prepare for the oncoming food, as well. Motility of the digestive tract also shifts into gear (hence your growling stomach).

Alright already! Bring on the food! Prehension[10] of food varies among domestic animals, depending on the structure of the mouth. Because dogs, cats, and ferrets are carnivorous, their teeth are designed for shearing and tearing of meat from a carcass. We mentioned this earlier when we discussed dentition. But what do they do with the meat once it's in their mouths? In the wild, pieces of meat are torn from the carcass and swallowed. Very little, if any, mastication (chewing) takes place. Domestication has provided dogs, cats, and even ferrets with preformed kibbles and other such forms of food. Although not necessary, the instinctive prehensile

---

[10]Prehension (pre-hen'shun); from [L. *prehensio*]; the act of seizing or grasping; clinically refers to the act of taking food into the mouth.

activity may still be exhibited, in the gulping and shaking of food taken into the mouth. Alas, domestication has progressed such that some dogs and cats do masticate the food (even dry kibble), though their mouths are poorly designed for it. Prehension by our herbivores depends, in part, on the structure of their muzzles, especially the lips. Compare the muzzles of sheep and goats with that of cattle. Sheep and goats have cleft lips, allowing them to nibble on grasses until there is nothing left but stubble in the dirt. Cattle, on the other hand, do not have such agile muzzles. Consequently, they require taller grasses that they need to sweep their heads through and then drag grasses into their mouths with their tongues. Needless to say, if a herd of sheep grazed on a pasture before a herd of cattle, the cattle probably would not be able to feed well, if at all. (Do you see why some of the range wars took place between cowboys in the old west?) Horses have an amazing prehensile ability. They have what we refer to as prehensile lips. The lips of a horse can selectively discern between the best little nuggets of grain or the most-lush leaves of grass or alfalfa. Although each of our domestic herbivores may have different prehensile abilities, one thing they all do well is chew their food. (Mom always said, "Chew your food!") Mastication increases the surface area of the food so that the digestive process can work more effectively on that food. We've already talked about the importance of this in ruminants. Boy, ruminants are mastication masters! Mastication also serves to mix the food with the saliva, making a moist, slippery food bolus to slide through the esophagus. That is the principal role of saliva, to moisten the food and to stick the particles together so that the food may be formed into a manageable bolus for deglutition. (On a trivial note, cattle produce and swallow *gallons* of saliva per day.) Unlike human saliva, the saliva of domestic animals does not contain enzymes to initiate digestion. Domestic animal saliva has two components, an aqueous (watery) part for moistening the food and a viscous (thick and stringy) part to aid in the formation of the food bolus. It also contains some electrolytes, like potassium. Ruminants also have salivary buffers that aid in the health of the microenvironment of the rumen.

In our monogastric animals, during deglutition, the tongue and muscles of the pharynx will force the food bolus into the esophagus and then peristaltic activity of the esophagus will transport the food bolus to the stomach. (In ruminants, remember, the food will be carried to the rumen for microbial fermentation, then pass through the reticulum and omasum before reaching the abomasum. The abomasum does have glandular tissue, but far less than is discussed here for a monogastric stomach. Still, as you read about the monogastric stomach activity, simply consider the abomasum having similar activity, just on a much reduced scale.) When the food enters the stomach, it is tossed and turned by gastric contractions. The gastric motions pulverize the food further and mix it thoroughly with gastric secretions. Hydrochloric acid (HCl) and pepsin are the two principal secretions in the stomach. The hydrochloric acid is necessary to convert pepsinogen (the inactive form of the enzyme pepsin) into active pepsin. Pepsin is stored in an inactive form in the stomach to prevent autodigestion[11] of the stomach. Pepsin is a proteolytic[12] enzyme, for

---

[11]Autodigestion; *auto-*, a prefix meaning "self."

[12]Proteolytic (pro"te-o-lit'ik); *prote(o)-*, protein + *-lytic*, pertaining to destruction.

the initiation of protein digestion. We may be initiating protein digestion in the stomach, but the bulk of digestion is yet to come in the small intestine. The stomach serves more as a holding or storage tank, until the rest of the digestive tract can handle the food that has been consumed. (This is especially true for the abomasum.) Little by little, the stomach contracts and squirts small volumes of its liquefied contents through the pyloric sphincter into the duodenum. Gastric/abomasal emptying must be controlled and gradual, to ensure that digestive enzymes and bile in the duodenum will be proportional to the food it is presented with.

The duodenum is where digestion really gains momentum. Bile from the liver (especially concentrated bile from the gallbladder) is secreted into the duodenum through the common bile duct. The bile and bile salts are important for the emulsification of fats. When fats are emulsified, more lipid surface area is created for the pancreatic enzymes to work on. (Emulsification is nothing more than taking a large oil slick and turning it into manageable, smaller globs of fat. This is sort of the way Dawn dish soap works. It "gets grease out of your way.") Bile salts are also important for aiding in the absorption of fatty acids and some lipid-soluble vitamins. (Remember, our ruminants produced tons of volatile fatty acids through microbial fermentation. These fatty acids will provide those animals with tremendous energy. And the bile salts will help them absorb that energy source.) The pancreas also secretes its digestive juices into the duodenum. Three of the primary pancreatic enzymes are lipase, amylase, and trypsin (trip'sin; one of many proteolytic pancreatic enzymes). As the ingesta is mixed by the small bowel, the enzymes break down substances into usable, absorbable nutrients.

Peristalsis carries the ingesta through the duodenum and the jejunum. Throughout these sections of bowel, the enzymes continue to work. Nutrients released by the digestive process are absorbed by the duodenum and jejunum. Most nutrients are absorbed by active transport. While some water may be absorbed through osmosis here, most of the water contained in the ingesta at this point will remain in the enteric lumen until it reaches the colon.

Where do the absorbed nutrients go? Hepatoportal circulation is sort of a mass transit system that will direct their travels. Most of the nutrients absorbed throughout the intestinal tract, except lipids, make their way into the mesenteric veins. These veins carry the blood to the liver, entering the liver via the portal vein. While the blood percolates through the liver, hepatic macrophages remove bacteria and other organisms from the blood. The liver also detoxifies the blood, metabolizes (burns) some of the nutrients, and stores others. Eventually, the blood leaves the liver by way of the hepatic vein and flows back to the heart through the caudal vena cava. In the normal animal, any blood returning to the heart from the abdominal viscera must pass through the liver first. (If bypassed by a portocaval shunt, an accessory vessel directly connecting the portal vein and caudal vena cava, mild to severe disease signs may be seen in the animal. Detours are unacceptable in this system and are not tolerated well. Severity of disease depends on the size of the shunt and how much "filthy" blood is actually making its way into general circulation. Disease signs will be most severe during the postprandial period.)

Lipids or fats are absorbed and transported to the bloodstream by a different route. Lipids must be digested into smaller-sized molecules called fatty acids. Fatty acids can readily diffuse across the cell membranes of the enteric epithelium. This is because cell membranes are composed largely of lipids. As a fatty acid passes through the endoplasmic reticula and Golgi apparatus of the enterocyte, it is packaged with protein. This new fatty acid–protein compound is called a chylomicron.[13] Chylomicrons are then absorbed by the lacteals. (Yes, the chylous fluid does appear white. That's why the lacteals are so aptly named.) Once in the lacteals, the chylomicrons flow with the rest of the lymphatic fluids. They finally make their way to the bloodstream by passing through a structure called the thoracic duct. The thoracic duct provides a portal between the lymphatic system and the circulating blood. Eventually, the liver and body tissues remove the chylomicrons from the blood and use or store their components. Fatty acids provide a tremendous energy source for the body. Following a meal, because most animal diets will contain at least small amounts of fat, postprandial lipemia is normal. This is due to all of the circulating chylomicrons. As soon as they have been used or tucked away for storage, the lipemia will resolve. (In thoracic trauma cases, the thoracic duct may be damaged, resulting in leakage of the chylous fluid into the thoracic cavity and creating a chylothorax.)

Wait a minute. Until now we have only talked about digestive activity through the jejunum. What about that small section of ileum? Well, it's small so let's be brief. The ileum is most important for reabsorption of bile and bile salts. That's right, it's a recycling center. Recycling may be popular in today's society, but the ileum has been recycling bile and bile salts for millennia.

Peristaltic activity continues to carry the remaining liquid material past the cecum and into the ascending colon of our carnivores. Remember, the cecum, in dogs and cats, is a vestigial structure that contributes little, if anything, to the digestive process. In the pig, the cecum has a modest job, and bowel contents will flow through it before reaching the colon. For all of our horses, rabbits, and guinea pigs, don't forget the enormity of the cecum and its importance for microbial fermentation. In these animals, those roughages will spend a great deal of time in the cecum before being sent on to the colon. Once the ingesta is in the colon, it passes slowly through all of the colonic twists and turns. Microbial fermentation will continue through much of the proximal portions of the colon for our hindgut fermentors. Segmentation, rather than peristalsis, is the predominant muscular activity of anyone's colon. The haustrations, combined with segmentation, slowly mix and turn the bowel contents, like spading the earth as we mentioned earlier. This exposes a tremendous amount of surface area, to permit absorption of water and electrolytes from the ingesta. Hindgut fermentors will absorb some of the B vitamins and volatile fatty acids here too. Approximately 25% of those fermentative by-products will be lost in the manure. The more time spent in the colon and rectum, the drier the fecal material will become. If too dry, constipation may result. Of course, if we speed up transit time, less water will be removed and diarrhea will result. The intention is

---

[13]Chylomicron (ki″lo-mi′kron); *chyl(o)-*, juice + [Gr. *micron*, a small thing]; chyle is the milky white fat-laden fluid absorbed by the lacteals.

for the fecal material to be stored in the rectum for a reasonable period of time, until the animal voluntarily defecates.

Actually, defecation is partly an involuntary act and partly a voluntary act. Pressure of feces within the rectum stimulates involuntary relaxation of the internal anal sphincter. This puts all of the pressure on the external anal sphincter, which the conscious mind must now cause to constrict. The external anal sphincter is relaxed only when the animal chooses to do so for defecation. At this time, most of the haustrations in the colon and rectum disappear, making it easier for peristaltic actions of the mass movement to evacuate the bowel. It should be noted that very young animals have not yet developed the voluntary control mechanisms involved with the external anal sphincter. Particularly when training a puppy in its elimination habits, the owner should be aware that the puppy experiences a gastrocolic reflex for defecation approximately 15 to 30 minutes postprandial. Because the puppy may not have full anal sphincter control, it would be wise for the owner to take the pup outside to eliminate within that time period. It will save the owner having to clean up "accidents."

Nutrients

We've talked about digesting and absorbing nutrients. However, we really haven't discussed what those nutrients are. The basic classifications of nutrients are (1) water, (2) carbohydrates, (3) lipids, (4) proteins, (5) vitamins, and (6) minerals. Those nutrients that provide sources of energy are the carbohydrates, lipids, and proteins.

Water is a very important nutrient. Approximately 70% of the body weight is from water. Animals and people may be able to live for periods of time without food, but without sufficient volumes of water, an animal dehydrates and eventually dies. (Remember, answers to important physiologic and health questions are often water or liver.)

Carbohydrates provide the most easily digested nutrients for energy. They are basically compounds made of simple and complex sugar molecules. When digested, it is the simple sugar molecule that is readily absorbed and used by the body. Carbohydrates in the diet usually come from various grains, like wheat or corn. These grains, fed as supplements to our herbivores, are referred to as concentrates. Why concentrates? Because those little grains contain an abundance of energy from carbohydrates and fats in a very tiny, compact, concentrated package.

Lipids provide the most concentrated form of energy. Lipids are jam-packed with calories. Comparing lipids with carbohydrates, in terms of energy, is like comparing premium, high-octane gasoline with regular unleaded. They both provide usable fuel to burn, but performance is much better with the high-octane. For those animals who are under excessive physical demands, like herding and tracking dogs or performance horses, additional fats in the diet help meet their energy needs without their having to consume excessively large volumes of food. Plus, fats will provide a sustained "burn," unlike the "flash in the pan" provided by carbohydrates. Lipids are also necessary components of many cellular membranes, as are proteins.

Proteins can also be used for energy. The digestive process needed to achieve usable energy from protein is complex. Protein molecules are huge and need to be broken down to an amino acid size to be used for many things. Another important use of proteins, beyond providing an energy source, is to provide building blocks (amino acids) for ongoing tissue growth and repair. Protein in the diet must be of good quality to supply the needs of the body. Old boot leather or rawhide does not contain high-quality protein and essential amino acids for domestic animals. High-quality protein must come from good meats, dairy products, or some plants (particularly legumes, like soy and alfalfa hay—the later the cutting of hay, the higher the protein content). Cats are unique in that they require the essential amino acid taurine in their diets. In addition, cats require higher amounts of protein in their diets than do most other domestic animals. This is because cats are true carnivores and are designed to derive large amounts of energy from meat protein.

Vitamins are organic compounds found naturally in many different sources of food. They are required for many of the normal metabolic processes of the body. Vitamins are classified as either water soluble or lipid soluble. Water-soluble vitamins include vitamin C and the B complex vitamins. Vitamin C is found naturally in many fruits and other plants. Unlike people, most domestic animals do not require dietary supplementation of vitamin C because their bodies synthesize the compound. One common pet that does require vitamin C supplementation is the guinea pig. Vitamin C is an unstable vitamin that is easily destroyed by oxidation or by exposure to heat or light. Consequently, fresh sources of vitamin C must be provided for guinea pigs. These sources include citrus fruits, cabbage, tomatoes, potatoes, and leafy green vegetables. Vitamin C is important for numerous metabolic processes and particularly for the production of connective tissues. B complex vitamins are found in numerous meats, fruits, vegetables, and grains. B vitamins, remember, are one of the principle by-products of microbial fermentation in our herbivores. B vitamins are important for normal cellular metabolism. Lipid-soluble vitamins include vitamins A, D, E, and K. Each of the lipid-soluble vitamins can be stored in large amounts by the liver, except vitamin K; only limited amounts of vitamin K may be stored there. Because the body can store lipid-soluble vitamins, over-supplementation with them could result in toxic side effects. Vitamin A is readily found in eggs, fish, liver, dairy foods, and vegetable sources. Many animals, including humans, can synthesize vitamin A from beta-carotene (found in yellowish fruits and vegetables). Cats lack this ability, however, and must be provided with vitamin A directly from their food. Vitamin A is important for healthy eyes. Vitamin D also is synthesized by the body on exposure to sunlight. Vitamin D is important for the growth and maintenance of healthy bones. Dietary vitamin D is found in milk, eggs, and fish. Vitamin E helps maintain healthy hematopoietic and reproductive systems. It is found in eggs, liver, and many grains. It is considered to be an antioxidant because it tends to bind readily to oxygen, preventing oxidation of other compounds, like vitamins A and C. Vitamin K is important for the production of clotting factors for the blood and is found in eggs as well as many green, leafy plants, like spinach.

Minerals are inorganic elements and compounds, like iron, phosphorus, calcium, and so on. Iron is critical for the oxygen-carrying ability of the blood. Calcium and phosphorus are important for bone homeostasis. Calcium is poorly absorbed from the digestive tract, whereas phosphorus is readily absorbed. Inappropriate amounts or an inappropriate Ca/P ratio has a deleterious impact on bone growth and maintenance. Selenium is a trace mineral required in the diets of herbivores that is important for muscle integrity. Plants grown in selenium-rich soils will contain this essential nutrient. So, forages fed to horses and ruminants from these plants will contain sufficient selenium. In selenium-deficient areas, feeds for our hoofstock must be supplemented with selenium (usually through trace mineral salts). Michigan is an example of a selenium-deficient state.

Fortunately for small animal pet owners, dietary formulation has been simplified. Pet food companies formulate and package foods to meet the nutritional needs of domestic dogs and cats. Each prepackaged diet is completely balanced, including just the right amounts of carbohydrates, lipids, proteins, vitamins, and minerals to meet the pet's needs. Different formulations have been developed for young, middle-aged, active, and geriatric animals. Still other formulations have been developed specifically to help manage particular companion animal diseases. Provided an owner selects a name-brand diet appropriate for the age, activity level, and species of his or her pet, the commercial food should meet the nutritional needs of the pet. Supplementation usually is not required and in many situations is not advisable. The notion that dogs and cats need dietary variety is untrue. In fact, abrupt dietary changes usually result in gastroenteric upset and diarrhea. Abrupt dietary changes for horses usually result in either colic (abdominal pain) or laminitis (a serious foot condition to be discussed in the integumentary chapter) or both. Both colic and laminitis can be life-threatening to the horse. In dairy cattle, an abrupt dietary change could result in a life-threatening displaced abomasum. Gradual dietary changes and control of excesses are essential practices for any animal. Excesses lead to disease, like obesity, which may lead to other diseases, like diabetes, degenerative joint disease, or even cancer. Excesses can also lead to life-threatening disease like rumen bloat in ruminants, when they consume large quantities of grain at one time. Think "excess within control," when it comes to feeding anything beyond an animal's principal diet. In companion animals, that principal diet should be a well-balanced commercial food. In herbivores, that principal diet should be roughages. In all animals, a readily available, fresh water supply is also essential.

Digestive Pathophysiology and Disease

Periodontal Disease

Periodontal disease is a progressive disorder of the mouth. It is the most common oral disease of dogs and cats and it is one of the leading contributors to cardiac and renal disease in these animals. Periodontal disease begins with the accumulation of plaque (plak), which is an invisible film of saliva, food, and bacteria that coats the teeth and mucous membranes. The bacteria in plaque, if left unchecked, etch away the enamel and inflame and destroy periodontal tissues. Gingivitis is the first symptom of periodontal disease. Plaque is easily removed by brushing or by abrasives in the diet. If the plaque is removed and gingivitis is eliminated, periodontal disease will be stopped dead in its tracks. If plaque is allowed to build up, it begins to thicken into a more solid substance called tartar or calculus. (No, this calculus has nothing to do with mathematics.) It takes only 12 hours for plaque to begin to harden into tartar. Tartar buildup along the gingival margin and in the gingival sulcus begins to force the gingiva away from the neck of the tooth. Bacteria continue their vandalism under the protective covering of the tartar, destroying gingival and periodontal attachments to the tooth. Even in the absence of tartar, proliferating bacteria will carry on their destructive work. The tartar merely provides a better environment for the bacterial activity. Calculus mineralizes into rock-hard concretions that continue to accumulate over the teeth, providing an even more protective cover for the destructive bacteria below. Gingivitis and periodontitis worsen. Painful ulcers may develop anywhere on the oral mucosa. Periodontal ligaments and jaw bone are slowly and progressively destroyed. As a result the gingiva recedes, exposing the sensitive roots and intensifying the oral pain. Teeth become loose and may be lost. Abscesses may develop around the roots, accelerating the destructive process. Because the roots of premolars 108 and 208 are so close to the maxillary sinus, periapical abscesses of these teeth often progress into sinusitis and abscessation of the sinus itself. A maxillary sinus abscess such as this may eventually rupture through onto the face, creating a nasty, purulent (pus-filled) draining wound just beneath the eye of the animal. Are you disgusted yet? You should be. Recognize that once periodontal disease sticks its grimy foot in the door, so to speak, there is no stopping it. Professional and home care may slow the disease process, but it will not be stopped once it's got a foothold. If periodontal disease is to be stopped, it must be stopped at the outset of gingivitis. As awful as this oral disease is, it does not restrict itself to the mouth. As if the dysphagia from the stomatitis is not bad enough, bacteria will enter the bloodstream through the inflamed oral tissues. From there, vital organs like the heart, liver, and kidneys will be under attack. Cardiac, hepatic, and renal disease will rob these animals of their health and well-being and lead to an early grave.

Periodontal disease can be prevented through appropriate oral hygiene. In general, on an annual basis, it is recommended that dogs and cats be examined and, if necessary, receive dental prophylaxis (pro"fĭ-lak'sis) provided by veterinary professionals. Some pets may require more frequent visits (particularly if they do not engage in home care). The prophylaxis includes close inspection of the oral cavity and careful charting of all abnormalities, including gingivitis, calculus accumulations, gingival recession, dental wear, fractures, carious lesions, and tooth mobility. Gingival sulci are measured to determine the condition of the periodontal ligaments. Then, scaling (scraping off) of the tartar buildup from the crowns is performed. It is critical that the cleaning does not end here. One of the most important features of the professional cleaning process is polishing of the crowns and any exposed roots with an abrasive paste. The polishing is important to remove pits and grooves on the surface of the teeth (both natural and created by bacteria). The polished surfaces give future plaque and tartar less of a foothold. Oral care does not end here.

It is *essential* that owners play an active role in the prevention of periodontal disease. Their home care program should start as soon as they acquire a new puppy or kitten. The most basic home dental care program should include brushing. A soft toothbrush with veterinary toothpaste should be used. (Human toothpaste should not be used because it contains fluoride, which is toxic to pets.) Optimally, owners should brush their pets' teeth twice daily. Remember, it takes only 12 hours for plaque to begin to harden into tartar. Beyond brushing, owners have a plethora of options available to them to help them maintain oral health in their pets. There are a number of veterinary diets and treats that are designed for "tartar control." Of course, these require the pet to chew the food or treat. Veterinarians can prescribe various oral rinses and other applications that will help reduce bacterial populations. Certainly dogs who engage in "recreational" activities by chewing on toys and rawhides will aid in their own removal of plaque. No matter what additional activities, materials, or protocols are employed, *nothing* can replace the benefits of brushing. To use an old phrase, "an ounce of prevention is worth a pound of cure." Prevention of periodontal disease is the key to maintaining healthy teeth, mouths, and systemic health of our pets.

Gastroenteritis

Let's see, gastroenteritis. Can you say vomiting and diarrhea? (Well, the vomiting part can't happen in horses or ruminants. Oh, but they sure can have diarrhea and lots of it!) Inflammation may occur anywhere along the digestive tract. All of our domestic animals have a variety of infectious diseases that may inflame a portion or multiple portions of the GI (gastrointestinal) tract. From tiny bacteria and viruses to parasites and foreign bodies, there are a plethora of inflammatory etiologies (causes). "Who" the culprit is and where it is conducting its "dirty work" will determine some of the symptoms and severity of disease, as well as how we treat the patient. Yes, if we inflame the digestive tract, we have two main responses—vomiting and diarrhea. But, do we have one or both? Is anorexia associated with it? Is there extreme abdominal pain, as is often the case with pancreatitis or hepatitis? So, in addition to our physical assessment of the patient, we may need to diagnostically determine the cause. Think about it. Treating a patient, who has melenic diarrhea caused by a small intestinal parasite, with antidiarrheal agents may help resolve some of the symptoms temporarily. However, it will not eliminate the cause. The melenic diarrhea will persist. Plus, to do so could potentially endanger the animal. Bloodsucking parasites like hookworms in small animals and strongyles in large animals can cause severe, even lethal, blood loss. (By the way, the feces in these animals is black due to the partially digested blood from the proximal digestive tract.) The same is true for an animal with mucoid, hematochezic diarrhea, due to the colitis from whipworms. We have to attack the worms before we can effectively resolve the diarrhea. Of course, you do realize that part of the diagnostic plan may include physically examining the feces. Eeeeuw! It's a dirty job, but somebody has to do it. So many clues may be not only in the material itself, but how it was deposited. It's like Crime Scene Investigation. Only, most of our "criminals" are microscopic. Ah, but they do leave telltale clues that we must pursue by asking and then answering many questions. Is the defecation urgent and a small volume, as is so characteristic of colitis? Is it melenic? Is it steathorreic? Is it mucoid? How does it smell? (Okay, I know what you're thinking ... none of it smells good.

True. But believe me, certain diseases create such distinctive, foul odors that they make you think something crawled up in there and died.) We might even be able to find parasites, grossly or microscopically (i.e., grossly, meaning visible with the naked eye, not disgusting). Yes, there are times when we cannot determine the specific cause. In such cases we simply have to give supportive care to replace fluids lost through emesis and diarrhea. (Dehydration is one of the most common causes of death in animals with gastroenteritis.) Antiemetics and antidiarrheals may also provide the animal with temporary relief from their misery, until the disease runs its course.

Gastric Dilatation Volvulus

Gastric dilatation volvulus[14] (GDV) or "bloat," as it is commonly called, is a life-threatening disorder that most often affects deep-chested dog breeds, like Great Danes, Doberman Pinschers, German Shepherds, and other such dogs. It is an emergency! We must act on these dogs quickly or they will die.

How does GDV develop? There are many things that may lead up to its development, but the following is the most common scenario. The dog consumes a large meal or large volume of water and then engages in physical activity, like playing.

The weight of the gastric contents makes the stomach more pendulous. Because of the large structure of the caudal chest and cranial abdomen, the pendulous stomach has room to move and may flip over on its own axis (volvulus). It's like twisting a candy wrapper at both ends. Nothing can enter or exit the stomach, because the gastroesophageal and pyloric openings are twisted shut. The classic presentation of such a dog is nonproductive retching. That is, they go through all of the agonizing motions of emesis, but nothing is evacuated from the stomach. Blood flow to the stomach and spleen is also impaired. Gas and toxins accumulate in the stomach, causing it to distend (bloat). The stomach continues to expand until it is so stretched it sounds like a basketball when tapped (i.e., tympany or a "ping"). The extreme pressures exerted by the overdistended stomach traps blood in the mesenteric and abdominal vessels, reducing the overall available blood volume and leading to hypovolemic shock. Cardiac arrhythmias frequently develop. The huge, distended stomach will also impair movement of the diaphragm. The animal will become dyspneic, hypoxic, and hypercapneic. (These dogs deteriorate *rapidly*.) The stomach of such a dog must be decompressed (i.e., pressure relieved) as soon as possible. Passage of an orogastric tube is generally attempted first. Unfortunately, the volvulus typically prevents passage of the tube. A trocar (often a large-bore needle) may then be used for temporary pressure relief, before taking the dog to surgery. Yes, surgery will be required to detorse (untwist) the stomach. If portions of the stomach have become necrotic, a partial gastrectomy may be performed. The spleen may be removed too, if it appears necrotic. Dogs who have experienced GDV once are more likely to experience it again. To reduce the risk of this occurring to the dog in the future, a gastropexy may be performed. Gastropexy is not foolproof.

---

[14]Volvulus (vol'vu-lus); from [L. *volvere*, to twist around]; gastric dilatation volvulus is a twisting of the stomach, accompanied by excessive dilation with gas.

The surgical attachments of the stomach to the abdominal wall can be broken, leading to another torsion (i.e., volvulus). The immediate postoperative (after surgery) period for these dogs is critical. The surgery may have been a success, but the dog could still die of peritonitis, cardiac arrhythmias, or a coagulopathy (i.e., disseminated intravascular coagulation). If the dog survives following the surgery, it will be very important for the pet owner to make some lifestyle changes for the dog. Otherwise, GDV may happen again. The next time, the dog may not be so lucky. So, some of the measures that will help prevent recurrence are (1) feeding smaller, more frequent meals; (2) discouraging drinking of large volumes of water, especially following a meal; and (3) prohibiting play or exercise for at least a couple hours postprandial.

Common Ruminant Diseases

Displaced abomasum (DA) is a syndrome that most often occurs in dairy cattle. As with GDV in the dog, there are a number of factors that may contribute to displacement of the abomasum. First, the patient is usually a cow who has recently given birth. If she is a high milk-producer, she is at greater risk because she will experience greater changes in critical electrolytes like calcium. Finally, to keep up with her new energy needs for milk production, the farmer may dramatically change her feed. (We said earlier that abrupt dietary changes are not good practice.) The combination of all of these factors will reduce abomasal motility and slow its emptying. Gases will easily accumulate in this flaccid abomasum. Before you know it, there is so much gas within it that the abomasum "floats" up from the ventral abdomen. Left displacement is the most common. Regardless which side it displaces to, the abomasum will no longer be able to have ingesta pass through it; the entrance and exit are effectively pinched tightly closed by the displacement and distention. Her symptoms at first will be subtle, including anorexia, decreased milk production, and reduced fecal volume. Ruminations will cease. (This is very bad because it will lead to the death of all of our happy microbes in the rumen.) The distended abomasum will cause a bulge in the paralumbar fossa. As with the GDV in the dog, tympany (a "ping") will be present when the area is percussed. Surgery is often required to replace the abomasum to its correct location on the ventral abdomen. The laparotomy will be performed with the cow standing. Yes, standing. A regional nerve block will provide anesthesia for the surgical entry through the flank. Excess gasses will be evacuated from the abomasum, before it is returned to the ventral abdomen. To help in preventing future displacement, either an abomasopexy or an omentopexy may be performed. Postoperatively, rumen function may need a "jump start," by taking rumen juices from a healthy cow and giving them to the recovering cow (through, more or less, an "orogastric" tube).

Another common problem in cattle is reticulitis or "hardware disease," as it is commonly called. What could hardware possibly have to do with cattle, you ask? Well, it's not hardware like wrenches and hammers that we're talking about. It's metal objects like nails and wire and such. We said earlier that ruminants may consume metal foreign bodies. If they do, we said that those heavy objects will frequently settle into the reticulum. Loose, sharp metal objects may be very irritating to the wall of the reticulum, leading to reticulitis. Big deal?

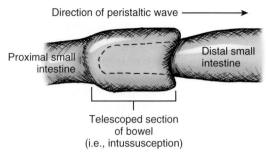

Direction of peristaltic wave ⟶

Proximal small intestine

Distal small intestine

Telescoped section
of bowel
(i.e., intussusception)

FIGURE 12-18   Intussusception schematic.

Yes, it can be. It can be a very big deal if those sharp objects penetrate the wall of the reticulum and migrate cranially. Look at Figure 12-13 again. Do you see what lies just cranial to the reticulum there in the thoracic cavity? That's right, the heart. Irritating or penetrating the heart with a sharp metal object under any circumstances is not good. Plus, there are critical nerve branches, like the vagus, that may also be irritated. If that happens, the cow may lose parasympathetic input to the digestive tract, permanently. Get the point? Hardware disease can be lethal. So, what can be done about it? Nothing may be possible once it happens. But we may be able to prevent it. Can we keep cows from consuming metal objects? Well, we can certainly minimize the hazards that they might consume around the barn. Even if a cow does consume a few nails or something, we can keep those objects from penetrating and migrating through the wall of the reticulum. How, you ask? By having the cow swallow a large magnet. (No, not one of those big horseshoe-shaped magnets like they have in cartoons. It's shaped more or less like a giant capsule—smooth, cylindrical, and rounded at the ends, usually a few inches long.) All of the little bits of metal that she's consumed will wind up stuck to the magnet in one large metallic blob. Blobs of metal are far less likely to severely traumatize the reticulum and certainly less likely to penetrate it or other structures. No, the magnet will not be removed. She gets to keep it for the rest of her life.

Bowel Obstruction

Thinking of foreign bodies, I can't think of a better way to obstruct the digestive tract of a puppy or kitten better than with a small rubber ball, rock, or knee-high stocking. Puppies and kittens explore their newfound worlds with their mouths. Many times they will ingest inappropriate objects. Unfortunately, those objects may obstruct the esophagus, pylorus, small intestine, or colon. If the object is big and significantly distends the bowel once it's wedged in, the tissues in the area may become necrotic. Sometimes, especially with linear objects like ribbon or a knee-high stocking, the natural peristalsis of the intestinal tract will wind up "walking" along the object until the bowel actually begins to envelope itself, creating an intussusception (Fig. 12-18). The intussusception will obstruct that section of bowel and necrosis of the tissues will occur. Removal of foreign bodies is essential if they are obstructing or have a high potential of obstructing. How the removal is approached depends on the condition of the patient and the location

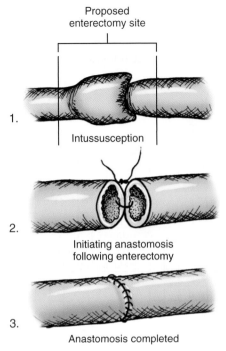

Proposed
enterectomy site

1.

Intussusception

2.

Initiating anastomosis
following enterectomy

3.

Anastomosis completed

FIGURE 12-19   Anastomosis schematic.

of problem. For instance, if a little rubber ball is in the stomach, gastroscopy would be the most efficient and least traumatic way to remove the ball. Unfortunately, if the object is not within reach of an endoscope, a laparotomy will be required. Obviously, there is far more risk of complications, like peritonitis, from an enterotomy than an endoscopic procedure. That risk increases if the section of necrotic bowel requires an enterectomy or colectomy. Once the diseased section is removed, an anastomosis[15] will join the two healthy free ends of intestine together (Fig. 12-19). Great care must be taken by the surgeon to ensure that the anastomosis does not leak bowel contents into the abdomen. Wow, that's a lot of work, expense, and endangerment of the pet. Can't things like this be prevented? You bet they can. All the owners have to do is pet-proof the home.

Prevention—what a great concept. There are innumerable digestive diseases in our domestic animals. Many of them can be prevented. Infectious viral diseases can be prevented through vaccination. Appropriate nutrition can prevent a plethora of diseases, far beyond the digestive tract itself. Most of the disorders discussed in this chapter are preventable. Can we prevent all disease of the digestive system? No, that's not realistic. But we sure can make a big dent in disease, if we just use a little common sense and educate our clientele.

---

[15]Anastomosis (ah-nas″to-mo′sis); from [Gr. *anastomosis*, opening, outlet].

SELF-TEST

Using the previous information in this chapter, complete the following crossword puzzle using the most appropriate medical term(s). Do not use abbreviations or common names unless requested.

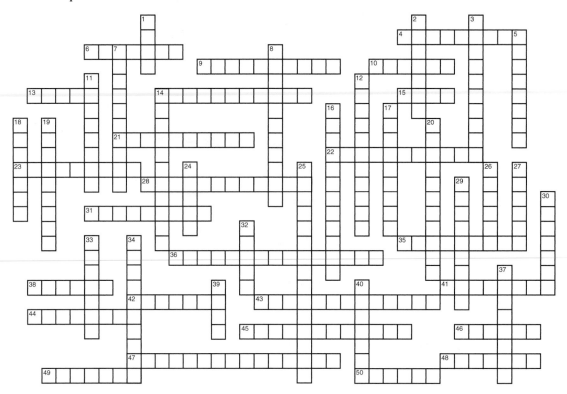

ACROSS

4	Difficulty eating
6	A state of fatty blood
9	Beneath the tongue
10	Resembling mucus
13	The largest fermentative chamber of a bovine stomach
14	Muscular contractions of the bowel that move ingesta along
15	The substance produced by the liver that helps emulsify fats in the digestive process
21	A drug that deters vomiting
22	Fixation of the abomasum to the peritoneal wall
23	Inflammation of the tongue
28	After a meal
31	Surgical removal of a portion of the colon
35	An abnormally large colon
36	Inflammation of the stomach and intestines

38   The hardest substance of the body that covers the crowns of carnivorous teeth
41   The proximal-most segment of small intestine
42   A starch enzyme
43   Excessive salivation
44   Twisting of a portion of bowel
45   The microbial process of the equine cecum and bovine rumen that produces by-products such as methane, CO_2, and volatile fatty acids
46   A suffix indicating surgical removal of a part
47   Telescoping of bowel onto itself
48   The "gums"
49   Pertaining to black feces
50   A fat enzyme

DOWN
1   A suffix meaning "to cut"
2   The distal sphincter of the stomach
3   Abdominal incision
5   The fourth chamber of a ruminant stomach; the "true" stomach
7   _____ enzymes, such as amylase, lipase, and trypsin that are secreted into the small bowel for digestion
8   Surgical connection between two hollow structures, such as loops of bowel
11   A state of no appetite
12   A surgically created hole in the stomach
14   Pertaining to surrounding teeth
16   Bloody feces
17   Inflammation of the liver
18   Pertaining to the tongue
19   The valve located between the ileum and the cecum
20   Eating feces
24   A suffix indicating creation of an opening or "mouth"
25   A hepatic function in which new sugars are produced
26   Pertaining to the cheek
27   The porous bony material of a tooth surrounding the pulp cavity
29   The "honeycombed" chamber of an ovine stomach
30   The longest portion of small intestine
32   A suffix meaning "to view"
33   Jaundice
34   A tube that is passed from the mouth to the stomach, for delivery of medication or for evacuation of the stomach
37   Pertaining to dead tissue
39   A suffix indicating surgical fixation (suturing) of a structure
40   A lymphatic vessel of a villus used for fat absorption

CHAPTER 13

The Urinary System

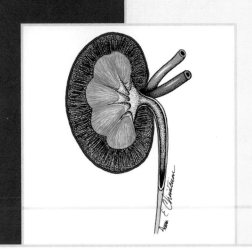

GOALS AND OBJECTIVES

By the conclusion of this chapter, the student will be able to:

1. Recognize common root words, prefixes, and suffixes related to the urinary system.
2. Divide simple and compound words into their respective parts.
3. Recognize, correctly pronounce, and appropriately use common medical terms related to the urinary system.
4. Demonstrate an understanding of urinary anatomy.
5. Demonstrate an understanding of renal physiology, with regard to urine production, water homeostasis, waste excretion, and electrolyte homeostasis.
6. Demonstrate familiarity with common urinary diseases and their pathophysiology.

Note: It is strongly recommended that the hematopoietic, respiratory, cardiovascular, and neurology chapters be completed before this chapter.

INTRODUCTION TO RELATED TERMS

Divide each of the following terms into its respective parts ("R," root; "P," prefix; "S," suffix; "CV," combining vowel).

1. **Renal** (adj.)   (R) _____ (S) _____
   renal (re'nal; pertaining to the kidney)

2. **Prerenal** (adj.)   (P) _____ (R) _____ (S) _____
   prerenal (pre-re'nal; pertaining to before the kidney)

3. **Postrenal** (adj.)   (P) _____ (R) _____ (S) _____
   postrenal (post-re'nal; pertaining to after the kidney)

4. **Retroperitoneal** (adj.)   (P) _____ (CV) _____ (R) _____ (S) _____
   retroperitoneal (re"tro-per"ĭ-to-ne'al, ret"ro-per"ĭ-to-ne'al; pertaining to behind the peritoneum)

5. **Cystitis** (n.)   (R) _____   (S) _____
   cystitis (sis-ti′tis; inflammation of the bladder; i.e., inflammation of the urinary bladder)

6. **Nephritis** (n.)   (R) _____   (S) _____
   nephritis (ně-fri′tis; inflammation of the kidney)

7. **Pyelonephritis** (n.)   (R) _____   (CV) _____   (R) _____   (S) _____
   pyelonephritis (pi″ě-lo-ně-fri′tis; inflammation of the kidney and its pelvis)

8. **Intravenous** (adj.) **pyelogram** (n.) (P) _____   (R) _____   (S) _____
                                          (R) _____   (CV) _____   (S) _____
   intravenous pyelogram (in″trah-ve′nus pi′ě-lo-gram″; pertaining to within a vein/to record the pelvis; clinically refers to a radiographic procedure in which intravenous radiopaque dye is used to visualize the renal pelvis and other urinary structures; abbr. IVP)

9. **Cystography** (n.)   (R) _____   (CV) _____   (S) _____
   cystography (sis-tog′rah-fe; recording of the bladder; i.e., clinically refers to a radiographic procedure in which contrast media is used to visualize the urinary bladder)

10. **Pneumocystogram** (n.)   (R) _____   (CV) _____   (R) _____
                                           (CV) _____   (S) _____
    pneumocystogram (noo″mo-sis′to-gram; a record of air of the bladder; i.e., clinically refers to a radiographic procedure in which air is injected into the urinary bladder)

11. **Retrograde** (adj.) **urethrocystogram** (n.)   (P) _____   (CV) _____   (S) _____
                                               (R) _____   (CV) _____   (R) _____
                                               (CV) _____   (S) _____
    retrograde urethrocystogram (ret′ro-grād u-re″thro-sis′to-gram; a backward recording of the urethra and bladder; i.e., clinically refers to a radiographic procedure in which radiopaque dye is injected through the urethra to visualize both the urethra and the urinary bladder)

12. **Cystocentesis** (n.)   (R) _____   (CV) _____   (S) _____
    cystocentesis (sis″to-sen-te′sis; puncture of the bladder; refers to the clinical procedure in which urine is withdrawn from the bladder using a syringe and needle, by puncture through the abdominal wall)

13. **Urethritis** (n.)   (R) _____   (S) _____
    urethritis (u″re-thri′tis; inflammation of the urethra)

14. **Urolithiasis** (n.)   (R) _____   (CV) _____   (R) _____
                                           (CV) _____   (S) _____
    urolithiasis (u″ro-lĭ-thi′ah-sis; a condition of urinary stones)

15. **Hematuria** (n.)   (R) _____   (R) _____   (S) _____
    hematuria (hem″ah-tu′re-ah, he″mah-tu′re-ah; a condition of bloody urine)

16. **Cystotomy** (n.)   (R) _____   (CV) _____   (S) _____
    cystotomy (sis-tot′o-me; to cut the bladder; clinically refers to a surgical procedure in which the bladder is incised)

17. **Polyuria** (n.)   (P) _____   (R) _____   (S) _____
    polyuria (pol″e-u′re-ah; a condition of much urine; clinically refers to passage of a large volume of urine in a given period of time)

18. **Oliguria** (n.)   (P) _____ (R) _____ (S) _____
    oliguria (ol″ĭ-gu′re-ah; a condition of small urination; clinically refers to a small volume of urine in relation to fluid intake)

19. **Pollakiuria** (n.)   (P) _____ (CV) _____ (R) _____ (S) _____
    pollakiuria (pol″ah-ke-u′re-ah, pol″ak-ĭ-u′re-ah; a condition of frequent urination)

20. **Dysuria** (n.)   (P) _____ (R) _____ (S) _____
    dysuria (dis-u″re-ah; a condition of difficult urination)

21. **Anuria** (n.)   (P) _____ (R) _____ (S) _____
    anuria (ah-nu′re-ah, an-u′re-ah; a condition without urination)

22. **Nephrotoxic** (n.)   (R) _____ (CV) _____ (R) _____ (S) _____
    nephrotoxic (nef″ro-tok′sik; pertaining to a kidney toxin [poison])

23. **Uremia** (n.)   (R) _____ (R) _____ (S) _____
    uremia (u-re′me-ah; a condition of [urea] in blood; clinically refers to retention of nitrogenous wastes in the blood that should be excreted by the kidneys and the systemically toxic condition produced)

24. **Azotemia** (n.)   (R) _____ (R) _____ (S) _____
    azotemia (az″o-te′me-ah, a-zo-te′me-ah; a condition of nitrogen in the blood; clinically refers to excess urea and other nitrogenous compounds in the blood)

25. **Proteinuria** (n.)   (R) _____ (R) _____ (S) _____
    proteinuria (pro″te-in-u′re-ah; a condition of protein in the urine)

26. **Glycosuria** (n.)   (R) _____ (R) _____ (S) _____
    glycosuria (gli″ko-su′re-ah; a condition of glucose in the urine)

27. **Uropoiesis** (n.)   (R) _____ (CV) _____ (R) _____ (S) _____
    uropoiesis (u″ro-poi-e′sis; the process of producing urine)

28. **Urethrostomy** (n.)   (R) _____ (CV) _____ (S) _____
    urethrostomy (u″re-thros′to-me; to create a "mouth" in the urethra; clinically refers to a surgical procedure in which a permanent opening is made in the urethra to facilitate urination)

29. **Glomerular** (adj.)   (R) _____ (S) _____
    glomerular (glo-mer′u-lar; pertaining to a glomerulus; [L. *glomerulus,* dim. of *glomus,* ball])

30. **Peritubular** (adj.)   (P) _____ (R) _____ (S) _____
    peritubular (per″ĭ-tu′bu-lar; pertaining to around a tubule)

31. **Nocturia** (n.)   (R) _____ (R) _____ (S) _____
    nocturia (nok-tu′re-ah; a condition of night urine; i.e., frequency of urination at night)

32. **Cystalgia** (n.)   (R) _____ (R) _____ (S) _____
    cystalgia (sis-tal′jah; a condition of bladder pain)

33. **Hydronephrosis** (n.)   (R) _____ (CV) _____ (R) _____
                                     (CV) _____ (S) _____
    hydronephrosis (hi″dro-nĕ-fro′sis; a condition of a watery kidney; i.e., distention of the kidney with urine, usually from obstruction of a ureter or the urethra)

34. **Hypertonic** (adj.)   (P) _____ (R) _____ (S) _____
    hypertonic (hi″per-ton′ik; pertaining to excessive tonicity; i.e., osmotic pressure)

35. **Hypotonic** (adj.)   (P) _____ (R) _____ (S) _____
    hypotonic (hi-po-ton′ik; pertaining to low tonicity; i.e., osmotic pressure)

36. **Isotonic** (adj.)   (P) _____ (R) _____ (S) _____
    isotonic (i″so-ton′ik; pertaining to equal tonicity; i.e., osmotic pressure)

37. **Isosthenuric** (adj.)   (P) _____ (R) _____ (R) _____ (S) _____
    isosthenuric (i″sos-the-nu′rik; pertaining to equal strength urine [Gr. *sthenos,* strength];
    i.e., urine that has the same osmotic pressure as plasma, because the urine has not been
    concentrated by the kidneys)

URINARY ANATOMY AND PHYSIOLOGY

Urinary System Anatomy

The kidneys are amazing little "water treatment plants." Let's begin by taking a look at their plumbing. The kidneys lie retroperitoneal, near the dorsocranial abdominal cavity (Fig. 13-1). The right kidney tends to be on the right dorso-lateral abdomen, slightly caudal to or partially under the last rib. It is typically attached fairly tightly along the dorsum. The left kidney is usually found on the left dorsolateral abdomen, slightly more caudal than the right kidney. It also tends to be more loosely attached than the right kidney, making it easier to palpate in companion animals. An easy phrase to help keep the positioning of each kidney straight is "righty tighty, lefty loosey and last." Each kidney receives blood supply through a renal artery. The arterial blood is full of impurities that the kidneys will need to filter out. This process will be discussed later. Then the renal veins carry "purified" blood back into general circulation.

Obviously, there needs to be plumbing connected to the treatment plant, to carry away the dirty "wastewater" to a holding tank. So, attached to each kidney is a ureter. These fine, small tubes carry urine to the urinary bladder (see Fig. 13-1). The urinary bladder is found in the caudal abdominal cavity, very near the pelvis. When the bladder is empty, it is found in the pubic area. As the bladder becomes full, it becomes more pendulous and progressively falls in a cranioventral direction in the peritoneal cavity. The bladder itself is composed of smooth muscle, and its interior is lined with stratified squamous epithelium. At the neck of the bladder is a sphincter, used to control evacuation of urine.

The urethra is a tube connecting the urinary bladder with the external environment (Figs. 13-2 and 13-3). As the urethra leaves the bladder it passes dorsal to the pelvis before progressing to its distal point, the urethral orifice. In male dogs, the urethra must pass through a bony structure in the penis (i.e., the os penis[1]). In addition, the prostate gland (a part of the male reproductive tract in all animals) surrounds the proximal urethra. This area, as well as the os penis and the curvature over the pelvis, creates natural areas for potential stricture,

---

[1]Os penis (os pe′nis); from [L. *os,* bone + penis].

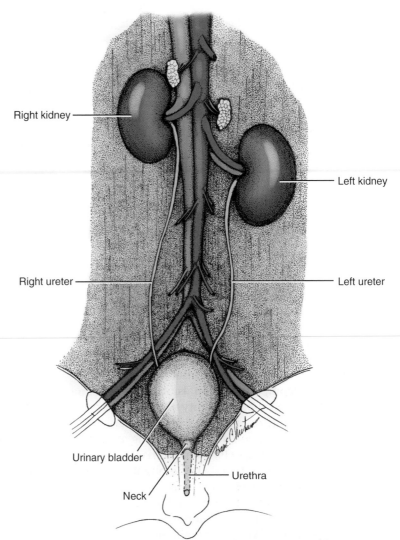

FIGURE 13-1   Urinary system (ventrodorsal view).

especially in animals prone to urolithiasis. Comparatively in male cats, the narrow, curved distal urethra commonly obstructs with uroliths. Urolithiasis will be discussed later in this chapter.

Renal Anatomy

Okay, now we get to take a close look at the intricate plumbing of the water treatment plant itself. The kidney is encased in a renal capsule, composed of tough, fibrous connective tissue (Fig.13-4). The renal cortex,[2] which is closest to

[2]Renal cortex (re'nal kor'teks); cortex from [L. *cortex,* shell].

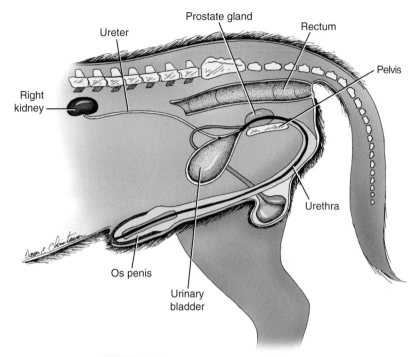

FIGURE 13-2 Canine male urinary tract.

the renal capsule, is the outermost functional portion of the kidney. The renal cortex contains billions of nephrons, the functional filtration units of the kidney. The renal medulla[3] is at the core of the kidney, surrounded by the renal cortex. The medulla is composed of numerous tubules that communicate with the other portions of the nephrons in the cortex and the collecting ducts, which lead to the renal pelvis (Figs. 13-4 and 13-5). Nephron components will be discussed in the next section. The renal pelvis merely serves as a large "funnel" to collect all of the urine from the numerous tubules and ducts to be passed onto the ureter.

Nephron and Uropoiesis

Here is where the "rubber meets the road," so to speak. To be in keeping with our analogy of the water treatment plant, we need to look at each functional component of the operation. As stated earlier, the nephron is an individual functional unit of the kidney (see Fig. 13-5). The ultimate purpose of each nephron is to purify the blood, ensure adequate chemical contents (e.g., water and electrolytes), and efficiently discard wastes. Each nephron is structured as a series of filters and tubes that serve to keep essential elements for the body and excrete potentially toxic wastes (particularly nitrogenous wastes like ammonia and urea). Failure to filter such wastes will result in azotemia and eventually uremia. Fresh, oxygenated blood arrives at the kidney and is pumped

---

[3]Renal medulla (re′nal mĕ-dul′ah); from [L. *medulla*, inmost part].

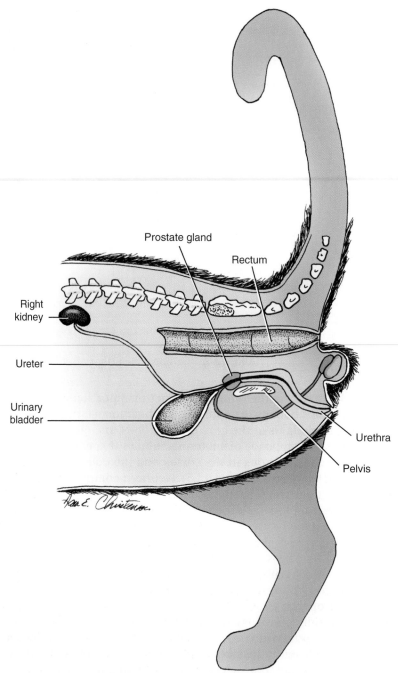

FIGURE 13-3 Feline male urinary tract.

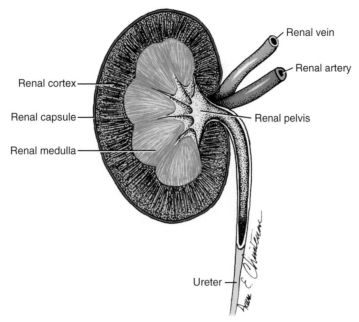

FIGURE 13-4   Sagittal kidney.

through billions of glomeruli. A glomerulus is simply a twisted bundle of highly permeable capillaries between an afferent and an efferent arteriole, and is surrounded by a spheroid structure called Bowman's capsule. The glomerulus is a filter that relies largely on hydrostatic pressure[4] to make it work. That's right, sufficient blood pressure is absolutely critical for this first component of our water treatment facility. Too great a pressure (i.e., hypertension) will actually progressively destroy glomeruli, just as hypotension may cause the glomeruli to shut down. Both extremes in blood pressure can result in renal failure. In a normal glomerulus, sufficient blood pressure will result in filtration of the blood.

Is blood pressure a constant? No. So, what happens with fluctuations in blood pressure that may actually reduce filtration? There is an automatic, internal response mechanism that will compensate for reductions in arterial pressure. First, sensory devices will perceive a reduction in filtration. Immediately, vasodilation of the afferent arteriole will be stimulated. Then, the enzyme renin will cause a plasma protein (angiotensinogen) to form angiotensin I. Angiotensin I will rapidly be converted to angiotensin II. Big deal? Yes, it is a big deal! Angiotensin II is a vasoconstrictor that will stimulate constriction of the efferent arteriole. Vasoconstriction of the efferent arteriole causes blood to back up into the glomerulus. Voilà! We just increased glomerular hydrostatic pressure. This will give us a relatively stable filtration rate, in spite of fluctuations in arterial pressure. Other factors that influence glomerular filtration are plasma osmotic pressure and hydrostatic pressure of Bowman's capsule. How, you ask? Let's consider osmotic pressure first. Plasma

[4]Hydrostatic pressure (hi″dro-stat′ik); [*hydr(o)-*, water + Gr. *statikos*, standing]; hydrostatic pressure is the force exerted by a liquid to maintain a state of equilibrium.

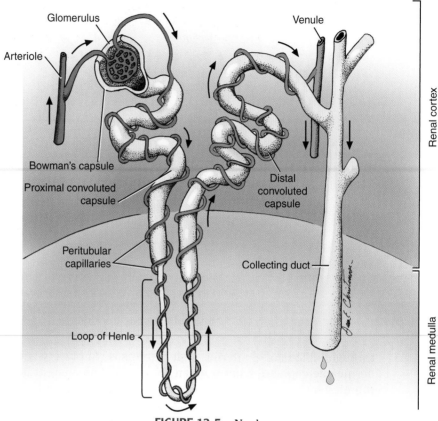

FIGURE 13-5   Nephron.

proteins basically give the blood "suck power," which is a tremendous, attractive force, like a huge sponge that keeps water in the bloodstream. Remember, plasma is mostly water. All of the plasma proteins act like little sponges to keep enough water in the plasma. So, strong osmotic pressure, as is seen in dehydration, will reduce the filtration through the glomerulus. In contrast, hypoproteinemia affords the plasma little "suck power," so hypoproteinemic animals will tend to produce more filtrate. So, hypoproteinemic animals may be polyuric.

Now, what about this hydrostatic pressure business with Bowman's capsule? Think about it. Bowman's capsule is sort of like a sink, and, in the case of glomerular function, filtration will dramatically slow if the sink is full, because there's no place to put the wastewater. Unlike the sink, however, Bowman's capsule within the kidney can't simply overflow onto the floor. A backup in the urinary plumbing will accumulate filtrate within the confines of the kidney and renal capsule. That makes it pretty obvious that if we simply obstruct the plumbing that drains the billions of Bowman's capsules (anywhere typically along a ureter or the urethra) we will have no place to put filtrate. So, rather than rapidly create hydronephrosis, we'd better significantly slow the production of filtrate. Isn't it great that there are built-in checks and balances to try to keep the body functioning normally? Well, let's carry on with normal renal function, shall we? The filtrate created is only the first step in the purification and recycling process. The glomerulus is a relatively nonselective purification filter. Large items like blood cells and plasma proteins cannot escape from normal glomeruli. (That's why proteinuria is such a big deal; it points to some significant renal problems if protein was able to escape.) Water and numerous dissolved substances (e.g., glucose, urea, electrolytes) will escape each glomerulus into Bowman's capsule. Leading from Bowman's capsule is an amazing plumbing creation. Okay, so it's just a series of pipes (tubes). Oh, but these are no ordinary tubes. Nearest Bowman's capsule is the proximal convoluted[5] tubule. Aha! Now we really go to work on the recycling process. The proximal convoluted tubule is important for reabsorption of water and sodium. Of course, the water is reabsorbed by osmosis into the peritubular capillaries. The sodium needs the active transport mechanism of the sodium pump. Most other things, like phosphate, sulfate, calcium, potassium, and glucose, have limited active transport capacities. Glucose reabsorption is limited by the active transport mechanism and blood glucose concentrations. When plasma glucose concentrations are elevated, the renal threshold for glucose reabsorption is altered, making fewer active transport vehicles available. The result is glycosuria. Patients receiving intravenous fluid therapy with glucose-containing fluids should be expected to have glycosuria. As soon as the fluid therapy is stopped, no glucose should be passed in the urine. In the absence of such therapy, glycosuria is an abnormality that may point to a disease like diabetes mellitus (to be discussed in Chapter 15).

Moving on from the proximal convoluted tubule, we find a structure that looks much like the "elbow" of the "trap," a section of drain pipe under a sink. (Go look under the sink. I'll wait.) This elbow of our nephron is referred to as the loop of Henle, named after Fredrich Gustav Jakob Henle, a German anatomist. (Boy, discover something and they'll name a body part after you. At least they used only his last name.) The loop of Henle is *very* important for reabsorption of sodium. A key point to make about sodium is that, as sodium is reabsorbed, things like water and negatively charged ions (like Cl$^-$) tend to follow. (Let's see, NaCl and water reabsorbed? Hmm, that could be a problem if we have edematous fluid to get rid of. Now, do you see why low-sodium diets are important for cardiac patients?) Of course, this gives the kidney a tremendous concentrating effect for the urine that is being produced. But what if we really do need to get rid of excess water from the body (e.g., pulmonary edema or ascites from congestive heart failure)? We target the loop of Henle! That's right, it's the loop of Henle that is targeted by loop diuretics,[6] like Lasix (furosemide). Loop diuretics inhibit reabsorption of sodium and water from the loop of Henle. This makes these drugs very useful for treating patients with edematous fluids from congestive heart failure. They really increase the volume of urine produced, making the patients polyuric. (Unfortunately, loop diuretics also tend to inhibit reabsorption of critical electrolytes like potassium. So, potassium levels should be carefully monitored.)

---

[5]Convoluted (kon′vo-lūt-ed); from [L. *convolutus*, coiled].
[6]Diuretic (di″u-ret′ik [Gr. *diouretikos*, promoting urine]); a diuretic is any agent that causes increased urine production.

Getting back to our nephron's anatomy, the loop of Henle leads to the distal convoluted tubule. On average, in a normal individual, most of the urine entering the distal convoluted tubule tends to be rather hypotonic. Well, you say, that's easily fixed by just reabsorbing more water and concentrating the urine like the loop of Henle did. That's easier said than done. You see, the distal convoluted tubules are rather impervious to water. Not to worry! In the presence of ADH (antidiuretic hormone), the distal convoluted tubules readily reabsorb water, provided there is a need. What kind of need, you ask? Well, in cases of decreased water in the blood (like in dehydration) or decreased blood volume or pressure, ADH will be secreted. The end result will be conservation of water for the body and production of hypertonic urine. In the absence of ADH, urine will be more dilute. (ADH will be discussed again in Chapter 15.)

All of the distal convoluted tubules converge at collecting ducts, which lead to the renal pelvis. Of course, from there the urine will pass through the ureters and into the urinary bladder. Did you know that the ureters actually have muscular walls that move the urine into the bladder with peristaltic action? That's right, just like peristalsis along the intestines (Chapter 12). No gravity needed here. That urine will spurt right into the bladder. When the bladder becomes stretched, the internal urethral sphincter will relax and muscles in the bladder wall should contract. Thankfully, there is an external urethral sphincter that is under conscious control. (Yes, just like the external anal sphincter discussed in Chapter 12.) Alas, just like conscious control of the external anal sphincter must be learned, so too must control of the external urethral sphincter be learned. In most puppies and kittens, this kind of learned bladder control doesn't become well developed until about 6 months of age. Until then, pet owners will probably have to clean up numerous puddles. Of course, geriatric pets may lose urethral sphincter control, leading to urinary incontinence.[7] I should mention that in humans too, the external urethral sphincter muscles may become weak with age. That's right, humans go from diapers to Depends, all on account of external urethral sphincter control or lack thereof. Well, some geriatric pets are not far behind in the urinary incontinence department either.

So, what exactly is in normal urine? Well, water of course, in varying amounts. Even in concentrated urine, water is still its largest component. We measure the concentrating ability of the kidneys by evaluating the urine specific gravity. (Distilled water has a specific gravity of 1.000. Normal dogs, cats, and horses should produce urine with a specific gravity between 1.020 and 1.040 or a little higher. A specific gravity of 1.010 is considered isosthenuric. Animals receiving isotonic intravenous fluids are often isosthenuric. In the absence of intravenous fluid administration, isosthenuria may point to problems with renal concentrating ability. Polyuric animals will tend to have lower urine specific gravity, and oliguric patients will tend to have higher urine specific gravity (Fig. 13-6). What exactly is concentrated in the urine? Urea is one thing. Urea is a nitrogenous compound formed from amino acid metabolism that will be found in urine. Probably half of the urea produced by the body will be excreted in the urine. (Gee, do you suppose

---

[7]Incontinence (in-kon′tĭ-nens [L. *incontinentia*]); inability to control excretory functions, such as urination and/or defecation).

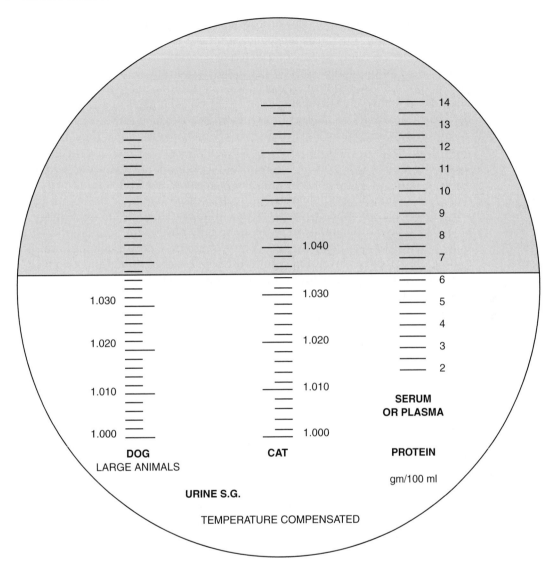

FIGURE 13-6 Specific gravity using a refractometer.

that's how urine got its name?) Uric acid, a product of nucleic acid metabolism, is excreted by the kidneys too. Finally, there are all sorts of electrolytes that may be found in varying concentrations in urine. Actually, some of the peritubular capillaries can aid in active tubular secretion of things like histamine, creatinine, certain drugs, and ions like potassium and hydrogen. The latter of these is very important in helping regulate acid–base balance in the body. In acidosis, more hydrogen ions will be secreted into the urine, making the urine more acidic. At times, for instance during the postprandial alkaline tide[8] (resulting from hydrogen ions being used for

---

[8]Postprandial alkaline tide (post-pran'de-al); from [*post-*, after + *prandi(o)-*, meal + *-al,* pertaining to]; the transient alkalinity of the body after a meal.

gastric secretions), the kidneys will conserve hydrogen ions for the body, making the urine alkaline. Other substances filtered from the glomerulus that may be in urine include calcium, phosphate, sulfate, and sodium. Some of these ions (trace minerals) may combine to form larger molecules. In the right environment, they may even precipitate to form crystals or even uroliths. Many crystalline precipitates can be controlled and even eliminated through changes in diet and alteration of the urine pH. We'll talk more about this when we discuss urolithiasis.

The kidney—how amazing is that?! Why, kidneys even play a role in red blood cell production, by secreting the hormone erythropoietin. That's an endocrine discussion we'll save for Chapter 15. Uropoiesis itself is an amazing feat! Renal filtration, osmosis, and secretion of additives into that fluid we know as urine really do sound very similar to the processes used by water treatment plants. Why, reverse osmosis is a principal way that commercial bottlers purify municipal drinking water. Most water commercially bottled for consumption in the United States is produced by just such a method. These concepts are really nothing new, from a physiologic point of view. After all, the kidneys have been doing those things long before it was used commercially.

Renal Pathophysiology and Disease

Let's begin our disease discussion with urinalysis. Many wellness programs for veterinary patients include urinalysis as part of an annual patient assessment. Certainly, if a patient is having obvious urinary problems, such as pollakiuria or dysuria, urinalysis will be part of the diagnostic workup. Nocturia commonly causes owners to bring their dogs in (it is such an annoyance for them to have to get up frequently overnight to let the dog out or to find numerous puddles in the house the next morning). A simple urinalysis can reveal much about renal function, health of the urinary tract, and overall health of the animal. Urinalysis may be performed on voided, catheterized, or cystocentesis specimens. Cystocentesis will provide the most sterile specimen possible. So, if a bacterial cystitis is suspected, cystocentesis would be the collection method of choice, not only for the urinalysis but for the culture and sensitivity testing as well. Regardless of how the sample is collected, the urinalysis procedure is the same. First, gross characteristics are noted, including things like color and turbidity. Normal urine from most domestic animals should be some shade of yellow (the more concentrated the urine, the darker the shade). Redness in the sample may indicate hematuria or hemoglobinuria. Turbidity (cloudiness) increases with crystals, cells, and other particulate matter suspended in the urine. (Horses tend to have very turbid urine normally, due to the presence of a significant number of calcium carbonate crystals.) All suspended items will be evaluated closely under the microscope.

Chemically, using urine "dipsticks," we can screen for solutes and certain suspended items that are contained in the urine (such as glucose, protein, bilirubin, ketones, urobilinogen, and blood). The pH is a very important part of the chemical screening. Remember, the kidney helps regulate acid–base homeostasis for the body through either active secretion or conservation of hydrogen ions. The more hydrogen ions are secreted, the lower the pH will be. Hydrogen ion conservation will result in more alkaline urine being produced. Not only does the pH tell us something about the patient's acid–base homeostasis, it may also give us clues as to the types of precipitates that may form. (Formation of many crystals is pH dependent. For example, struvite crystals tend to form in alkaline urine, whereas calcium oxalate [dihydrate] crystals tend to form in acidic urine.)

Certainly, the specific gravity will give us clues as to the renal concentrating ability and patient hydration. This is optimally tested on a centrifuged sample. That way suspended particles won't interfere with the refractometer. Once the sample is centrifuged, the supernatant is used for specific gravity determination, and the sediment at the bottom of the tube must be evaluated under the microscope. Urine sediments, even from normal animals, may contain epithelium, some crystals, fat droplets, sperm (in intact male urine), and mucus. Red blood cells should not be present. However, they could be an artifact from a cystocentesis. Abnormal conditions that may create hematuria include bacterial cystitis, urolithiasis, and cancer. White blood cells are most frequently seen with bacterial cystitis along with the bacteria creating the cystitis. Of course, hematuria and pyuria can be produced by disease problems more proximal along the urinary tract, such as nephritis or pyelonephritis. The presence of casts in the urine sediment (formed in the renal tubules) may offer just the evidence needed to warrant further diagnostics. (Remember the secreting ability of the renal tubules? Some of those secretions may actually harden and form a casting of the tubule. Sometimes cells may become caught up in the matrix of a cast, such as erythrocytes or leukocytes. Such cellular casts could be very revealing of something like nephritis.) Serum chemistries may be ordered to evaluate the patient for azotemia or uremia.

Of course, the investigation does not end with simply determining through blood work that the patient is uremic. That finding raises even more questions, as to whether the uremia is prerenal, renal, or postrenal in origin. Cardiovascular diagnostics may pursue prerenal causes. Renal and postrenal etiologies will require further evaluation of the urinary tract itself. Radiographically, various portions of the urinary tract can be systematically evaluated for structural abnormalities. Intravenous pyelograms offer a fabulous look at the renal cortex, medulla, and pelvis. Certainly, the dye can then be followed down the ureters and into the bladder. Generally, if the lower urinary tract is of concern, some form of cystography will be performed. The dye may be introduced via a retrograde urethrocystogram. If inconclusive, a second contrast study using a pneumocystogram may reveal abnormalities with the bladder wall or uroliths within the bladder. Such abnormalities may be elusive without the double contrast studies (i.e., dye and air). Urolithiasis is a common cause of postrenal azotemia and uremia, especially when the uroliths cause obstruction of a ureter or the urethra.

Urolithiasis plagues both dogs and cats. Certainly the presence of uroliths can create symptoms of cystitis, due to cystalgia from bladder wall trauma. The pollakiuria, dysuria, and straining may be compounded by urethritis. Unfortunately, uroliths can and frequently do lead to urethral obstruction. This can be a very painful and lethal condition. Tomcats develop urethral obstructions more frequently than male dogs. If you look back at the male feline urethra, you can see that it won't take much to obstruct its narrow, curved lumen. In fact, many male cats will become obstructed with such small uroliths that they actually look more like sand than stones. (Male dogs who develop obstructions usually have a urolith become wedged in the os penis.) Regardless of whether it is a dog or a cat, urethral obstruction is an emergent condition. The obstruction must be removed. The dog owner will probably take prompt action after observing the dysuria with little to no urine produced by the effort. This is particularly evident if the dog cries out during the obvious attempt to urinate. With male cats, it is a little more difficult to recognize the urinary problem. Male cats, unlike dogs, do not lift their legs to urinate, making it difficult to see exactly what they're doing. They squat in the litter box to urinate, much like they do when they defecate. So, just how do most cat owners interpret the male cat visiting the litter box frequently, squatting, and crying out as if in pain? They think the cat is constipated. Every seasoned veterinary professional gets chills when they receive a phone call from a male cat owner wondering what to do about the cat's constipation. Ding, ding, ding, ding! Alarms go off, or at least they should. Any such cat owner should be told that the cat needs to be seen immediately. The cystalgia that these animals bear must be incredible. Imagine your bladder stretched to the point of bursting like a water balloon and you can't relieve it. Ouch! The longer the obstruction exists, the more probable a postrenal azotemia and eventually uremia will develop. Remember, we said earlier that arterial blood was full of nitrogenous impurities. Now that the waste water plumbing is blocked, those impurities have nowhere to go. Uremic animals will often be clinically ill from the accumulated toxins in their bloodstream (depression, confusion, anorexia, nausea, vomiting, etc.). The obstruction must be relieved as quickly as possible. With urethral catheters and techniques like retropulsion[9] to wash uroliths back into the bladder, the current obstruction can be relieved. But future obstructions will likely occur. The question now is: how do we prevent a repeat episode? Encouraging adequate water consumption may help "flush the plumbing." That means keeping lots of fresh water available at all times. Some cats like their water so fresh that they drink straight from the tap! Depending on the composition of the uroliths, scheduled feeding and/or dietary changes may help. If the uroliths creating the obstruction form only in alkaline urine, dietary changes that will acidify the urine may prevent future problems. For stones currently in the bladder, prescription diets are available to dissolve certain uroliths. Other uroliths may need to be removed through a cystotomy. For animals who repeatedly experience urethral obstruction, the urethra may become so stenotic from scar tissue that, even in the absence of uroliths, bladder evacuation is difficult. For these animals, a urethrostomy may be the only solution. This is a permanent anatomic change that will surgically access a larger-diameter point along the urethra and create a new urethral orifice there. In dogs, a prescrotal[10] urethrostomy is most frequently performed,

---

[9]Retropulsion (ret"ro-pul'shun; [*retro-*, backward + *pulsion*, pushing]); a method to remove urethral obstruction, using a viscous solution to flush the stone back into the bladder.
[10]Prescrotal (pre-skro'tal; [*pre-*, before + *scrotum* + *-al*, pertaining to].

placing the new urethral orifice caudal to the penis and cranial to the scrotum. Because of the cat's anatomy, perineal[11] urethrostomies are most frequently performed. Yes, both of them will have to urinate "like girls," but the important point is that they will be able to urinate.

Thus far, we've mentioned cardiac disease as a potential prerenal cause of renal failure. Remember, the kidneys rely on sufficient blood pressure for glomerular function. During a crisis, such as hypovolemic shock, glomeruli will cease to function and may never regain function if the hypovolemia is prolonged. We've just discussed urolithiasis and urethral obstruction as a postrenal etiology for uremia. What about a renal cause? The most common renal causes of renal failure that result in azotemia and uremia are direct insults to the kidneys, like glomerulonephritis (often stemming from periodontal disease) or nephrotoxins. The most common nephrotoxic agent in veterinary patients is antifreeze (ethylene glycol).

Ethylene glycol is deadly and attractive. What? Yes, ethylene glycol is attractive because it has a very sweet smell and taste. So, animals and children may be enticed to drink it. Unfortunately, it takes very little of the stuff to kill an animal. As little as a teaspoon could kill an 8-pound cat. For an average 40-pound dog, only about 2.5 ounces may be deadly. The prognosis for an animal relates directly to the amount of antifreeze consumed and how quickly the animal is treated. Time is of the essence, if an animal is to be saved. Even if a pet owner merely suspects that the animal may have ingested some antifreeze, immediate veterinary care should be sought. If medical care is not initiated, the pet will likely die of acute renal failure. Such a death will happen in a matter of days. How does this happen, you ask? Ethylene glycol is rapidly absorbed by the gastrointestinal tract and rapidly metabolized. Its metabolite, oxalic acid, combines with calcium to form calcium oxalate monohydrate crystals. It is these crystals that for all practical purposes "plug up" the glomeruli and renal tubules. Tubular necrosis often occurs. Crystals may even collect in small vessels of other organs as well, leading to multisystemic failures. In anuric renal failure patients, there is little hope of recovery. Oliguric patients have only a slightly better outlook. The key to survival is prompt medical intervention. Even then, there may be a guarded prognosis. Frankly, the best course of action is to prevent ethylene glycol ingestion in the first place. Owners should be aware that this chemical poses a threat to animals and people alike. Innocent children and animals are the typical, unfortunate victims. For anyone using ethylene glycol, it should always be stored out of reach of children and pets, and any spills should be promptly cleaned up.

Another common nephrotoxin for dogs is the grape. What?! Grapes are toxic to dogs?! Yes, they are. So, while you might think that grapes or raisins would be good healthy snacks for your dog, don't feed them. The actual mechanism behind the acute renal failure after dogs eat grapes is unknown. Tubular necrosis is often observed at necropsy, but how it develops is unknown. How fast might it occur? Nearly as rapidly as ethylene glycol toxicity, following consumption of even just a few ounces of grapes. Until the true mechanism of the grape-induced nephrotoxicity can be determined, the safe play is to not feed any grapes to any dogs.

---

[11]Perineal (per″ĭ-ne′al; [Gr. *perineos*]); the perineum is the region between the anus and genitals.

Renal failure is no picnic, whether it is caused by nephrotoxins or other etiologies. Let's face it. We and animals can't live without functional kidneys. Just like the modern world cannot survive without fresh, clean water supplies, animals cannot live without their personal little wastewater treatment plants—the kidneys. Yes, there are rare opportunities for kidney transplants and dialysis. But for the average animal, renal failure (especially acute renal failure) will be a death warrant. As veterinary professionals, it is our duty to help owners prevent renal diseases. And for those animals who suffer from renal disease, we must offer the best possible diagnostic and treatment plans available.

SELF-TEST

Using the previous information in this chapter, complete the following crossword puzzle using the most appropriate medical term(s). Do not use abbreviations or common names unless requested.

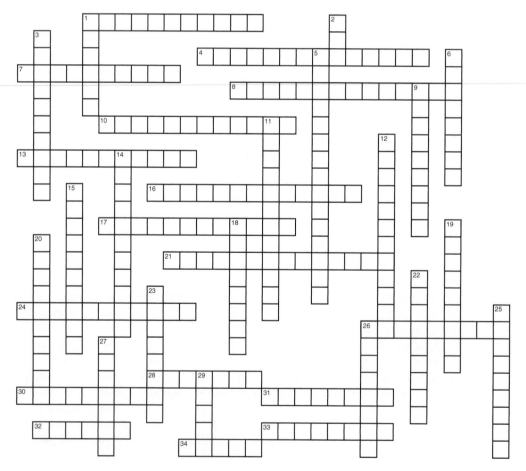

ACROSS

1	The substance that causes vasoconstriction of the efferent arteriole in the kidney
4	Inflammation of the renal pelvis
7	Pertaining to high osmotic pressure
8	Two words for the nephrotoxic agent antifreeze
10	Pertaining to urine that is the same strength as plasma
13	Protein in the urine
16	Puncture of the bladder, usually for sterile urine collection
17	A condition of urinary stones
21	A condition in which water accumulates in the kidney
24	Frequent urination
26	A surgical operation cutting into the bladder
28	A collective, functional unit of the kidney
30	Blood in the urine
31	Having to urinate at night
32	A serious clinical condition of nitrogenous compounds like urea accumulating in the blood due to renal malfunction making the animal systemically ill
33	Small volumes of urine
34	Pertaining to the kidney

DOWN

1	A condition without urine
2	Abbreviation for the hormone that promotes water reabsorption from the distal convoluted tubule
3	Glucose in the urine
5	A radiographic procedure in which air is infused into the bladder
6	Excessive urine
9	Bladder pain
11	Inability to control urination, resulting in dribbling
12	A surgical procedure in which a new urethral orifice is created
14	Pertaining to something that is poisonous to the kidney
15	The capillary "filter" of the kidney
18	A condition of nitrogen in the blood
19	Inflammation of the kidney
20	To go backward
22	After the kidney
23	Before the kidney
25	Pertaining to low osmotic pressure
26	Inflammation of the bladder
27	Difficult urination
29	The renal loop targeted by loop diuretics like furosemide

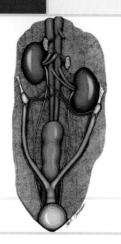

CHAPTER **14**

The Reproductive System

GOALS AND OBJECTIVES

By the conclusion of this chapter, the student will be able to:

1. Recognize common root words, prefixes, and suffixes related to the reproductive system.
2. Divide simple and compound words into their respective parts.
3. Recognize, correctly pronounce, and appropriately use common medical terms related to the reproductive system.
4. Demonstrate an understanding of reproductive anatomy (male and female).
5. Demonstrate an understanding of reproductive physiology as it relates to estrus; gestation; parturition; lactation; and, in the male, spermatogenesis.

Note: It is very important to have completed all previous chapters before completing this one.

INTRODUCTION TO RELATED TERMS

Divide each of the following terms into its respective parts ("R," root; "P," prefix; "S," suffix; "CV," combining vowel).

1. **Cryptorchid** (n.)   (R) _____ (R) _____
   cryptorchid (krip-tor'kid; hidden testicles; clinically refers to an animal whose testes have not yet descended into the scrotum)

2. **Orchiectomy** (n.)   (R) _____ (S) _____
   orchiectomy (or"ke-ek'to-me; excision of the testes; i.e., castration; cf. orchidectomy)

3. **Spermatogenesis** (n.)   (R) _____ (CV) _____ (R) _____
                                         (CV) _____ (S) _____
   spermatogenesis (sper"mah-to-jen'ĕ-sis; the process of sperm production)

292

4. **Ovariohysterectomy** (n.)   (R) _____ (CV) _____ (R) _____ (S) _____

   ovariohysterectomy (o-va"re-o-his"ter-ek'to-me; excision of the ovaries and the uterus; cf. spay)

5. **Pyometra** (n.)   (R) _____ (CV) _____ (R) _____

   pyometra (pi"o-me'trah; pus in the uterus)

6. **Mastitis** (n.)   (R) _____ (S) _____

   mastitis (mas-ti'tis; inflammation of the breasts/mammary tissue)

7. **Gestation** (n.)   (R) _____ (S) _____

   gestation (jes-ta'shun; the state of bearing; clinically refers to the stage of the reproductive cycle in which the female is carrying young in utero)

8. **Parturition** (n.)   (R) _____ (S) _____

   parturition (par"tu-rĭ'shun; the state of birthing)

9. **Lactation** (n.)   (R) _____ (S) _____

   lactation (lak-ta'shun; the state of milking)

10. **Postparturient** (adj.)   (P) _____ (R) _____ (S) _____

    postparturient (post-par"tūr're-ent; pertaining to after birthing; cf. postpartum)

11. **Dystocia** (n.)   (P) _____ (R) _____ (S) _____

    dystocia (dis-to'se-ah; the process of difficult birth)

12. **Neonatal** (adj.)   (P) _____ (R) _____ (S) _____

    neonatal (ne"o-na'tal; pertaining to newly born)

13. **Mutagenic** (adj.)   (R) _____ (R) _____ (S) _____

    mutagenic (mu"tah-jen'ik; pertaining to change producing; clinically refers to anything that alters the DNA to create genetic abnormalities)

14. **Teratogenic** (adj.)   (R) _____ (CV) _____ (R) _____ (S) _____

    teratogenic (ter"ah-to-jen'ik; pertaining to monster producing; clinically refers to anything that causes physical defects in the developing embryo/fetus)

15. **Proestrus** (n.)   (P) _____ (R) _____

    proestrus (pro-es'trus; before estrus; clinically refers to the period of the reproductive cycle before sexual receptivity)

16. **Metestrus** (n.)   (P) _____ (R) _____

    metestrus (met-es'trus; beyond/after estrus; clinically refers to the period of the reproductive cycle after sexual receptivity)

17. **Anestrus** (n.)   (P) _____ (R) _____

    anestrus (an-es'trus; absence of estrus; clinically refers to the period of the reproductive cycle in which the female animal is in sexual quiescence; cf. diestrus—the period between metestrus and the next proestrus)

18. **Monestrous** (adj.)   (P) _____ (R) _____ (S) _____

    monestrous (mon-es'trus; pertaining to one estrus; clinically refers to those animals who experience one estrous cycle in a sexual season)

19. **Polyestrous** (adj.)   (P) _____ (R) _____ (S) _____
    polyestrous (pol"e-es'trus; pertaining to much [many] estrus; clinically refers to those
    animals who experience numerous estrous cycles during a sexual season)

20. **Pseudocyesis** (n.)   (R) _____ (CV) _____ (R) _____
    pseudocyesis (su"do-si-e'sis; false pregnancy)

21. **Metritis** (n.)   (R) _____ (S) _____
    metritis (me-tri'tis; inflammation of the uterus [womb])

22. **Prostatitis** (n.)   (R) _____ (S) _____
    prostatitis (pros"tah-ti'tis; inflammation of the prostate)

23. **Endometrium** (n.)   (P) _____ (R) _____ (S) _____
    endometrium (en"do-me'tre-um; within the uterus; the endometrium is the interior lining
    of the uterus)

24. **Episioplasty** (n.)   (R) _____ (CV) _____ (S) _____
    episioplasty (ĕ-piz'e-o-plas"te, e-pēz'e-o-plas"te; to repair/reform the vulva [Gr. *plassein,*
    to form]

25. **Mastectomy** (n.)   (R) _____ (S) _____
    mastectomy (mas-tek'to-me; to cut out the breast; i.e., surgical removal of the breast)

REPRODUCTIVE ANATOMY AND PHYSIOLOGY

Female Reproductive Anatomy

Well, before we can talk about the "birds and bees," we need to know something about the anatomy involved. Any hormones associated with the reproductive tract will be discussed in Chapter 15. Let's begin with female anatomy. Female animals have a pair of ovaries, located near the dorsum of the abdominal cavity (Figs. 14-1 and 14-2). They are firmly attached to the body wall with fibrous connective tissue (suspensory ligaments). In the mature female, the ovaries contain oocytes[1] at various stages of development. Oocytes are created by meiosis[2] from primary ovarian cells. Each egg contains half of the genetic information found in the parent cell (half that required to produce offspring). Some chemicals and other agents can have mutagenic effects on the primary ovarian cells. Oocytes produced from these altered cells produce genetically abnormal offspring.

The ovaries are held close to the uterine horns by the proper ligaments. At ovulation,[3] oocytes are deposited into the infundibulum[4] of each uterine horn. Unlike humans, many animals tend to produce multiple offspring from a single

---

[1]Oocyte (o'o-sīt); from [Gr. *oon,* egg + -*cyte*].
[2]Meiosis (mi-o'sis); a special method of cell division of sex cells, in which daughter cells receive only half the chromosomes of the parent cell.
[3]Ovulation (o"vu-la'shun); the release of an oocyte from the ovary.
[4]Infundibulum (in"fun-dib'u-lum); from [L. *infundibula,* funnel]; the infundibulum of the uterine horn is a funnel-shaped structure designed to "catch" the oocyte on ovulation.

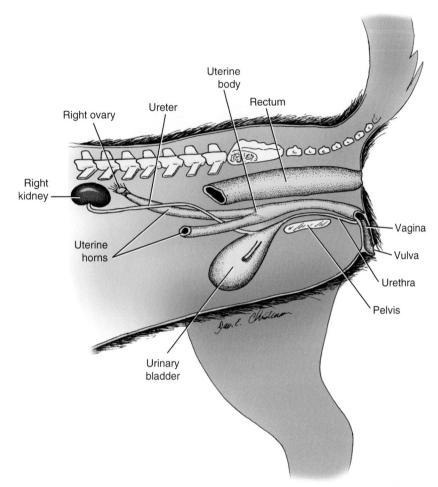

FIGURE 14-1   Canine female reproductive tract (lateral view).

pregnancy. Therefore, the uterus is subdivided into two horns. This makes it much easier to carry multiple young during gestation. The broad ligaments, which are basically folds of peritoneal tissue, support the uterine horns. Ovarian and uterine arteries lie within the supportive connective tissues. Why is all of this minute anatomy important? Veterinary surgeons and the technicians who assist them in the operating room must be familiar with these anatomic structures during ovariohysterectomies and caesarean sections. While we're on a surgical topic, look at Figures 14-1 and 14-2. Notice that the ureters lie very near the uterus. Care must be taken to ensure that the ureters are not inadvertently ligated[5] with uterine vessels during an ovariohysterectomy. (It's always a good idea to make sure that a female can still urinate following an ovariohysterectomy.) The uterine horns converge caudally at the uterine body. The cervix

---

[5]Ligate (li′gāt); to tie or bind with a ligature ([L. *ligatura*]; e.g., suture).

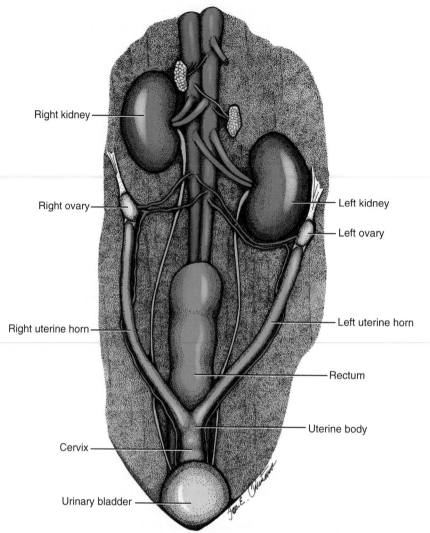

FIGURE 14-2   Canine female reproductive tract (ventrodorsal view).

(ser′viks), a strong sphincter, demarcates the uterus from the vagina. The vagina (vah-ji′nah) serves as a passageway for not only the reproductive tract, but also the urinary tract. The urethral orifice is found along the ventral floor of the vagina, in the caudal third of the passage. The endometrium and the vagina are lined with stratified squamous epithelium. Cytologic analysis of vaginal epithelium in dogs can be helpful in determining where the animal is with regard to the estrous cycle. We'll talk about that momentarily. To finish the gross anatomy, the labia (la′be-ah) of the vulva (vul′vah) provide some protection for the vaginal opening and tissue. You might think that the vulva is of little importance. When its conformation is abnormal, it can be very important. Mares with poor vulvar conformation (tilted such that feces may easily enter the vagina) may require an episioplasty to minimize risk of vaginitis or metritis. Episioplasty may also be performed in dogs with inversion of the vulva. The folds of an inverted vulva promote bacterial growth, leading to chronic vulvar dermatitis.

Now although it is true that gross physical and behavioral changes will be seen with estrus, those factors may not be reliable for breeding in all females. Classically, dogs will experience vulvar swelling and a vaginal discharge, as well as exhibiting flirtatious behaviors (like "flagging" their tails). But these changes may be present before, during, and after estrus. For those female dogs who are not conceiving when bred, vaginal cytology can help the breeder determine exactly when estrus occurs. (It is very important to note that a series of vaginal swabs over a period of days is essential in most cases. The cytologic changes are dynamic and must be seen in progression to make the best recommendations for breeding.) The epithelium is most important for determining the stage of estrus (Fig. 14-3). Oh dear, here we go with that cellular stuff again! Yes we are, but it's really not as difficult to understand as you might think. First of all, think of the stratified epithelium as being stacked up like a bunch of eggs. Yes, chicken eggs (the yolk being the nucleus and the white being the cytoplasm with a cellular membrane). On and near the bottom (the basal epithelial layer) we have boiled eggs—plump, rather round (we'll call these small round epithelial cells or parabasal[6] cells). No matter how you look at them, they are quite plump and perky, like little pillows. Parabasal cells are the youngest cells we may see in our cytology. During diestrus we may see quite a few parabasal cells (they are small and darkly staining because they are so plump).

As we move up into the transitional layer of epithelium, we find poached eggs. They are still rather plump, but not as plump as a parabasal cell. (Lay a boiled egg next to a poached egg on the counter top. Looking from the side, the boiled egg is very plump and tall, whereas the poached egg is a bit thinner or shorter. Looking at them from the top, the boiled egg is still very plump, but the poached egg appears bigger because it's had the chance to spread out more.) In the epithelial world, that poached egg is transitional epithelium, sometimes referred to as a large round or transitional epithelial cell. These transitional cells are older. They've been around awhile, moving up through the stratification. Just like we get that middle-aged spread, transitional epithelium gets a bit wider too (wider yes, but not sagging). During diestrus, proestrus, and metestrus we'll see many large round epithelial cells. Their numbers will progressively taper off during proestrus and begin to reappear and increase in numbers during metestrus and diestrus. At the top of our stack of eggs are the fried eggs, some with yolks, some with broken yolks, and some without yolks at all. These are the superficial epithelial cells or "squames." Compared with the others, they are broad, flat, and flabby. (Yes, we get flabby and wrinkled with age too.) The margins of these cells are irregular because they wrinkle and fold up on themselves.

These superficial epithelial cells are key to determining estrus in the dog. They are so critical to pinpointing estrus that we actually subdivide them into non-cornified squames (superficial intermediate epithelium) and cornified squames

---

[6]Parabasal (par-ah-ba'sal); from *para-*, near + *basal*, pertaining to the base.

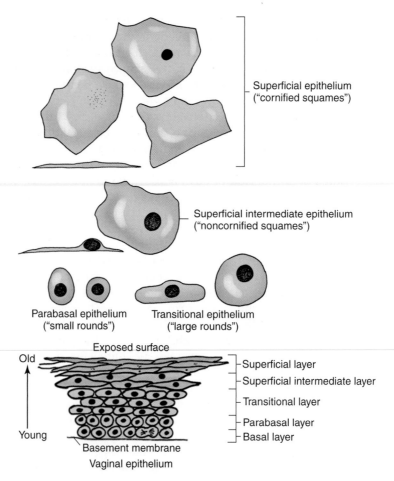

Superficial epithelium ("cornified squames")

Superficial intermediate epithelium ("noncornified squames")

Parabasal epithelium ("small rounds")

Transitional epithelium ("large rounds")

Exposed surface

Old

Superficial layer
Superficial intermediate layer
Transitional layer
Parabasal layer
Basal layer

Young

Basement membrane

Vaginal epithelium

FIGURE 14-3   Canine vaginal epithelium.

(superficial epithelium). Noncornified squames are big, flabby, and folded, but they still have happy, plump nuclei (sunny-side up yolk). Cornified cells are the oldest, crustiest, most superficial of the epithelial cells (like that dried, flaky skin that comes off when our hands dry out from washing them too much with harsh detergents). Cornified cells have very pyknotic (shriveled, disintegrated) nuclei, if they have nuclei at all (i.e., shrunken, broken yolks or no yolks at all). During proestrus, we'll begin seeing more and more squames, first with a predominance of noncornified cells and then more and more cornified cells. By the time we reach estrus, we should see 100% cornified squames. Like birds of a feather, cornified squames tend to clump together during estrus. Time to breed! As we begin to progress into metestrus, we'll still have a large number of cornified squames, but noncornified and transitional epithelium will begin to enter into the mix. By the time we're well into diestrus, we'll be back to mostly transitional and parabasal cells.

Yes, there are other cells that may help us in determining which stage of the estrous cycle the dog is in, but they are not as reliable because of variances among dogs and other factors that may artificially increase their numbers. For instance, erythrocytes may be seen on our vaginal cytology. In a normal female we would expect to see red blood cells (RBCs) during proestrus. However, in some females we may still have some RBCs in estrus. And if we traumatize the vaginal tract when taking the swab, we can create hemorrhage during any stage. Leukocytes may also be seen in vaginal cytology. We may see moderate numbers during proestrus and many of them during metestrus and diestrus (somebody needs to clean things up and protect the reproductive tract). We certainly don't want any white blood cells (WBCs) present during estrus. Why, they'd attack and destroy most if not all of the sperm that came by. Unfortunately, if the dog has vaginitis, WBCs may be present in large numbers in any stage. The same is true for bacteria. So, if the other cytologic features and gross characteristics of the dog seem to fit the progression of the epithelium, great! If not, focus your attention on the epithelium exclusively to determine where she is in the estrous cycle. Because we're talking about breeding, we'd better talk about the male too. She can't breed without him.

Male Reproductive Anatomy

The testes/testicles of mature male animals are suspended by the spermatic cord in the scrotum[7] (Figs. 14-4 and 14-5). The testes of immature males actually originate in the abdominal cavity. During the maturation process, the testes will eventually descend through the inguinal ring and into the scrotal sac. Abnormal retention of one or both testes in the abdomen is referred to as cryptorchidism. (It is very important when performing a preoperative examination on an orchiectomy patient to ensure that both testicles have descended. If one or both have not, a decision may be made to postpone the surgery. If surgery is still a "go," our surgical prep and approach will be dramatically altered from a scrotal or prescrotal site to an abdominal prep for a laparotomy.) The spermatic cord and testes are covered by a fibrous connective tissue sheath (the vaginal tunic). Within the vaginal tunic of the spermatic cord are the ductus deferens[8] and the testicular artery and vein. Some males have a well-developed cremaster muscle within the spermatic cord (e.g., bulls). Contraction of the muscle draws the testes closer to the body to keep them warm when it's cold outside. During warm weather the muscles relax, allowing the testes to drop well into the scrotum and away from the body. (Many rodents can actually withdraw the testes completely into the abdomen as well as extrude them from the abdomen voluntarily!) Of course, to prevent some undesirable behavioral problems, as well as physical problems like prostate enlargement or cancer, many male animals

---

[7]Scrotum (skro'tum); from [L. *scrotum,* bag]; the scrotum is a pouch of skin that contains the testes.

[8]Ductus deferens (duk'tus def'er-enz [L. *deferens,* different]); the ductus deferens are vessels that transport sperm from the testes to the urethra.

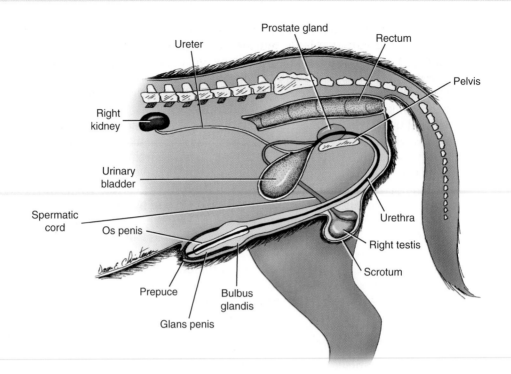

FIGURE 14-4   Canine male reproductive tract.

have orchiectomies. The vaginal tunic of the spermatic cord is important during castrations. During a "closed" orchiectomy, the vaginal tunic will remain intact. The entire spermatic cord will be ligated collectively, with the ligature placed and tightened over the vaginal tunic. During an "open" orchiectomy the vaginal tunic is incised, allowing for ligation of individual vessels within the spermatic cord. Obviously, the open orchiectomy affords better hemostasis in males with well-developed testicular vessels. (However, it also provides an open pathway into the abdomen, especially if skin closure of the surgical site breaks down.)

The spermatic cord passes through the inguinal rings from the abdominal cavity. The ductus deferens ultimately terminate at the proximal urethra, near the prostate gland. The prostate (pros'tāt) gland encircles the proximal urethra and is a reproductive structure responsible for contributing a transparent fluid to semen. The urethra in males serves a dual purpose: (1) as a passage for urine from the bladder during urination, and (2) as a passage for semen during copulation.[9] The urethra is centrally located in the penis. Among domestic animals, the male dog is unique in that he has a bony structure called the os penis, through which the urethra passes. The penis is composed of highly vascular, sponge-like erectile tissue. During copulation, the penile tissue becomes engorged with blood, creating a somewhat rigid structure. In a relaxed state, the penis is covered by a moist mucous membrane and protected by the prepuce

[9]Copulation (kop"u-la'shun); sexual union between a male and a female animal.

(pre'pūs). There are some unique penile anatomic differences among domestic animals. The bulbus glandis, located at the proximal end of the canine penis, is one of the notable differences. During copulation, the bulbus glandis enlarges tremendously and is responsible for the "tie."[10] Bulls also have unique penile structure, with a sigmoid flexure (an S-shaped curve) approximately halfway the length of the penis. This flexure reduces the overall length of the penis in a relaxed state so that it may be completely protected by the prepuce. Boars have a less pronounced sigmoid flexure that lies more proximal on the penis. The most unique feature of the boar's penis is the spiral-like twist at the exposed end. The male cat is unique in that his penis is not positioned along the ventral midline of the abdomen, as it is in all of our other domestic animals. The penis of the male cat is directed caudally (Fig. 14-5). In addition, it is covered with numerous barb-like projections.

Spermatogenesis

The testes are structured for continuous production of sperm (Fig. 14-6). Spermatogenic cells throughout the testes continually develop new sperm via meiosis. Temperature extremes can adversely affect spermatogenesis. That's why the cremaster muscle, mentioned earlier, is important. As the sperm develop, they collect in the seminiferous tubules,[11] which are coiled throughout the testes. Eventually, they pass into the ductus deferens of the epididymis[12] for a period of maturation. Ultimately, mature sperm cells make their way through the ductus deferens of the spermatic cord and through the urethra for insemination of the female. Insemination can occur via natural copulation or artificial insemination (AI—not be confused with artificial intelligence). If artificial insemination is to be performed, all of the equipment used for collection and delivery must be clean, dry, and warmed to body temperature. The presence of chemicals, water, and temperature extremes (especially cold) may be lethal to the sperm. The same conditions must be provided if semen quality is to be evaluated too (i.e., looking at numbers, motility, and morphology). Temperature of the microscopic slides is most important for motility evaluation.

Spermatozoa contain only half of the genetic information required to create a new animal of that species. Their basic structure facilitates active mobility (Fig. 14-7). Each sperm has a head that is partially covered by a small cap called the acrosome (ak'ro-sōm). The head is the actual nucleus of the sperm cell, containing the chromosomes. The acrosome contains lysosomal enzymes to facilitate penetration and fertilization of the oocyte. Only one sperm cell is permitted entry into any one oocyte. Adjacent to the head is the neck or midpiece, which

---

[10]The "tie" is the period of copulation between a male and female dog during which the two animals are physically locked together. The male cannot completely dismount until the bulbus glandis reduces in size.

[11]Seminiferous tubules (se"mĭ-nif'er-us, sĕ"mi-nif'er-us); from [L. *semen,* seed + *ferre,* to bear + *-ous,* pertaining to]; the seminiferous tubules are tiny channels throughout the testes in which spermatozoa develop and through which they leave the glandular tissue.

[12]Epididymis (ep"ĭ-did'ĭ-mis); from *epi-,* upon + [Gr. *didymos,* testis].

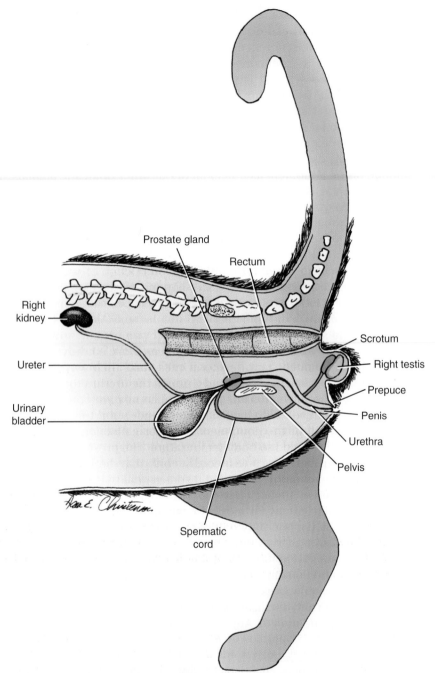

FIGURE 14-5   Feline male reproductive tract.

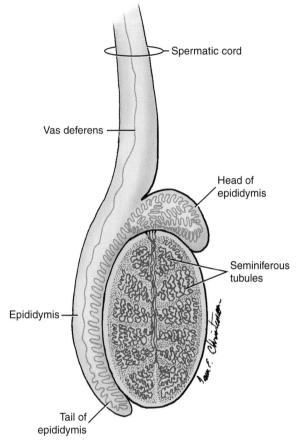

Spermatic cord

Vas deferens

Head of
epididymis

Seminiferous
tubules

Epididymis

Tail of
epididymis

FIGURE 14-6 Testis cross section.

contains numerous mitochondria. The tail of the sperm cell is a long, slender structure that contains a temporary energy store for the cell. This energy is required for the whipping movement of the tail that propels the sperm. On fertilization of the ovum, the sperm cell loses its midpiece and tail. When evaluating the morphology of sperm, abnormalities are conveniently divided into head, midpiece, and tail problems.

Estrous Cycle

Female domestic animals differ widely with regard to the length and frequency of their estrous cycles. Some are monestrous, whereas others are polyestrous. Some dogs tend to be monestrous, meaning the females will typically experience estrus once during the year followed by a long period of anestrus. (Many dogs may be biestrous, cycling twice during the year.) Polyestrous animals (i.e., cycling throughout the year) include cattle and pigs. Those animals that are seasonally polyestrous (meaning they will cycle numerous times during a given "season" of the year, and that season will be followed by a long anestrous

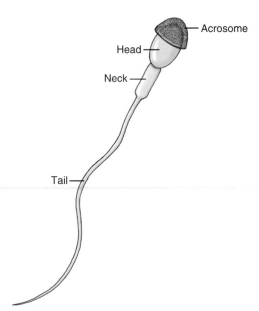

FIGURE 14-7   Spermatozoon.

period) include horses, sheep, goats, and cats. Horses and cats tend to come "in season" in the late winter/early spring. Sheep and goats, on the other hand, tend to cycle in the fall. Regardless of the frequency or length of the estrous cycle, each animal progresses through the same stages of estrus. Proestrus is the stage in which the female animal prepares for conception. Ovarian follicles form with ready oocytes, and the endometrium begins to engorge with blood in preparation for embryonic/fetal development. Estrus is that stage of the cycle in which the female is receptive to the male and can conceive. Depending on the animal, estrus could last only a matter of hours to days. Cows' and sows' average length of estrus is only about 18 hours. In contrast, dogs may be in estrus for several days. Ovulation for most animals is hormonally dependent. Cats are unique in that they are "induced ovulators." In other words, the queen will not ovulate unless stimulated by the male during copulation. Metestrus is the period immediately following estrus. If conception has not taken place, the ovarian follicles regress and the uterine wall returns to a more normal state. Anestrus or diestrus is the period of sexual quiescence in the female. Behavioral changes during each of these stages of the estrous cycle are variable among each of the domestic species. The single most consistent behavior exhibited by domestic animals in estrus is acceptance of the male. Estrus is the only time during which the female animal accepts the advances of a male and is able to conceive.

Conception and Gestation

On copulation of a female in estrus, millions of sperm "swim" through the female's reproductive tract in search of oocytes. (Many female domestic animals release multiple oocytes during estrus. This facilitates the production of multiple offspring from a single breeding. Dogs and cats are most inclined to produce litters of young. Of course, remember that cats are induced ovulators. So, theoretically, a queen could produce a litter of kittens conceived from multiple fathers. Ewes frequently produce twins. Mares and cows usually produce single offspring.) Each oocyte encountered along the reproductive tract is surrounded by sperm. Each sperm begins to attempt penetration of the oocyte by using proteolytic enzymes found in the acrosome. Vigorous tail lashing propels the sperm. Only one sperm is permitted entry. As soon as one sperm penetrates the ovum, the cell wall of the ovum becomes impermeable to any other sperm. The fertilized egg is now referred to as a zygote. The combined DNA of the sperm cell and the oocyte provide complete information for the creation of a new being. The zygote undergoes mitosis and implants on the endometrium. The placenta develops, providing a highly vascular, stable attachment for the developing embryo. Hormones produced by the ovarian follicle and the placenta maintain the pregnancy. All blood and nutrients pass from the mother through the placenta to the developing embryo/fetus, and all wastes from the offspring are transported back to the mother for elimination. Because of this shared arrangement, it is important to avoid administration of potentially teratogenic agents to the mother during the pregnancy. Even the administration of some immunizations during gestation could have teratogenic effects. (Feline panleukopenia virus is a good example of such a vaccine. If given to a queen late in pregnancy, some or all of the kittens could be born with cerebellar hypoplasia as a teratogenic effect of the vaccine.) Before anything is given to a pregnant female, a veterinarian should be consulted.

The gestation period varies from species to species. Refer to Table 14-1 for average gestation periods for each of the domestic species.

TABLE 14-1   Average Gestation Periods

Species	Gestation Period (Days)	Average No. of Young
Bovine	280–290	1
Canine	60–65	8–10
Equine	330–340	1
Feline	60–65	8–10
Ovine	140–150	1–2

Parturition

Parturition is the actual birthing process. Hormonal changes signal the onset of parturition. Domestic animals exhibit behavioral changes before the onset of physical labor. Most females appear anxious and restless and engage in preparturient "nesting" behaviors. Once the cervix has sufficiently dilated and uterine contractions intensify, the fetus is forced from the uterine horn through the uterine body and into the birth canal (vagina). Continued contractions force the fetus from the body of the female. The most common presentation of young is with the fetus positioned in sternal recumbency with the forefeet and head caudal in the mother (i.e., the forefeet and head to be presented first). Malpositioning of the fetus or excessively large fetuses often result in dystocia. (Dystocia caused by a large calf may produce postparturient paraparesis in the cow, due to obturator nerve damage. Obturator nerve paralysis is most commonly seen in cows.) As soon as the neonate is born, the mother begins to remove the fetal membranes from it. She severs the umbilical cord, usually by chewing through it. Shortly after giving birth to the neonate, placental attachments break down, and uterine contractions expel the placenta. This is often referred to as the "afterbirth." Many female animals consume the afterbirth. This is a protective mechanism, so that predators are not as readily attracted to her and her young. (Evidence is eliminated.) In animals who produce multiple offspring, it is important to account for a placenta for each neonate. A retained placenta could result in postparturient complications, such as metritis.

Lactation

Hormones usually stimulate lactation a number of hours or even days before parturition. The mammary glands become laden with milk and may even leak small amounts from the teats/nipples before parturition. The first milk produced by the female is called colostrum (ko-los'trum). It contains large quantities of maternal antibodies that provide the neonate(s) with temporary immunity. It is extremely important for neonates to suckle as soon as possible postpartum. The colostrum is contained only in the first milk produced, and the neonates can readily absorb the antibodies only during the first hours of life. In most domestic animals, absorption of colostral antibodies drops significantly after 12 hours postpartum. The maternal antibodies in the colostrum will provide passive immunity for the neonates. Failure of passive transfer of these antibodies will leave the young at grave risk of infectious diseases. Milk produced after the initial colostrum is much richer in milk fats, providing a better energy source for the young. The female continues to lactate, provided she is stimulated through natural suckling or mechanical milking. In those species that tend to produce multiple offspring, each neonate tends to select a specific teat from which it will nurse. Subsequent feedings are likely to be from the same teat as the first. The time of weaning varies from species to species and female to female. On average, however, most young are weaned between 3 and 6 weeks of age. If mastitis develops, the young must be weaned earlier or bottle-fed with a milk replacer until an appropriate weaning time can be achieved. Of course, dairy calves are fed milk replacers in lieu of milk from the cow, so that the milk can be marketed. Calves are bottle-fed colostrum (usually stored frozen until needed for a neonate). Careful milking practices and husbandry of dairy cattle are important to prevent mastitis. Mastitis in dairy cattle can have a profound economic impact on the dairy operation and the industry. Because the dairy industry is so important to food animal practice, it is very important that veterinary professionals understand the structure and function of the bovine mammary glands (i.e., udder; Fig. 14-8).

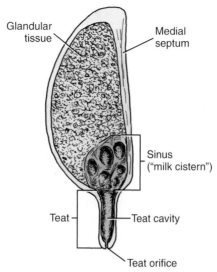

Glandular tissue

Medial septum

Sinus ("milk cistern")

Teat

Teat cavity

Teat orifice

FIGURE 14-8 Individual bovine quarter.

The udder of a cow is actually subdivided into four quarters. Each quarter is distinct and separate from the others. (This is important with regard to mastitis. It is very possible to have one mastitic quarter, while the other three quarters remain healthy and functional.) Suspensory ligaments help support and subdivide the quarters. On physical examination, the suspensory apparatus is one feature to be evaluated. With a strong, healthy suspensory apparatus, the udder should have a deep, well-defined cleft between each of the quarters, and the udder should be carried high. The ventral aspect of the udder and the teats, ideally, should be above the level of the tarsus. Cows whose udders hang lower are at greater risk of teat and udder injury. Cleanliness of the udder is of utmost importance in the prevention of mastitis. Housing and bedding areas must be kept as clean as possible, to minimize contamination of the udder while the cows are lying down. (Never discard milk into the bedding when collecting samples for analysis. This provides bacterial growth media in the bedding.) Whenever handling the udder and teats for collection of milk samples, it is important to clean the udder and teats before collection. The cleaning process serves two purposes: (1) it removes potential contaminants, and (2) it promotes milk letdown. To collect the sample, it is useful to understand the internal anatomy of the mammary gland (see Fig. 14-8). Once milk letdown has occurred (stimulated too by bumping the gland with your hand, much like the calf would do when suckling), you must trap the milk in the teat cavity before you can milk it out. The easiest way to do this is to grasp the base of the teat (nearest the udder) by wrapping your thumb and forefinger around it snuggly. While maintaining that grasp, the teat may be emptied by progressively applying pressure with the remaining fingers in sequence (i.e., third, fourth, and then fifth digits). Through this entrapment and applied pressure, milk should be forced through the teat orifice. If you fail to trap the milk in the teat cavity, the milk will simply be forced back up into the larger gland sinus (also called the milk cistern). It takes practice, so don't be disappointed if you cannot extract milk on your first attempt. Following any milking procedure, it is important to apply a bacteriostatic agent to the teats.

Pseudocyesis and Related Issues

Pseudocyesis occurs most commonly in dogs. Hormonal and physical changes in this female's body follow a typical gestation period. The only trouble is, she's not pregnant. She may develop mammary enlargement and may even lactate briefly. Psychologically, the female is inclined to behave with maternal instincts. She may exhibit preparturient nesting behaviors, just like a normal pregnancy. Of course, there will be no parturition in the dog experiencing pseudocyesis. No puppies? No problem. In the absence of puppies, she may nurture stuffed toys or other such objects. The incidence of metritis and pyometra is much greater in cases of pseudocyesis, and therefore these animals should be watched closely for signs of disease. Ovariohysterectomy (spay) is the best means of preventing pseudocyesis and its potentially lethal "cousin"—pyometra. When performed before a dog's or cat's first estrous cycle, an ovariohysterectomy can reduce the animal's risk of mammary cancer to almost zero. (It is a myth that every dog and cat should have one litter before she is spayed.) Even older females will benefit from reduced risk of mammary cancer, although the older she gets as an intact female, the greater her risk of serious, potentially life-threatening diseases like pyometra and cancer. A mastectomy in a dog or a cat is extremely invasive and traumatic. Remember, their mammary tissue extends from the pubic area, over the abdomen, and onto the ventral thorax. Just imagine the length of that incision line. Then imagine the painful recovery from the mastectomy—a surgery that may have been prevented by an ovariohysterectomy performed when the animal was a puppy or a kitten.

Of course, the importance of ovariohysterectomy and orchiectomy surgeries for population control in the United States goes without saying. It is an ugly truth that millions of unwanted dogs and cats are put to death every year by animal control agencies and humane societies. Veterinary professionals have an obligation to society and the animals they serve to promote spaying and neutering of pets, in the interest of animal health and in the interest of curbing the overpopulation problem.

SELF-TEST

Using the previous information in this chapter, complete the following crossword puzzle using the most appropriate medical term(s). Do not use abbreviations or common names unless requested.

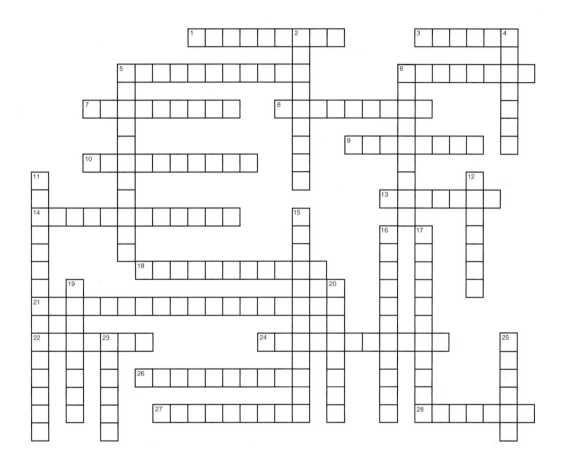

ACROSS

1   Something that causes physical defects in a developing fetus
3   The phase of the reproductive cycle when the female is receptive to the male and can conceive
5   Inflammation of the prostate gland
6   Pus in the uterus
7   The first milk containing maternal antibodies
8   The process of milk production
9   The period of reproductive quiescence in a female—synonym diestrus
10 Surgical removal of mammary tissue
13 Something that alters DNA

14	"Plastic surgery" of the vulva
18	The interior lining of the uterus
21	Surgical removal of the ovaries and uterus
22	The _____ cycle is the complete reproductive cycle of the female
24	An animal with retained testes
26	Females who have only one reproductive cycle per year
27	The phase of a female's reproductive cycle immediately following estrus
28	A newborn

DOWN

2	Pregnancy
4	The sac that contains the testes
5	Females who have multiple reproductive cycles during the year
6	The stage of the reproductive cycle immediately preceding estrus
11	The production of sperm
12	The process of creating eggs and sperm
15	A false pregnancy
16	Castration/surgical removal of the testes
17	The process of giving birth
19	Inflammation of the mammary tissue
20	A difficult birth
23	An egg cell
25	A fertilized oocyte

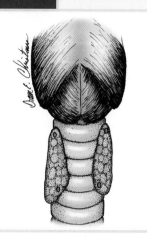

CHAPTER 15

The Endocrine System

GOALS AND OBJECTIVES

By the conclusion of this chapter, the student will be able to:

1. Recognize common root words, prefixes, and suffixes related to the endocrine system.
2. Divide simple and compound words into their respective parts.
3. Recognize, correctly pronounce, and appropriately use common medical terms related to the endocrine system.
4. Demonstrate an understanding of endocrine anatomy.
5. Demonstrate an understanding of endocrine physiology with regard to hormones and negative feedback.
6. Demonstrate an understanding of endocrine physiology and pathophysiology with regard to principal functions and effects of each of the major endocrine organs.

Note: It is advisable that this chapter be attempted only after Chapters 1 through 14 have been successfully completed. Assumptions of anatomic and physiologic knowledge of previous body systems are made throughout this chapter.

Introduction to Related Terms

Divide each of the following terms into its respective parts ("R," root; "P," prefix; "S," suffix; "CV," combining vowel).

1. **Adrenal** (adj.)   (P) _____ (R) _____ (S) _____
   adrenal (ah-dre′nal; pertaining to near the kidney; clinically refers to the adrenal glands, which are located close to the kidneys)

2. **Adrenergic** (adj.)   (R) _____ (R) _____ (S) _____
   adrenergic (ad″ren-er′jik; pertaining to adrenal working; clinically refers to activity stimulated by adrenaline [epinephrine])

3. **Endogenous** (adj.)   (P) _____ (R) _____ (S) _____
   endogenous (en-doj'ĕ-nes; pertaining to inside/inner production; i.e., produced within the body)

4. **Exogenous** (adj.)   (P) _____ (R) _____ (S) _____
   exogenous (ek-soj'ĕ-nes; pertaining to outside/outer production; i.e., originating from outside the body)

5. **Adrenocorticotropic** (adj.)   (R) _____ (CV) _____ (R) _____
                                    (CV) _____ (R) _____ (S) _____
   adrenocorticotropic (ad-re"no-kor"tĭ-ko-tro'pik; pertaining to adrenal cortex stimulating/influencing; cf. adrenocorticotrophic)

6. **Endocrinopathy** (n.)   (R) _____ (CV) _____ (S) _____
   endocrinopathy (en"do-krĭ-nop'ah-the; a disease of the endocrine system)

7. **Hyperadrenocorticism** (n.)   (P) _____ (R) _____ (CV) _____
                                    (R) _____ (S) _____
   hyperadrenocorticism (hi"per-ă-dre"no-kor'tĭ-siz-em; a condition of excessive adrenal cortex; i.e., excessive secretion of adrenal cortex hormones)

8. **Adenohypophysis** (n.)   (R) _____ (CV) _____ (P) _____
                                    (CV) _____ (S) _____
   adenohypophysis (ad"ĕ-no-hi-pof'ĭ-sis; growth of a gland below; clinically refers to the glandular, anterior portion of the pituitary gland)

9. **Neurohypophysis** (n.)   (R) _____ (CV) _____ (P) _____
                                    (CV) _____ (S) _____
   neurohypophysis (nu"ro-hi-pof'ĭ-sis; growth of nerves below; clinically refers to the neural, posterior portion of the pituitary gland)

10. **Parathyroid** (n. or adj.)   (P) _____ (R) _____
    parathyroid (par"ah-thi'roid; beside the thyroid)

11. **Hypothyroidism** (n.)   (P) _____ (R) _____ (S) _____
    hypothyroidism (hi"po-thi'roid-izm; a state of low thyroid; clinically refers to deficient levels of hormones produced by the thyroid gland)

12. **Hyperthyroidism** (n.)   (P) _____ (R) _____ (S) _____
    hyperthyroidism (hi"per-thi'roid-iz-em; a condition of excessive thyroid; i.e., excessive thyroid hormone secretions)

13. **Antidiuretic** (adj.)   (P) _____ (R) _____ (S) _____
    antidiuretic (an"tĭ-di"u-ret'ik; pertaining to being against urination)

14. **Hypoglycemia** (n.)   (P) _____ (R) _____ (R) _____ (S) _____
    hypoglycemia (hi"po-gli-se'me-ah; a state of low glucose in the blood)

15. **Hyperglycemia** (n.)   (P) _____ (R) _____ (R) _____ (S) _____
    hyperglycemia (hi"per-gli-se'me-ah; a state of excessive glucose in the blood)

16. **Polydipsia** (n.)   (P) _____ (R) _____ (S) _____
    polydipsia (pol"e-dip'se-ah; a condition of much thirst [Gr. *dipsa*, thirst])

17. **Hypocalcemia** (n.)   (P) _____ (R) _____ (R) _____ (S) _____
    hypocalcemia (hi″po-kal-se′me-ah; a condition of deficient blood calcium)

18. **Somatotropic** (adj.)   (R) _____ (CV) _____ (R) _____ (S) _____
    somatotropic (so″mă-to-tro′pik; pertaining to body influencing [Gr. *tropos,* turn, influence])

19. **Gonadotropic** (adj.)   (R) _____ (CV) _____ (R) _____ (S) _____
    gonadotropic (go″nă-do-tro′pik; pertaining to gonad influencing)

20. **Prolactin** (n.)   (P) _____ (R) _____ (S) _____
    prolactin (pro-lak′tin; before milk; prolactin is the hormone that stimulates milk production)

21. **Oxytocin** (n.)   (P) _____ (R) _____ (S) _____
    oxytocin (ok″se-to′sin; a quick birth [Gr. *oxys,* quick + *tokos,* birth]; oxytocin is the
    hormone associated with labor)

22. **Erythropoietin** (n.)   (R) _____ (CV) _____ (R) _____ (S)_____
    erythropoietin (ĕ-rith″ro-poi′e-tin; a red producer [Gr. *poien,* to make]; i.e., the hormone
    responsible for stimulating red blood cell production)

Endocrine Anatomy and Physiology

Before we begin to discuss the endocrine system in detail, I must preface the discussion. There will be times you will probably think that I am talking in circles. The fact of the matter is, you will probably be right. There is no way around it. When it comes to the hormones produced by this system and the influence that they exert on the body, it is much like Sir Isaac Newton said when discussing his theory on physics: "For every action there is an equal and opposite reaction." You must think of the endocrine system as an internal communication network. The only difference is, this communication system does not use tangible devices like intercoms and telephones. Instead, the endocrine system uses chemicals called hormones.[1] Rather than communication between people in a relationship, the endocrine system provides communication between organs and tissues, helping them maintain their mutual relationships. So, will we talk in circles? Yes, we will. As in any relationship and the communication used to maintain that relationship, there must be a give and take. There must be open lines of communication—giving and receiving of information and ideas. Feedback is necessary. Without feedback, be it positive or negative, how can we know that actions taken in the relationship are in everyone's best interest? Complex? Yes. Isn't every relationship complex? Ah, but the efforts put forth in open communication are worth it, by maintaining a well-balanced (i.e., homeostatic) relationship.

Let us begin by looking at those principle organs of the endocrine system, briefly touching upon the hormones produced by each. Then we will delve into that delicate dance of communication that this system provides for homeostasis.

---

[1]Hormone [Gr. *hormaein,* to set in motion]; hormones are chemicals of the body that stimulate various bodily activities.

Unlike other chapters in which the normal anatomy and physiology was discussed before any disease syndromes, the normal and abnormal physiology will be discussed together. In this complex system, it is often easier to understand normal function by immediately looking at ways that it can be broken.

Endocrine Organs

Pituitary Gland (Hypophysis)

The pituitary is the master gland. Endocrinology "command and control central" is right here. Why, its location alone gives the impression that it is significant. Where is it? The hypophysis is located on the ventromidline of the brain, beneath the hypothalamus (Fig. 15-1). A small depression in the floor of the cranial vault cradles the tiny pituitary gland. It may be small, but it is mighty in its function. The gland itself is subdivided into two distinct lobes: the anterior pituitary or the adenohypophysis, and the posterior pituitary or the neurohypophysis. As the names indicate, the adenohypophysis is truly glandular tissue, whereas the neurohypophysis is actually specialized neural tissue (specialized because it secretes hormones). Why is the hypophysis "pilot in command," so to speak? Well, the hypophysis tells most of the other major glands and organs what to do. Somebody has to be in charge, otherwise we'd have systemic chaos. Its neighbor, the hypothalamus, is sort of the "first mate." Between the hypothalamus and the hypophysis, we can coordinate most of the body's activities. The major hypophyseal hormones are noted in Table 15-1.

What does each of these hormones do? Well, for some, their names give their function away. Take growth hormone (GH), for instance. It has tremendous somatotropic effects, to promote (what else?) growth. Ah, but the need for GH does not end when one reaches adulthood. In response to injuries, GH is necessary to stimulate an increased rate of cellular reproduction for the repair of those tissues. Another hormone named by its function is thyroid-stimulating hormone (TSH). There are a plethora of hypophyseal hormones. We'll address the rest of the hormones later. First, let's look at the rest of our endocrine organs.

Thyroid Gland

The thyroid gland is located on the ventrolateral aspect of the trachea, slightly caudal to the larynx (Fig. 15-2). In most of the domestic animals, the thyroid is found as two lateral lobes of glandular tissue that, depending on the species, may or may not be connected by an isthmus. Let's see, we said that the adenohypophysis secretes TSH. Guess what! TSH stimulates the thyroid gland to secrete its hormones! (No rocket science there.) Two of the thyroid hormones produced are thyroxine (thi-rok'sin; T_4—because its molecule has four atoms of iodine), and triiodothyronine (T_3).[2] Both T_3 and T_4 control the body's metabolic rate. In the presence of these thyroid hormones, cellular activity and, consequently, metabolism increase. Okay, time to get a little "loopy" (i.e., discuss

---

[2]Triiodothyronine (T_3); (tri-i″o-do-thi′ro-nēn); so named because its molecule has three atoms of iodine [*tri-*, three + *iod(o)-*, iodine + *thyr(o)-*, thyroid + *-ine*].

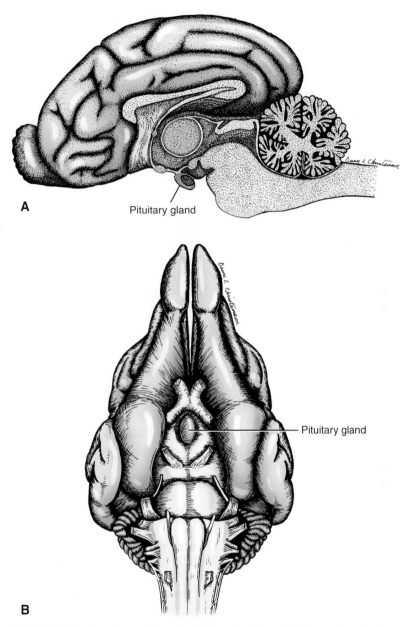

FIGURE 15-1   Pituitary gland. **A,** Midsagittal view. **B,** Ventrodorsal view.

feedback loops). Ready or not, here we go! The hypothalamus detects low levels of T_3 and T_4; the hypothalamus then stimulates the adenohypophysis to secrete TSH (this is our first mate calling to the captain to respond to a problem; this captain responds with TSH); in the presence of TSH, the thyroid gland secretes T_3 and T_4; with sufficient levels of T_3 and T_4 the hypothalamus stops stimulating

TABLE 15-1 Major Hypophyseal Hormones	
Hormones of the Adenohypophysis	**Hormones of the Neurohypophysis**
Adrenocorticotropic hormone (ACTH)	Antidiuretic hormone (ADH)
Follicle-stimulating hormone (FSH)	Oxytocin (OT)
Growth hormone (GH)	
Luteinizing hormone (LH)	
Prolactin (PRL)	
Thyroid-stimulating hormone (TSH)	

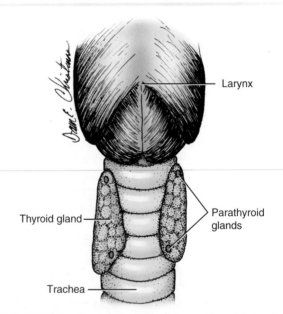

FIGURE 15-2   Canine thyroid and parathyroid glands.

the adenohypophysis and, in turn, TSH is no longer secreted. It's as though in our communication network the hypothalamus perceives that our "glass is full" and says, "Whoa! Hold it, Captain! We've got enough!" That's what we refer to as negative feedback. It's negative because it stops the glandular secretory activity. It is really no different from pouring soda into a glass. When you see that the glass is full, you stop pouring. Of course, that's the way negative feedback works if we're normal.

There are times when this wonderful feedback loop can be broken. In cases of hypothyroidism, either the adenohypophysis fails to secrete TSH or the thyroid gland fails to respond adequately to TSH. Either way, in hypothyroidism we have insufficient T_3 and T_4 to adequately control the body's metabolic rate. Hypothyroidism is one of the more common endocrinopathies in dogs. Having reduced metabolic activity, these dogs will tend to be obese and lethargic. Providing exogenous thyroid hormones through oral replacement therapy can improve their metabolic rates and overall well-being. Dogs receiving replacement therapy can effectively lose weight and experience renewed energy and vitality. On the flip side of the coin, hyperthyroidism is quite common in cats. The appearance of these cats is just the opposite of our hypothyroid dogs. These cats may eat like kings, yet remain incredibly thin. They're like supercharged Energizer bunnies. Unfortunately, having a body metabolically on the go-go-go takes its toll. Conditions like hypertrophic cardiomyopathy often accompany feline hyperthyroidism. That can have deadly consequences. So, therapy for these cats is aimed directly at the thyroid gland to reduce its secretions of T_3 and T_4.

Calcitonin (kal″sĭ-to′nin), also produced by the thyroid gland, helps control concentrations of calcium and phosphorus. In the presence of calcitonin, blood levels of calcium and phosphate ions are lowered. How? Well, calcitonin inhibits osteoclastic activity, reducing the rate at which calcium and phosphate ions leave the bone. Calcitonin also increases renal exretion of these ions. Okay, this is a good time to talk about another one of those feedback loops in our communication network. Let's see. The first question that comes to mind is: what makes the thyroid secrete calcitonin in the first place? Look at the name of the hormone and think about what it does—that's right, it's going to involve calcium concentrations. In hypercalcemia, the thyroid will secrete calcitonin. Calcitonin will effectively reduce the calcium and phosphate released from the bone and increase renal excretion of these ions. But wait, we need an "off switch," right? So, what inhibits calcitonin secretion? When blood calcium levels reach a reasonable, normal range, we stop secreting calcitonin. See how the give and take works? For every action there is an equal and opposite reaction, to maintain homeostasis.

Parathyroid Glands

We cannot discuss calcium, phosphorus, and bone without looking at the parathyroid glands. The parathyroid glands are found in pairs on the surface of each of the thyroid gland lobes (see Fig. 15-2). The four parathyroid glands are small in comparison with the thyroid. Now, let's name the hormone produced by the parathyroid glands. Keep it simple. That's right, the parathyroid glands secrete parathyroid hormone (PTH, also called parathormone). Why do we need PTH, if we have calcitonin from the thyroid gland? Think about it. All calcitonin can do is reduce blood calcium concentrations. Don't we need a way to increase calcium concentrations? Yes we do. That's where PTH comes into our give-and-take communication picture. The parathyroid glands are "free agents," seizing the opportunities to "play" when those opportunities present themselves. What kind of opportunity are we talking about? How about hypocalcemia? In neurology, we talked about the importance of calcium concentration. It must be maintained in just the right concentration for appropriate neuromuscular function. Hypercalcemia will depress neurotransmission, and hypocalcemia will permit neurons and muscles to depolarize with little to no stimulus. Of the two abnormal calcium concentrations, hypocalcemia is far more common. Let's put that into perspective, shall we? Take a postparturient cow. She'll have a sudden high demand for calcium because of lactation. (Prolactin from the adenohypophysis facilitates the lactation.) Demand for calcium may far exceed the ready supply in the bloodstream, creating a hypo-calcemic state. In an attempt to maintain homeostasis, the hypocalcemia should stimulate the parathyroid glands to secrete PTH. As a result, osteoclastic activity will increase calcium and phosphate release from the bone. Plus, the renal tubules will respond to PTH by conserving calcium and increasing excretion of phosphate. PTH will even indirectly increase the absorption of calcium from food, by influencing the metabolism of vitamin D into its active form. Active vitamin D is the necessary transport mechanism for absorption of calcium from the digestive tract. If normal, all of these PTH-influenced activities will increase blood calcium concentrations to normal. If the hypocalcemia is severe enough, the cow may actually be clinically ill, with agitation and body-wide muscle tremors. More severe hypocalcemic ("milk fever") cows may become anorexic, tachycardic, and quadriparetic from the tremendous, acute calcium depletion (and other electrolyte imbalances), leaving very little calcium available for the presynaptic bulbs and myofibrils. Serum calcium levels in these animals could drop to as low as 2 mg/dL from a normal level of approximately 10 mg/dL. Needless to say, that doesn't facilitate very good neuromuscular function. This extreme state is beyond anything the parathyroid glands can correct. This requires medical intervention. Exogenous calcium will need to be administered, usually intravenously, to correct the imbalance. Of course, the treatment itself can be risky. If given too rapidly, calcium can be cardiotoxic, leading to potentially lethal arrhythmias. If given at an appropriate rate, most of these cows recover rapidly. Once a normal state is reestablished, with appropriate nutritional support and management practices, thyroid hormones, and PTH should be able to maintain homeostasis as far as calcium levels are concerned.

Do you see the intricate web that we are weaving in endocrinology? One thing leads to another. We can't simply talk about one of the endocrine glands as its own separate entity, because the hormones produced by it may impact a plethora of other organs and tissues directly and indirectly. That can make this system seem very overwhelming. To add to the frustration of learning about endocrinology, we can't *see* it work. I mean, it's not like talking about the relationship of a muscle to a joint. Make the muscle contract and we can see the joint move. Why, we can even feel the muscle contract. We can't see or touch hormones. Sure we can perform serology to check hormonal levels, but that doesn't really let us "see or touch" them. All we can see or feel are the results of hormonal work through reactions of the body to the various hormones. Fortunately, some of those reactions and responses can be profound. That is so true when we look at adrenal function.

Adrenal Glands

We touched on the adrenal glands briefly, when we discussed fight or flight in the neurology chapter. Talk about profound body reactions to hormones! There is nothing subtle about epinephrine—a powerful, sympathomimetic hormone that is secreted by a couple of the smallest endocrine glands of the body. Why adrenal? The prefix *ad-* means toward or near, and you already know what renal means. Well, the adrenal glands were so named because they lie near the kidneys (Fig. 15-3). How's that for simplicity in a complicated system? These

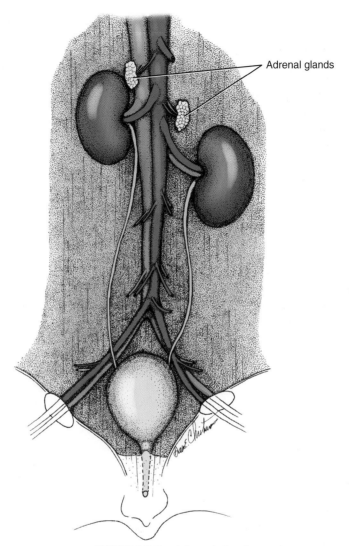

FIGURE 15-3   Adrenal glands.

two small glands are structurally similar to the kidneys, in that they have an adrenal cortex and an adrenal medulla. Each of these areas secretes different hormones. The adrenal medulla secretes epinephrine and norepinephrine. Epinephrine is the more powerful and significant of the two. Okay, time to look at another loop. Which branch of the autonomic nervous system innervates the adrenal medulla? That's right, the sympathetic branch. Under sympathetic control, epinephrine is constantly secreted. So, what about those "power surges" of epinephrine? If you recall, the epinephrine stress response (fight or flight) was set into motion by exposure to sensory stimuli. Remember, it could be visual, tactile, auditory, or olfactory stimuli that set off the sympathetic branch. Yes, those profound sympathetic impulses will directly cause the mydriasis, bronchodilation, peripheral vasoconstriction, and positive inotropism, as well as turn off the digestive tract. But neurologically, that's not enough. The nervous system cannot sustain those responses. By stimulating massive secretion of epinephrine, we can sustain sympathomimetic support of the responses that the nervous system originally kicked into gear. It's the adrenergic effects of epinephrine that permit us to fight or flee. How long will we continue to secrete those increased volumes of epinephrine? As long as the stimulus is present and we have a conscious brain to perceive the threat. Once the stimulus is removed, sympathetic fibers will no longer increase the rate of neurotransmission to the adrenal medulla. Adrenal function will return to its normal, ready state. What happens if we administer exogenous epinephrine to an animal? The very same responses occur. Except, in this case, we have artificially created those responses without stimulating the sympathetic fibers or the adrenal gland. But the exogenous epinephrine will bind to the same alpha- and beta-adrenergic receptors[3] as the endogenous hormone would. So, the results are the same. Okay, I know what you're thinking. Why would we want to artificially induce such profound responses in the body? Well, how about anaphylaxis, hypovolemia, or, better yet, asystole? Yes, it's typically critical situations that cause us to pull out the "big guns," like epinephrine. Thankfully, we have exogenous big guns available to help those critical animals.

The stress story does not end with the adrenal medulla and fight or flight. We still have an adrenal cortex that we haven't discussed. This time, we'll use pure hormonal triggers. That's right. Here's where adrenocorticotropic hormone (ACTH) comes into play. ACTH is another one of those hormones secreted by the adenohypophysis. When ACTH stimulates the adrenal cortex, cortisol[4] is secreted. Probably the most familiar and popular effect of cortisol is its antiinflammatory activity. We capitalize on the antiinflammatory properties of glucocorticoids (corticosteroids) with allergic conditions. Corticosteroids, whether exogenous or endogenous, can really suppress immune reactions. Vascular permeability will be reduced and antibody production will diminish in the presence of cortisol. That's very useful therapeutically in hypersensitive animals. Okay, that makes sense. But inflammation due to allergic conditions can't be the only reason cortisol exists. Why else would we need to secrete endogenous cortisol? In the presence of chronic disease or stress, ACTH stimulates cortisol secretion. This glucocorticosteroid (glucocorticoid) stress response[5] is a protective mechanism intended to promote rapid mobilization of amino acids and fatty

---

[3]Alpha- and beta-adrenergic receptors; the response of an organ to epinephrine depends on the numbers of alpha- and beta-receptors. Some organs may have only one type of receptor. Alpha-receptors tend to predominate in areas like peripheral vasculature, to facilitate vasoconstriction. Think: "beta is better." Strategically located beta-receptors give us the stimulatory effects of epinephrine, like mydriasis, bronchodilation, positive inotropism, and vasodilation to major muscles.

[4]Cortisol (kor'tĭ-sol); a corticosteroid produced by the adrenal cortex; also called hydrocortisone.

[5]Glucocorticosteroid stress response (glu"ko-kor"tĭ-ko-ster'oid); a process in which cortisol is secreted in large amounts to reduce inflammation and provide energy, in the form of glucose, for the body. This response is usually associated with chronic disease or injury.

acids from energy stores in the body and to stimulate gluconeogenesis by the liver. It also promotes a better appetite. But even if food is not available, the glucocorticoid stress response is one way that the body manages to maintain normal blood glucose levels. It's a way that, when the going gets tough, we can be tough and keep going. Of course, there are undesirable effects of corticosteroids. That reduced vascular permeability we mentioned earlier? Well, that's a problem when neutrophils and monocytes can't exit the vasculature to battle pathogenic organisms in the tissues. Suppressed immunity from corticosteroids? Well, we might as well just open the door for infectious diseases to ravage the body. Wounds won't heal as rapidly as they should either. (Wound healing will be discussed in Chapter 16.) What kind of stress are we talking about that leads to this response? It could be physical or emotional. Physical problems could be things like chronic pain of osteoarthritis, cardiac disease, or cancer. Emotional stresses may include overcrowding of animals, moving to a new home, or surrender of a dog or cat to an animal shelter. Let's really combine the physical and emotional factors by shipping livestock to a crowded stockyard. These animals will be highly susceptible to disease. What you have to realize is that the immunosuppression from these stresses can be so great that even normal, commensal bacteria can overcolonize and cause disease. That's often what happens in shipping fever pneumonia in cattle. It may be the cattles' own *Pasteurella* bacteria that cause the pneumonia. Okay, so we've made a very good point of the significance of immunosuppression that may result from corticosteroids, be they endogenous or exogenous. So, what can we do about it? Good question. First, knowing what might trigger such a response enables us to take steps to prevent it. Simply knowing that the immunosuppression does occur is a very valuable piece of information. We can anticipate the immunosuppressive problems in the event of unavoidable stress or when an animal is treated with exogenous corticosteroids. Then steps can be taken to minimize the exposure of that animal to possible infectious diseases. We can anticipate that a surgical patient receiving corticosteroids will have a longer healing time. Therefore, its surgical wounds may be managed differently from the average surgical patient (e.g., leaving skin sutures in longer than normal). Knowledge is empowering.

While we're talking about side effects of corticosteroids, let's look at the problems of polyuria and polydipsia (PU/PD) that they typically cause. "So what," you say? What do you suppose would happen if we prescribed corticosteroids for a dog with an allergic condition and we did not tell the owner about these side effects? The owner would not anticipate the dog's need to urinate more during the day. So, the owner will likely come home to numerous accidents in the house after work. Not understanding the cause of the problem, the owner may wrongly reprimand the dog. Then, when the owner realizes that the dog is actually drinking more too, he or she may decide to reduce or withhold water to solve the problem. This is no solution. The dog will still be polyuric, in spite of the reduced water intake. What will this lead to? Dehydration. We have discussed numerous times the consequences of dehydration. What's the point to be made here? That the empowering knowledge of corticosteroids causing PU/PD is worthless unless we educate the owner about those side effects. Just as it would be worthless if we did not share with the owner that this dog will be more susceptible to infectious diseases while taking the drug. What good does it do to remedy the allergic symptoms if the dog becomes extremely ill or dies of an infectious disease or dehydration? Another thing to remember with the administration of exogenous glucocorticoids is that we totally bypass the negative feedback loop. You see, under normal circumstances the hypothalamus (in response to external or internal stress stimuli) turns on the adenohypophysis to secrete ACTH. Once the adrenal cortex has produced enough cortisol, both the hypothalamus and the adenohypophysis "step down" and cease their activities. Exogenous corticosteroids, especially with chronic and higher doses, can result in hyperadrenocorticism (Cushing's disease). These animals will typically be polyphagic, polyuric, and polydipsic; lose hair; and develop thin skin. The other adverse effects discussed earlier (i.e., immunosuppression and prolonged healing) will also be present. Our whole negative feedback system will be lulled into a state of poor responsiveness or unresponsiveness. The adrenal cortex, like a muscle that is not exercised, may atrophy. In fact, if exogenous corticosteroids are abruptly withdrawn, the animal could be placed into an acute hypoadrenocortical (addisonian[6]) crisis. Exogenous corticosteroids must be withdrawn very gradually at a reduced dose over time. This permits all of the players in this feedback loop (hypothalamus, adenohypophysis, and adrenal cortex) to work slowly back up to a fully functional state.

Glucocorticoids are not the only hormones produced by the adrenal cortex. Mineralocorticoids are also produced, the most important of which is aldosterone. Unlike cortisol, aldosterone is not produced in response to ACTH. Factors involved with the secretion and use of aldosterone really revolve around the kidney. So, let's go back and review a little renal function, shall we? Remember in Chapter 13 when we discussed the effects of angiotensin on the rate of filtrate production? Well, we left out a few pieces to that puzzle. Now, we'll discuss the rest of the story. Let's start the story with a decrease in arterial pressure. In response to the decreased blood pressure, the kidney will secrete renin, which stimulates the release of angiotensin I. Angiotensin-converting enzyme (ACE) will change angiotensin I into angiotensin II. This will cause several simultaneous events. As we said in Chapter 13, angiotensin II will cause vasoconstriction of the efferent glomerular arteriole to improve hydrostatic pressure in the glomerulus. (In fact, it will even cause vasoconstriction in many areas of the body in an attempt to improve overall blood pressure.) Additional direct renal effects include reduced glomerular filtration and increased water absorption.

So what does all of this have to do with endocrinology? Increased levels of angiotensin II also stimulate the adrenal cortex to secrete aldosterone. In turn, aldosterone will reduce sodium excretion. Conservation of sodium will help us hold onto water, to improve blood pressure. Last but not least, increased angiotensin II levels will affect the hypothalamus, causing an increase in thirst. Plus, the hypothalamus will stimulate the neurohypophysis to secrete antidiuretic hormone (ADH). This will make the distal renal tubules more permeable to water so that it can be reabsorbed. What's the end result? Increased blood pressure. Woo hoo! What a team! All for one and one for all! Talk about cause and

---

[6]Addisonian; i.e., Addison's disease (hypoadrenocorticism).

effect! Do we have a negative feedback loop? You bet we do. In fact, I'll bet you can guess what initiates it. That's right, with the improved, normal blood pressure the kidney no longer secretes renin. With no renin, there is ultimately no excess angiotensin II, which in turn shuts off adrenocortical secretion of aldosterone and neurohypophyseal secretion of ADH. What a complicated scenario that was. It almost seems as though there are too many redundancies. Perhaps. Frankly, that's how important sufficient blood pressure is. In fact, it is so important that hypotension is not the only trigger for ADH secretion. In a developing state of dehydration, adequate blood pressure will be maintained by many compensatory cardiovascular mechanisms. Behind the scenes, the hypothalamus will sense increased extracellular osmolarity. This too will trigger the secretion of ADH from the neurohypophysis. Again, the distal convoluted tubules will respond by absorbing water. This conservation measure may be just enough to improve hydration before hypovolemia and hypotension develop. ADH secretion will stop as soon as extracellular osmolarity resumes a normal state. Aldosterone isn't simply secreted in response to angiotensin II either. Hyperkalemia will also stimulate aldosterone secretion, not only to conserve sodium but to excrete more potassium too. What a tangled web we weave in endocrinology! Do you see why, if one of these critical endocrine organs fails, the whole body may suffer? Take antidiuretic hormone, for instance. If the neurohypophysis fails to secrete ADH we lose a powerful water conservation mechanism and the affected animal is chronically polyuric and polydipsic. "What we've got here is a failure to communicate."[7] That is precisely the problem in diabetes insipidus (not be confused with diabetes mellitus, which is a pancreatic disorder). In diabetes insipidus the neurohypophysis fails to communicate with the kidney by not secreting ADH.

Of course, we cannot discuss renal function with regard to hormones without discussing erythropoietin. Let's see, what do red blood cells (RBCs) do? They transport oxygen, right? So, to set up a logical feedback system, let's rely on oxygen-carrying capacity. However, the kidney does not take a "head count" to know how many transport vehicles we have (i.e., RBCs). Instead, the kidneys rely on PaO_2 levels. In hypoxia, the kidneys will be stimulated to secrete erythropoietin. Once the bone marrow responds by manufacturing and releasing more erythrocytes into circulation, our oxygen levels (in the absence of cardiopulmonary disease) should return to normal. The amount of erythropoietin secreted should then diminish. (Remember, there is always a certain amount of turnover with regard to erythrocytes.) Shall we break our communication network here? Let's look at a patient with chronic renal failure. Renal failure patients will be prone to developing nonregenerative anemia, because they will lack the capacity to secrete erythropoietin. How will we know the anemia is nonregenerative? Polychromasia and reticulocytes will be absent.

Pancreas

What a remarkable organ the pancreas is. It's a "switch-hitter" among organs, because it has both exocrine and endocrine functions. The exocrine activity of the pancreas was discussed in Chapter 12. What does its endocrine "communication"

---

[7]Quote from the 1967 Oscar-winning movie, "Cool Hand Luke," starring Paul Newman.

revolve around? Glucose homeostasis is its forte. The pancreatic hormone insulin (in'su-lin) is responsible for lowering blood glucose concentrations. In the presence of insulin, active transport of glucose into cells is promoted. By facilitating active transport and use or storage of glucose, blood glucose concentrations are lowered. On reaching normal blood glucose concentrations, insulin secretion stops. Yes, it's another negative feedback loop. Okay, but what if the animal becomes hypoglycemic? No problem! The pancreas will simply secrete glucagon (gloo'kah-gon) to increase blood glucose concentrations. Glucagon stimulates the liver to convert glycogen into glucose and stimulates hepatic gluconeogenesis. Voilà! Blood glucose concentrations again return to normal (Yes, shutting off the secretion of glucagon). Compared with some of the other endocrinology we've discussed thus far, the pancreas seems pretty straightforward and simple. That may be true, but this simple scenario is one of the more frequently broken "communication" pathways. Diabetes mellitus is the most common communication breakdown. *Diabetes* in Greek indicates increased urine volume. The word *mellitus* in Greek means "sweet." In diabetes mellitus we have either reduced secretion of insulin or fewer functional insulin receptors on the cells of the body. Either way, we wind up with hyperglycemia (there's the sweet). Remember in Chapter 13 when we discussed the limited mechanism for absorbing glucose from the renal tubules? Well, then hyperglycemia will in turn create glycosuria. By the way, with the high osmolarity of renal filtrate (with all of that glucose) water will naturally follow (there's the diabetes). So, here is yet another possible cause of polyuria. Why does diabetes mellitus develop? Sometimes it's just a genetic predisposition. There are a number of potential contributing factors in this "failure to communicate," which may include obesity or chronic exogenous glucocorticoid administration. Fortunately, for most patients it is a manageable disorder, through proper diet, exercise, and perhaps the administration of exogenous insulin.

Reproductive Hormones

In our discussions of "the birds and the bees" in Chapter 14, we left out all of the hormonal influences. The male is pretty straightforward. The most abundant male hormone is testosterone (tes-tos'tĕ-rōn). Testosterone, produced by the testes, is important for spermatogenesis and for imparting all of the typical male characteristics in animals and people. The female has numerous hormones that guide her reproductive cycle and support pregnancy and lactation. Estrogen (es'tro-jen) is probably the most widely known female hormone. If you break down the word *estrogen*, it literally means estrus producing. (Actually, we would be more correct in saying "estrogens." There are a number of estrogen hormones, the most prominent of which is estradiol.) Estrogens are responsible for far more than simply the development of feminine characteristics. In Chapter 14 we looked at the estrous cycle, as well as gestation and parturition. Now, let's correlate those events with the hormonal influences that govern them.

Let's begin by having the adenohypophysis secrete two very important gonadotropic hormones: follicle-stimulating hormone (FSH) and luteinizing hormone (LH). As the female enters into proestrus, both FSH and LH are secreted. The FSH has a fairly gradual increase that does as its name implies and stimulates ovarian follicle development (i.e., promoting oocyte maturation within the follicles). As a follicle develops it secretes large amounts of estrogens. Those estrogens will stimulate endometrial hypertrophy, in preparation for ovulation and potential pregnancy. The estrogens will also, in a feedback loop, promote greater secretion of LH. Plus, estrogens will promote secretion of pheromones[8] to attract males for breeding. As we enter estrus, LH will peak, allowing for ovulation. LH levels will rapidly diminish following ovulation. Levels of both FSH and estrogens will taper off as the female heads into metestrus. By the time diestrus arrives, those hormones are gone and being replaced by progesterone. How? Well, the follicle that once contained the egg actually becomes a progesterone-secreting endocrine structure called the corpus luteum.[9] Particularly if fertilization occurred, the corpus luteum will secrete large amounts of progesterone. It is progesterone that will support the uterus and embryo during gestation (gee—it's *for* gestation…*pro*gesterone. Get it?).

How does the corpus luteum know that there is a developing pregnancy? Well, believe it or not the endometrium and the corpus luteum communicate. If scripted, the conversation would be something like: Corpus luteum: "How's it looking down there? Got anything, Maude?" Endometrium: "No, Ethyl! Nobody's home. Better luck next time!" Okay, so it's really not as whimsical as that. Honestly, the communication is rather boring. If there's no pregnancy, the endometrium secretes large amounts of prostaglandins that lead to regression of the corpus luteum (i.e., Ethyl shrivels up because she has nothing to do). If there is a pregnancy, very few prostaglandins will be secreted (more or less like a whisper from two counties away). The corpus luteum can't "hear" it. Therefore, it stays in full vigor, happily secreting progesterone. By the way, LH will continue to be secreted in moderation to support the corpus luteum's secretion of progesterone throughout the pregnancy. (On the flip side of this coin, the progesterone inhibits excessive secretion of LH so that no further ovulation will occur during the pregnancy. Negative feedback is a good thing.) Late in gestation, progesterone levels will decrease and secretion of estrogens will increase. This enhances activity of the myometrium in preparation for parturition. Once ready for parturition, the neurohypophysis will secrete oxytocin. The oxytocin does two things. First, it stimulates smooth muscle contractions in the uterus. Secondarily, it targets smooth muscle of the mammary glands to stimulate milk letdown (i.e., the milk is basically squeezed out of the glandular tissue into the cisterns and teats). Why wasn't milk produced during gestation? Progesterone during gestation ties up prolactin receptors. Late in gestation as the progesterone levels drop, prolactin has numerous available receptors to stimulate lactation. Plus, as parturition nears, the adenohypophysis really increases its secretion of prolactin. That way, once we've got a happy healthy neonate, there will be no need to ask, "Got milk?"

---

[8]Pheromones (fer′o-mōn); a substance secreted to the outside of the body that has a particular scent. These scents elicit certain behaviors in others of the same species.
[9]Corpus luteum (kor′pus lu′te-um); [L. *corpus,* body + *luteus,* yellow] the corpus luteum is a yellowish body formed after rupture of an ovarian follicle.

Wow! Are you exhausted from our discussions of endocrinology? There are so many twists and turns to these hormonal stories. Believe it or not, we've only scratched the surface. At least you have a minimal understanding of endocrinology in both health and disease. Hopefully, you'll feel empowered by the knowledge you've gained. Like hormones and the hypothalamus, with any luck these discussions will stimulate your "thirst" for more endocrinology. After all, in endocrinology the cause and effect of hormones tends to snowball. So too should your knowledge snowball. That's what lifelong learning is all about. That's a win-win situation. Most importantly, your veterinary patients will be the beneficiaries.

SELF-TEST

Using the previous information in this chapter, complete the following crossword puzzle using the most appropriate medical term(s). Do not use abbreviations or common names unless requested.

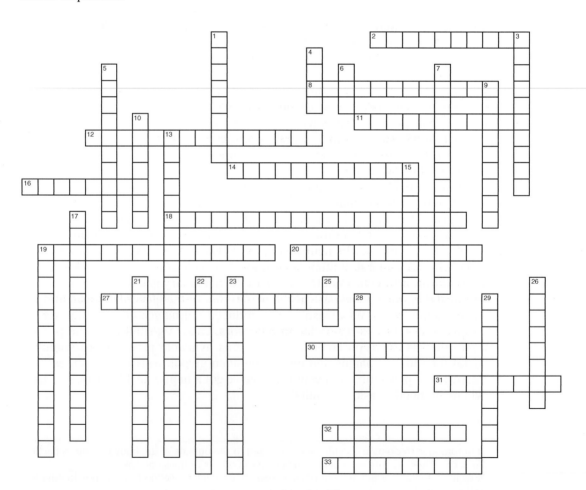

ACROSS

2	Glucose in the urine
8	The predominant male gonadal hormone
11	The adrenocortical hormone that stimulates renal retention of sodium
12	The anterior pituitary gland
14	The hormone of the corpus luteum that supports pregnancy
16	The most prominent glucocorticoid produced by the adrenal cortex
18	Pertaining to adrenal cortex influence
19	An endocrinopathy in which excess T_3 and T_4 are secreted
20	The posterior pituitary hormone that is "against urination"
27	The posterior pituitary
30	Pertaining to influence of the reproductive organs
31	The posterior pituitary hormone that stimulates "quick birth"
32	The hormone that stimulates milk production
33	Pertaining to something produced within the body

DOWN

1	The pancreatic hormone that elevates blood glucose concentrations
3	Pertaining to adrenal (gland) work; syn.: sympathomimetic
4	Abbreviation for adrenocorticotropic hormone
5	Increased thirst
6	Abbreviation for thyroid-stimulating hormone
7	The renal hormone that stimulates production of RBCs
9	Originating from outside the body
10	The pancreatic hormone that reduces blood glucose levels
13	Medical term for Cushing's disease
15	A disease of the endocrine system
17	A condition of insufficient thyroid hormones
19	A condition of excess blood glucose
21	_____ hormone; i.e., LH
22	Insufficient blood calcium
23	Pertaining to body influencing, like that of growth hormone
25	Abbreviation for follicle-stimulating hormone
26	Increased urine volume
28	The endocrine glands responsible for calcium and phosphorous homeostasis by producing PTH
29	The thyroid hormone that inhibits osteoclastic release of calcium and phosphorus from bone

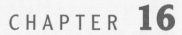

CHAPTER 16

The Integumentary System

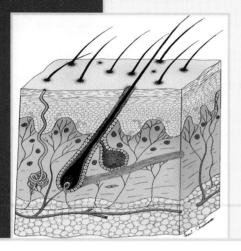

GOALS AND OBJECTIVES

By the conclusion of this chapter, the student will be able to:

1. Recognize common root words, prefixes, and suffixes related to the integumentary system.
2. Divide simple and compound words into their respective parts.
3. Recognize, correctly pronounce, and appropriately use common medical terms related to the integumentary system.
4. Demonstrate an understanding of integumentary anatomy.
5. Demonstrate a basic understanding of integumentary physiology and pathophysiology with regard to functions including hair growth, wound healing, and allergic dermatitis.

Note: Completion of all previous chapters is recommended.

INTRODUCTION TO RELATED TERMS

Divide each of the following terms into its respective parts ("R," root; "P," prefix; "S," suffix; "CV," combining vowel).

1. **Dermatitis** (n.) (R) _____ (S) _____
   dermatitis (der"mah-ti'tis; inflammation of the skin)

2. **Epidermal** (adj.) (P) _____ (R) _____ (S) _____
   epidermal (ep"ĭ-der'mal; pertaining to upon the dermis)

3. **Intradermal** (adj.) (P) _____ (R) _____ (S) _____
   intradermal (in"trah-der'mal; pertaining to within the dermis)

4. **Subcutis** (n.) (P) _____ (R) _____
   subcutis (sub-ku'tis; beneath the skin; cf. hypodermis; adj. subcutaneous)

5. **Erythematous** (adj.)   (R) _____   (S) _____
erythematous (er″ĭ-them′ah-tus; pertaining to erythema [Gr. *erythema*, flush upon the skin]; clinically, an erythematous lesion would appear reddened)

6. **Pruritus** (n.)   (R) _____   (S) _____
pruritus (proo-ri′tus; the state of itching)

7. **Melanocyte** (n.)   (R) _____   (CV) _____   (S) _____
melanocyte (mel′ah-no-sīt, me-lan′o-sīt; a black cell)

8. **Piloerection** (n.)   (R) _____   (CV) _____   (R) _____
piloerection (pi″lo-ĕ-rek′shun; hair erection)

9. **Fibroplasia** (n.)   (R) _____   (CV) _____   (R) _____   (S) _____
fibroplasia (fi″bro-pla′se-ah; the process of fiber forming)

10. **Circumoral** (adj.)   (P) _____   (R) _____   (S) _____
circumoral (ser″kum-o′ral; pertaining to around the mouth)

11. **Interdigital** (adj.)   (P) _____   (R) _____   (S) _____
interdigital (in″ter-dij′ĭ-tal; pertaining to between toes)

12. **Perianal** (adj.)   (P) _____   (R) _____   (S) _____
perianal (per″e-a′nal; pertaining to around the anus)

13. **Allergen** (n.)   (R) _____   (R) _____
allergen (al′er-jen; allergy producer)

14. **Carcinoma** (n.)   (R) _____   (S) _____
carcinoma (kar″sĭ-no′mah; a cancerous tumor; clinically, carcinoma refers to a type of malignant growth that originates from epithelial cells)

15. **Polydactyly** (n.)   (P) _____   (R) _____   (S) _____
polydactyly (pol″e-dak′tĕ-le; a condition of many "fingers"/toes [*poly-* + Gr. *daktylos,* finger + *-y*])

16. **Onychectomy** (n.)   (R) _____   (S) _____
onychectomy (on″i-kek′tĕ-me; surgical removal of a nail [Gr. *onychos*, nail + *-ectomy*])

17. **Pododermatitis** (n.)   (R) _____   (CV) _____   (R) _____   (S) _____
pododermatitis (po″do-dur″mă-ti′tis; inflammation of the foot skin; [Gr. *podos,* foot])

18. **Dermatophytosis** (n.)   (R) _____   (CV) _____   (R) _____   (CV) _____
(S) _____
dermatophytosis (dur″mă-to-fi-to′sis; a condition of skin "plants," i.e., fungus [Gr. *phyton,* plant]; cf. dermatomycosis)

19. **Pyoderma** (n.)   (R) _____   (CV) _____   (R) _____
pyoderma (pi″o-dur′mah; skin pus; i.e., a purulent skin disorder)

20. **Hyperkeratosis** (n.)   (P) _____   (R) _____   (CV) _____   (S) _____
hyperkeratosis (hi″per-ker″ĕ-to′sis; a condition of excessive keratin [Gr. *keratos,* horn]; i.e., hypertrophy of the cornified, superficial layer of the epidermis)

21. **Seborrhea** (n.)   (R) _____ (CV) _____ (S) _____
    seborrhea (seb"o-re'ah; flow of sebum [L. *sebum*, suet (fat) + *-rrhea*, flow]; excessive
    secretion of sebum)

22. **Laminitis** (n.)   (R) _____ (S) _____
    laminitis (lam"ĭ-ni'tis; inflammation of the lamina; i.e., inflammation of "quick" of a hoof;
    also called "founder")

23. **Cornuectomy** (n.)   (R) _____ (S) _____
    cornuectomy (kor"nu-ek'tem-e; surgical removal of a horn [L. *cornu*, horn]; i.e., dehorning)

24. **Epithelialization** (n.)   (R) _____ (CV) _____ (S) _____
    epithelialization (ep"ĭ-the"le-al-i-za'shun; the process of epithelial [growth]; e.g., for
    healing)

25. **Transdermal** (adj.)   (P) _____ (R) _____ (S) _____
    transdermal (trans-dur'mal; pertaining to across/through skin)

INTEGUMENTARY ANATOMY AND PHYSIOLOGY

What can be so special about skin? I mean, okay, we have it. Big deal, you say?
Yes, it is a big deal, a very big deal! Did you know that the skin is the largest
organ of the body? The skin is an organ? You bet it is! First, let's look at how
it's built. Sorry, but if you don't know the players, how can you understand the
game? So, let's begin by looking at the players and the roles that they play.

Epidermis

The epidermis is the most superficial of the skin layers (Fig. 16-1). It is composed of stratified squamous epithelium. Notice, as you look at Figure 16-1, that
there are no vessels or nerves or glands in the epidermis. How, you ask, does
an avascular structure survive? The epidermis draws its sustenance from interstitial fluids and the highly vascular dermis below. Generous neighbors, what
a blessing. What does the dermis get in return? Protection! You see, the keratinized layer of the epidermis (stratum corneum), in combination with sebum,
provides waterproofing for the skin. That's important for keeping environmental
water out (giving animals like otters and ducks the ability to simply let water
roll off their backs). More importantly, this epidermal waterproofing keeps the
body from dehydrating from evaporation. While we're on the subject of protection, the superficial layer of the epidermis actually gives the body its first
line of defense against entry of microorganisms. It even prevents absorption of
some chemicals. (Although, depending on the chemical makeup, it may easily
penetrate the skin. Pharmaceutical manufacturers must take into account the
structural characteristics of the epidermis, as well as dermal blood flow, when
they develop transdermal medications. Thanks to their research and development, transdermal application of analgesics like fentanyl are becoming common
in human and veterinary medicine.) A little deeper in the epidermis are melanocytes. The dark cytoplasmic granules of the melanocytes provide pigmentation

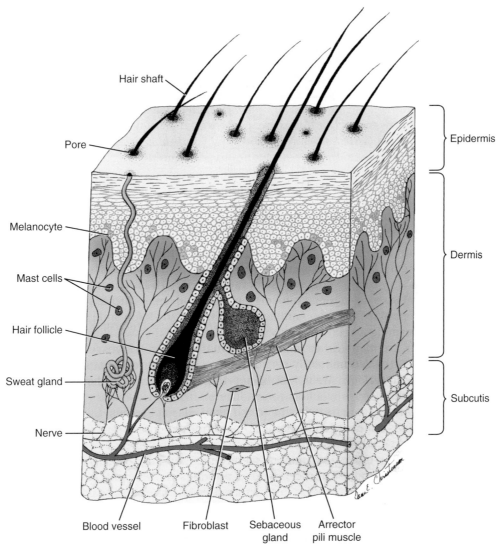

Hair shaft

Pore

Melanocyte

Mast cells

Hair follicle

Sweat gland

Nerve

Epidermis

Dermis

Subcutis

Blood vessel   Fibroblast   Sebaceous   Arrector
gland   pili muscle

FIGURE 16-1   Skin cross section.

to the skin by sharing their melanic granules with epithelial cells (Fig. 16-2). As those epithelial cells move up in the stratification of the epidermis, they keep the pigments with them. Superficial pigmentation provides protection of deeper tissues from the harmful effects of ultraviolet radiation. The melanic granules of the cells absorb light energy rather than permitting it to pass through to deeper layers of the epidermis or beyond. Animals with little or no pigmentation are more susceptible to the harmful effects of ultraviolet light and are more likely to develop diseases such as squamous cell carcinoma.

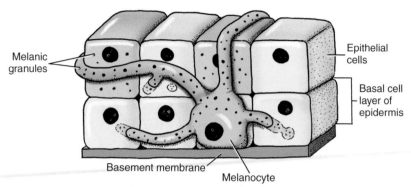

FIGURE 16-2   Melanocyte.

Dermis

Beneath the epidermis is the dermis. Here is the truly living, breathing part of this organ. The dermis is composed of fibroelastic connective tissue, making the skin a very tough yet elastic structure (see Fig. 16-1). The dermis is the thickest of the two skin layers, connected to the epidermis with finger-like projections called papillae.[1] These papillae interlock with the folds and ridges of the epidermis, forming a relatively strong bond between the two skin layers. Within the dermis are many other important structures, such as vessels and nerves. The nerves are predominantly sensory, many of which terminate at the epidermal–dermal interface. We'll talk about the importance of those nerve endings when we discuss wound healing. The intradermal capillary network provides nourishment for the dermis and the avascular epidermis. Clinically, the dermis also gives a means to check the color of our patients—mucous membrane color, that is. Yes, when you look at those mucous membranes, you're peering through a very thin, epidermal mucous membrane covering to see that glorious, highly vascular dermis. The dermis also provides an efficient mechanism through which body heat may be lost. Thermoregulation relies heavily on the dermis, in more ways than one. Vasodilation of these intradermal capillaries facilitates the loss of excess body heat and is clinically apparent as erythema. This is easily observed on the oral mucous membranes and any lightly haired areas, like the ear pinnae. For the ultimate in cooling, horses, of any of our domestic animals, have an abundance of sweat glands. By sweating, horses can cool through evaporation. (So, where did the phrase "sweat like a pig" come from? I've no idea, because pigs don't have sweat glands in the skin of their bodies to be able to sweat. That's why they wallow in mud.) When an animal needs to conserve body heat, dermal capillaries will constrict. Plus, those wonderful arrector pili (ah-rek'tor pi'li) muscles contract, fluffing up the fur or feathers for insulating dead space. The best we can do is develop goose bumps. Yes, it's the same muscular activity. Fortunately or unfortunately, depending on your point of view, we aren't fur covered to have the same insulating effects of piloerection. There is far more to the skin than meets the eye and we've only scratched the surface. Let's save the rest of those

---

[1]Papillae (pah-pil'e); plural of papilla (pah-pil'ah); a small, nipple-shaped projection.

dermal structures for later, shall we? Then we can make better sense of things like mast cells and fibroblasts, when we talk about issues like allergic dermatitis and wound healing. For now, let's move a little deeper and get under the skin.

Subcutis

The hypodermic layer of the subcutis is composed of adipose and loose connective tissues, loosely attaching the skin to underlying tissues and structures (see Fig. 16-1). The adipose tissue is important for providing insulation for the body. More importantly, its loose, flexible structure also permits the skin to easily glide freely over the underlying tissues. Have you ever lifted up on the skin of an animal, say over the neck? It tents up easily and snaps right back to its original location when released, right? No harm done. Between the elasticity of the dermis and the loose attachments of the subcutis, it is less likely that the skin will tear from light to moderate traumatic blows to the skin. This flexibility also makes the subcutis an excellent location for depositing subcutaneous fluids, medications, or vaccinations.

Accessory Skin Structures

Glands

No, glandular structures are not limited to the lymphatic or endocrine systems. Numerous exocrine glands are found in the dermis. Sebaceous glands[2] produce sebum,[3] an oily substance that keeps the skin and fur relatively soft, pliable, and waterproof. As I mentioned earlier, it's the sebum in combination with the stratum corneum that gives very good exterior protection. Normal sebum actually helps control colonization of commensal bacteria on the skin. That is a very important protective mechanism. Sebaceous glands are usually associated with hair follicles (see Fig. 16-1). Some sebaceous-type glands secrete scent markers called pheromones.[4] We communicate verbally, and animals, with their superior sense of smell, communicate through body language and pheromones. Pheromones are used by domestic animals for marking territory and for attracting mates. (As you may recall, I mentioned pheromones in the reproductive chapter.) Most pheromones are used as territorial markers. For instance, have you ever had a cat rub its chin and muzzle all over you? That cat wasn't being affectionate. It was saying: "Mine!" You were marked with the cat's circumoral glands. You've probably seen cats rub those glandular secretions on furniture and other objects. You may have bought the furniture, but the cat has claimed "squatters rights" to those possessions. Possession is nine tenths of the law, as they say. What about dogs? Have you ever observed dogs greeting one another? What do they usually do? They tend to sniff the other dog's perianal area. That's because dogs have numerous tiny perianal glands. "Fred, is that you?" (sniff) "Ah, good to see you again!" Aren't you glad people shake hands? Now, if you want to talk

---

[2]Sebaceous (sĕ-ba'shus); from [L. *sebaceus*, pertaining to sebum].
[3]Sebum (se'bum); from [L. *sebum*, suet].
[4]Pheromone (fer'o-mōn); scent marker that elicits certain behaviors in others of the same species.

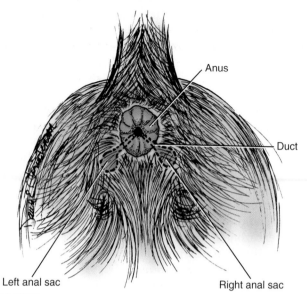

FIGURE 16-3   Schematic of canine anal sacs.

about some serious territorial marking, we need to talk about the anal glands (Fig. 16-3). Dogs and cats have a pair of anal glands, located at approximately the 4 o'clock and 8 o'clock positions around the anal opening. Every time the animal defecates, the anal glands will be expressed and their excretions deposited with the feces. They leave a "calling card," if you will. Those anal gland and perianal secretions let everyone else know that he or she was there. "Cross this line at your own risk." What about our hoofstock, do they have pheromone-secreting sebaceous glands too? Of course they do. Their glands are strategically located. Take animals with horns, like goats for instance. They have pheromone-producing glands near the base of their horns. That's why you may see them head butting and rubbing their heads on objects. Now, for our cloven-hoofed animals like sheep and goats to find their way, they have interdigital glands. These very efficiently mark their paths as they walk along. How convenient is that? (Much better than leaving a trail of bread crumbs.) While we're on the subject of sheep, we have to mention their lanolin glands. Yes, lanolin is a sebaceous secretion of sheep. (You'll probably never find a sheep farmer with dry, cracked hands, all because of the lanolin.) Sheep have a number of lanolin glands. Two of the more predominant ones are located in the inguinal region. When you set a sheep up, these two glands are easy to locate because of the thick, brownish secretions caking the area.

Sweat glands are quite different in their structure from sebaceous glands (see Fig. 16-1). Rather than a sac-like structure, sweat glands are sort of coiled tubes. They generally exit the surface of the skin through pores, rather than being associated with hair follicles. Sweat glands tend to produce watery secretions, rather than the oily secretions of sebaceous glands. Depending on the domestic animal in question, sweat gland numbers vary tremendously. As mentioned earlier, sweat glands are found in abundance over the entire body of horses. This provides an excellent cooling mechanism for the horse. Cattle also have large numbers of sweat glands over their bodies, although not quite as abundant as the horse. Still, cattle have enough to permit them to cool through sweating. In most other domestic animals, however, sweat glands are found in limited numbers. Pigs have very few, located on the plenum of the nose. In dogs and cats, for instance, appreciable numbers of sweat glands are found only in the foot pads. So, on a very warm day, you may see moist little paw prints left behind on the hardwood floor. Sheep and goats have very few sweat glands as well. I guess that makes sense. After all, what good would it do a sheep to sweat into its heavy wool coat? Obviously, pigs, sheep, goats, dogs, and cats cannot use sweating for thermoregulation. Minimizing activity, finding shade, wallowing in cool mud (for pigs), or panting are these animals' best defense against the heat.

Nails, Hooves, and Horns

Toenails, hooves, and horns are all formed from specialized keratinized epithelial cells. The stratum corneum that I mentioned with the epidermis becomes very thick and hardened in the wall of the nail, hoof, or horn. Figure 16-4 shows the hoof wall of a horse's foot. Growth of the hoof wall progresses down from the coronet or coronary band.[5] But if this is simply a variation on a theme of normal skin structure, isn't there more to this than simply a hoof wall? Yes, there is. In Figure 16-5, you can see that the hoof wall is only the outer "shell" surrounding the dorsum and sides of the foot. Just inside the hoof wall is the white line. This is also epidermal tissue. It's a little less dense and a bit more porous than that of the highly keratinized wall. In Figure 16-6, you can see in the cross section of the hoof that the epidermal tissue that makes up the white line actually has finger-like projections that laminate the epidermis to the dermis. Those finger-like projections of epidermal tissue are referred to as insensitive lamina, and the projections of the dermal tissue are referred to as sensitive lamina. It's the rest of the dermal tissue that connects the hoof to the distal phalanx of the foot. (We'll discuss the importance of these laminar tissues when we talk about laminitis later.) What about the sole? The outer surface of the sole is also made up of keratinized epithelium. However, it is not quite as rigid as the hoof wall. The sole is a bit more flexible, allowing it to conform a little when walking. Certainly, within the hoof, especially at the heels (and frog region of the horse's foot) there is an abundance of shock-absorbing digital tissue.

In dogs and cats, the shock-absorbing tissue is found in the digital, metacarpal, and metatarsal pads (Fig. 16-7). The nails grow in a similar fashion to the hooves, from the attachment of the skin at the nail base. The dermal tissue that you may be able to see through a white nail is often referred to as the "quick." Obviously when trimming nails, one tries to trim only the keratinized nail and avoid the quick. It is very important to keep the nails trimmed. If allowed to grow unchecked, the dog or cat will no longer walk on their pads as they should

---

[5]Coronary (kor'o-na-re); from [L. *corona*, pertaining to encircling].

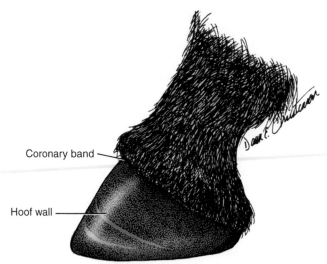

FIGURE 16-4   Equine hoof.

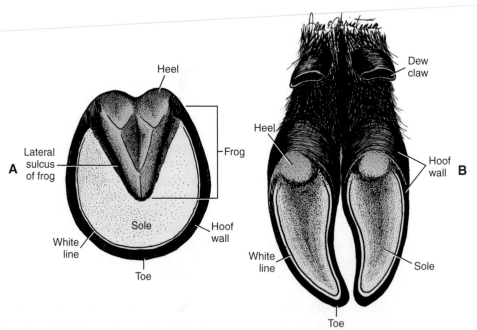

FIGURE 16-5   **A,** Equine foot: palmar view. **B,** Bovine foot: palmar view.

and may develop lameness as a result. Plus, the nails may curl right around and grow into the pads. That is a very painful experience. Now some cats, even if the nails are regularly trimmed, tend to be very destructive with their nails. (Imagine the destruction a cat with polydactyly could do.) Some cats refuse to use scratching posts. Some of those same cats pull off those soft latex covers

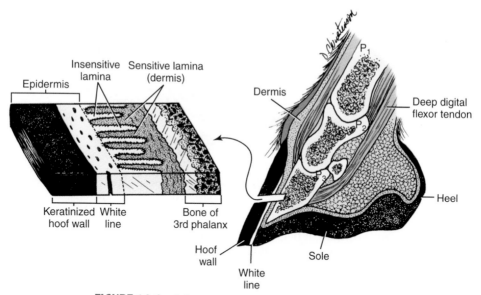

FIGURE 16-6 Schematic of equine foot.

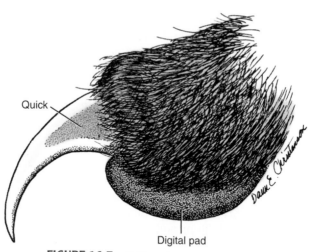

FIGURE 16-7 Feline claw.

that can be glued over the claws. Owners of such cats often resort to a forepaw tenotomy[6] or onychectomy. Incising the tendon that extends the claw is not always successful. Some cats learn to exert just the right amount of pressure on the digital pads to still facilitate claw extension. Therefore, they may still engage in destructive behaviors. During an onychectomy, the distal phalanx is completely amputated (Fig. 16-8). Obviously, this is an extreme measure to

---

[6]Tenotomy (tĕ-not'o-me); to cut a tendon.

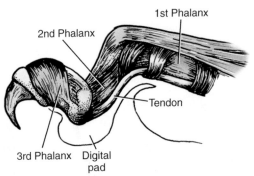

FIGURE 16-8   Feline claw in extension.

prevent destructive behavior (owing to debate over its practice). However for some owners, it becomes a decision between onychectomy and euthanasia. The onychectomy suddenly becomes the lesser of two evils.

Horns grow in much the same way as hooves and nails. The difference is in the early stages. You see, animals are not born with horns. Horns begin to grow as the animal matures. The horn actually begins as a small "bud" in the epidermis over the poll (i.e., the top of the head). As the animal grows and matures, the epidermal bud begins to grow. As time goes on, the skull beneath the growing horn bud will grow with it. Once fully mature, the horn will rest over a large boney protuberance of the skull. The frontal sinus will actually extend into the mature horn. (Go back to Chapter 8 to see this.) Needless to say, the optimal time to perform a cornuectomy is when the animal merely has a horn bud. Whether the dehorning is done early or late in the horn development, it is very important to remove enough of the skin surrounding the horn. The cornual growth area must be completely removed to prevent abnormal horn regrowth (called a "scur").

Hair and Hair Growth

Most domestic animals are covered in hair, or fur, if you will. Those coats vary tremendously, depending on the species and breed. In fact, some breeds (like the Chinese Crested dog) have very little in the way of a furry covering. Regardless, those hairs originate from follicles in the dermis (see Fig. 16-1). Each follicle is lined with epithelium and traverses the dermis and epidermis to the surface of the skin. Each follicle has an arrector pili muscle associated with it. As mentioned earlier, these muscles are responsible for piloerection. (By the way, piloerection may be used for thermoregulation or for dramatic displays. Yes, animals can be drama queens. Ever see a dog or a cat with its hackles up? That is one of those dramatic displays designed to make the animal look larger and more frightening to its opponent. While it might look impressive, it's often part of a fear response. When frightened, you may have experienced the hairs on the back of your neck standing up. It's the same thing.) The hair bulb, which gives rise to the hair shaft, is found at the base of the follicle. Just as nails and hooves developed from specialized epithelial cells, so do hairs. During hair growth periods, the hair bulb is large and has a vigorous blood supply (Fig. 16-9). As the hair shaft grows in length, the hair follicle begins to extend deeper into the dermis.

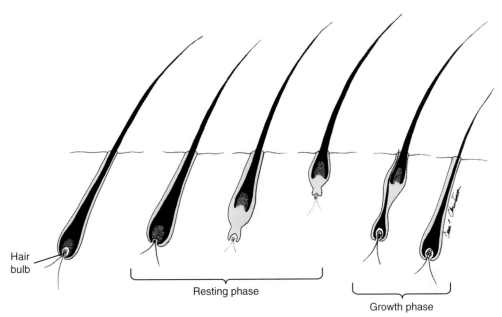

Hair
bulb

Resting phase

Growth phase

FIGURE 16-9 Hair growth.

On entering the resting phase of hair growth, the hair bulb regresses. Eventually, the hair follicle shrinks in length, forcing the now poorly attached hair shaft out. This normal cycle of hair growth and loss occurs on a seasonal basis. It is truly seasonal, because hair growth and loss are closely correlated with the amount of daylight. That is why most domestic animals, even if housed indoors, begin to shed heavily during late winter and begin to acquire thicker, more luxurious coats during the fall. Wait a minute, aren't there different types of hair that go through these cycles of growth and loss? Yes, there are. In fact, when you look at the mane and tail of a horse, most of those hairs are chronically in a growth phase. Ah, but during those transitions through the seasons of the year, horses and most other animals tend to develop or lose dense undercoats. How do we explain that? Look at Figure 16-10. That is what is referred to as a compound follicle. There is a principle follicle with a long guard hair surrounded by a whole bunch of smaller wool hairs. The wool hairs make up the dense undercoat. During those shorter daylight periods of the year (fall and winter), those accessory wool hairs will be growing in abundance. That provides tremendous insulation for the animal during cold winter months. Why are wool hairs so much softer than the guard hairs? In the cross section of the guard hair, there are three parts shown. It's the medulla that makes guard hairs a little more course and rigid. Wool hairs typically lack a medulla, making them thinner and softer. You can probably think of some breeds that have a predominance of wool hairs and fewer, if any, guard hairs. That's right, Rex cats and Poodles. Obviously, sheep are covered in wool hairs. (Get it?—wool?)

What about whiskers? Are they simply exaggerated guard hairs? Not exactly. Whiskers are actually referred to as tactile hairs (Fig. 16-11). They are extremely

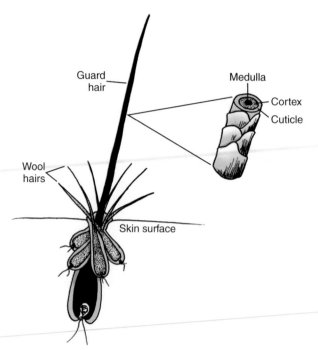

FIGURE 16-10   Compound follicle.

long and rigid. Surrounding the follicle of a tactile hair you'll find a very complicated network of capillaries and nerve endings. That specialized structure surrounding the follicle makes tactile hairs far more sensitive to touch. (Hence the
name—tactile hair.) These hairs are not exchanged as frequently as others.

What's different about alopecia,[7] compared with the normal growth and loss
cycle? Alopecia is abnormal loss. It usually results from a disease process. The
etiology may not even be a primary dermatologic disorder. Let's look at supply
and demand for a moment. Whether parasitized by intestinal worms or receiving
an inadequate diet, malnourished animals will typically have very thin, rough
hair coats. Why? The body has a choice to support critical organs and tissues
with the few available nutrients or to support hair growth. For survival, hair
growth must be sacrificed. Take some endocrine disorders, like hypothyroidism, discussed in Chapter 15. Endocrinopathies like that frequently result in alopecia. The unique feature of endocrine-induced alopecia is its symmetry. Many
dermatopathies result in asymmetric alopecia. Dermatophytosis (ringworm),
for instance, results in very focal, round areas of alopecia. (It's because of the
ring-like lesions that it is called ringworm. Remember, it's fungal in origin and
has nothing to do with worms of any kind.) Suffice it to say that many, many
things may result in alopecia. Only careful evaluation of a patient, perhaps both
internally and externally, will reveal its origin. A scar gives an immediate clue of

---

[7]Alopecia (al"o-pe'she-ah); abnormal hair loss from [Gr. *alopekia*, a disease in which the hair
falls out].

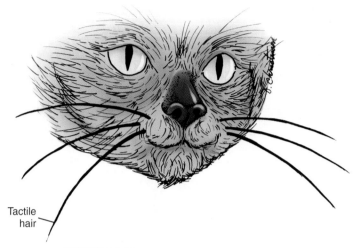

FIGURE 16-11   Tactile hairs.

past injury. Follicles do not typically regenerate in scarred tissue. Ah, but I am getting ahead of myself. First, we must understand the wound-healing process to even begin to understand how a scar is formed.

Wound Healing

Everyone has experienced minor scrapes and cuts, on themselves or animals. Certainly, surgical incisions are intentional wounds to the skin, albeit a means to an end. All of those injuries, whether accidental or intentional, had to follow the same sequence of events to heal. Let's subdivide that sequence of events into four distinct stages: the inflammatory stage, the debridement stage, the repair stage, and the maturation stage. For the purpose of simplifying the healing process, a simple laceration is used to demonstrate each of the stages (Fig. 16-12).

Immediately after a skin laceration, the inflammatory stage of the healing process ensues. There is hemorrhage from all of the intradermal and perhaps subcutaneous vessels. Bleeding is important to help cleanse the wound of contaminants. To prevent excessive blood loss, hemostatic mechanisms rapidly engage. Severed vessels constrict. Platelets aggregate and activate to form a platelet plug. Activated clotting factors secure the final thrombus with fibrin. This thrombus provides a weak matrix to hold the wound edges together for approximately the first 4 days. (Those fibrin strands also provide sort of scaffolding for fibroblasts to do their work during the initial repair stage.) Desiccation (drying) of the surface of the thrombus (i.e., scab) prevents entry into the wound of additional microorganisms and debris. Alright, you're probably wondering why this is called the inflammatory stage. Although the bleeding and hemostasis are important, the rest of our healing process is critically hinged on inflammation. Obviously, whenever tissue is injured inflammation quickly ensues, characterized by pain, edema, erythema, heat, and some loss of function of the body part. Inflammation was discussed in detail in Chapter 5. What

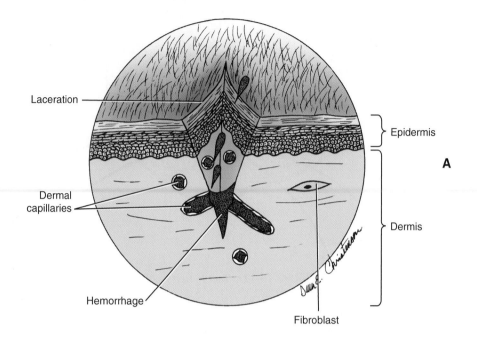

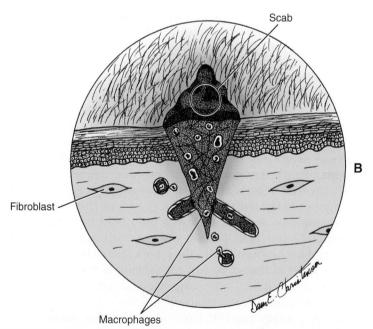

FIGURE 16-12   Wound healing. **A,** Inflammatory stage. **B,** Debridement stage.

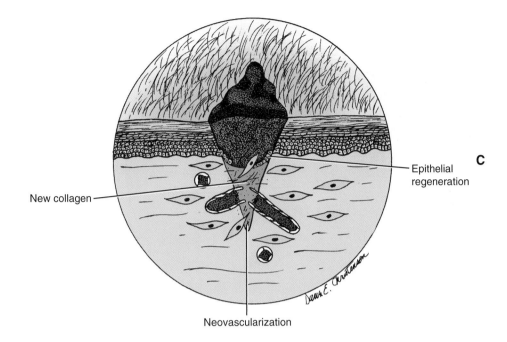

C

New collagen

Epithelial regeneration

Neovascularization

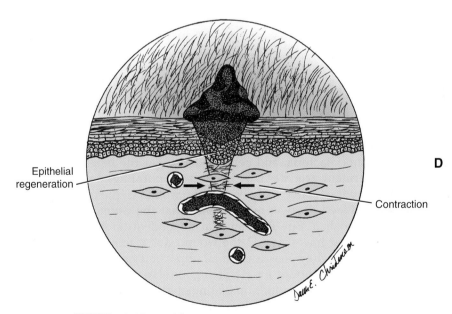

D

Epithelial regeneration

Contraction

FIGURE 16-12, cont'd   C, Repair stage. **D**, Late repair stage.

Continued

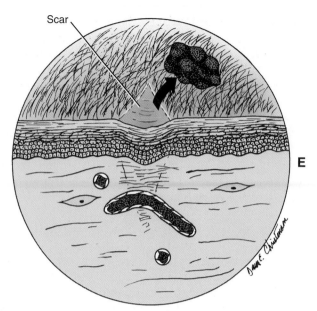

Scar

FIGURE 16-12, cont'd **E,** Maturation stage.

does it have to do with healing a wound? Inflammation releases tons of chemical mediators, right? Those inflammatory mediators provide for chemotaxis. Chemotaxis is critically important to gather macrophages for debridement of the wound. Without inflammation, the rest of our wound healing activities may not occur. (Now might be a good time to go back to Chapter 15 to review the effects of corticosteroids and the corticosteroid stress response. Healing will be significantly impaired in the presence of corticosteroids.)

Macrophages are responsible for debridement of the wound, during the second stage of wound healing. Initially available and called upon will be neutrophils. If you remember, neutrophils will tend to exacerbate inflammation with their sloppy phagocytic activities. Soon, monocytes will predominate the infiltration of the wound. What do these macrophages do? Well, they phagocytize contaminants, bacteria, and cellular debris. At the height of the debridement stage, a purulent exudate[8] may be seen suppurating (oozing) from the wound. The more contaminated and necrotic the wound is, the more purulent exudates will be produced. Okay, it makes sense that the wound should be cleaned up before we repair it. But is repair that dependent on it? Yes, it is! You see, the monocytes that have entered the wound don't simply debride. While they're busy debriding, they also secrete all important growth factors. Those growth factors will be important for attracting fibroblasts for dermal repair, for stimulating angiogenesis, and for stimulating epithelialization. Wow, that sounds like

---

[8]Purulent exudate (pu'roo-lent eks'u-dat); a purulent exudate contains pus; exudates are fluids that, in general, contain a high proportion of protein, cells, and cellular debris. Please note that pus or purulent exudate are the only appropriate ways to refer to this opaque fluid. "Pussy" is inappropriate for numerous reasons.

our whole repair stage is dependent on monocytic growth factors. You're absolutely right! (Again, I remind you of the adverse consequences of corticosteroids, with regard to neutrophil and monocyte migration from the vasculature into the wound. Aside from that, just think of the negative impact of a monocytopenia on healing. Sure, neutrophils could take care of the debridement, but those critical monocytic growth factors would be lacking for repair.)

Before we discuss the repair stage, let's quickly review skin structure. The skin is actually two separate layers, the dermis and epidermis, right? Those two layers are structurally very different, right? Okay, then we'll have to talk about the repair of each layer separately. What you'll need to remember is that in a simple laceration, these two layers will engage in repair simultaneously. Let's look at repair of the dermis first. Fibroblasts (attracted by monocytic growth factors) will slowly migrate to the wounded area. They will begin to deposit collagen (fibroplasia), the dense connective tissue of the dermis. Initially, the fibroblasts will use the fibrin strands of the clot to deposit their collagen on. As more and more fibroblasts enter the area, large amounts of collagen strands will be laid down and remodeled. Vessel walls will also be repaired (angiogenesis). The combination of new collagen and new vessels is what is called granulation tissue (because of its red, granular appearance). (In open wounds, granulation tissue provides a firm foundation on which the epithelium may rebuild the epidermis. Because its granulation tissue development may take several days, epithelialization will be delayed for days in open wounds.) Numbers of fibroblasts will begin to peak between 5 and 21 days following the wounding incident. In a normal individual, the fibroplasia will have laid down a strong enough collagen matrix to hold the wound edges together without any external support (like sutures or staples) by day 10. That's why most suture and staple removal is scheduled for 10 to 14 days after the injury or surgery. By day 15, the dermal strength at the wound site will be as good as it's going to get. Because it is not as elastic as the surrounding skin, this collagen scar will be about 20% weaker than normal skin.

Wait, we've only talked about fibroplasia in the dermis. What about the epidermis? Well, let's see, the epidermis is made up of epithelium, right? So, epithelialization must be the way the epidermis is healed. What exactly does that entail? At the margins of the wound, epithelial cells in the basal cell layer undergo mitosis. Progressively, the newly formed epithelial cells build a bridge of epithelium between the wound margins. Once a single layer of epithelium covers the dermis, the epithelial cells can proliferate upward to create stratification of the epidermis. Collagenase produced by the epithelium will dissolve any remaining fibrin attachments of the scab so that it may naturally fall off. By the way, do you remember that I mentioned some specialized nerve endings at the epidermal–dermal interface? Well, as those nerve endings are covered by epithelium, they can be stimulated. The sensation felt when they are stimulated is pruritus. Usually, in a simple laceration or surgical incision, the epithelium can fully cover the dermis within about 48 hours. That means that an animal may begin to bother its incision by 2 days postoperatively. Do we have any appreciable wound strength by 2 days postop? No. So, we may have to do something to keep the animal from disturbing the wound. If in these early stages of repair, the animal rips off the scab, it's going to rip off new epithelium, collagen, and vessels with it. Then, in terms of healing, we need to start from square one. Healing will be delayed and scarring will likely be greater. Worse yet, if the animal significantly stresses the wound, it may completely dehisce.[9] In an abdominal incision, dehiscence could be deadly. Until repair is complete, wounds (especially surgical wounds) need to be protected from self-inflicted trauma.

Toward the end of the repair stage, fibroblast numbers in the wounded area will diminish. Small numbers will be kept in the area to continue to contract and remodel the area, well into the maturation stage. During the maturation stage of wound healing, collagen fibers continue to be remodeled and contract. Maturation of the scar tissue may last for a year or more. During this time, the visible scar will become narrower (due to contraction) and flatter (due to remodeling). Remember, even a mature scar will be 15% to 20% weaker than the normal elastic skin.

Some horses are prone to a very abnormal healing process, known as "proud flesh." It typically develops on the distal extremities, where the skin is under tension. What is it? Proud flesh is exuberant granulation tissue. Yeah, right. What does that mean? To be exuberant is to be enthusiastic or excited, right? Didn't we say that, particularly in open wounds, it may take several days for granulation tissue to form? Well, in horses prone to proud flesh, their granulation tissue is so exuberant that it may form in less than 24 hours. It goes absolutely crazy (like fibroplasia on caffeine). The epithelium doesn't stand a chance of keeping up with the fibroplasia, let alone covering the granulation tissue. For some of these horses, the exuberant granulation tissue creates huge, tumor-like growths. These wounds will never heal. In a horse prone to proud flesh, when even minor lacerations occur, immediate veterinary intervention to close the wound will be best. In a closed wound, the epithelium has a fighting chance to cover the granulation tissue before it gets out of control.

Is it possible for fibroplasia to still be excessive even if the granulation tissue is covered by epithelium? Yes. That would describe a progressively enlarging scar commonly called a *keloid.* Keloids will tend to form in areas of skin under chronic tension. You see, under normal circumstances a mature scar or one that is months into the maturation stage has no need for large numbers of fibroblasts. But if we place the scarred area over a joint, it will be subjected to extreme tension—pulling and tugging at the stiff, weak scar. The only logical response is to keep more fibroblasts in the area. What is the intent? To bulk up the collagen fibers in an attempt to strengthen the scar. In the end, we wind up with a very thick, ugly scar (keloid).

Allergic Dermatitis

Allergic dermatitis is a frequent cause of erythema, pruritus, and urticaria[10] in companion animals. Yes, even inhaled allergens will typically cause dermatitis. Unlike humans, animals don't have as many mast cells in their airways. Domestic

---

[9]Dehisce (de-his′); [L. *dehiscere*, to gape]; dehiscence is a splitting open or separation of wound edges.
[10]Urticaria (ur″tĭ-ka′re-ah); from [L. *urtica*, "stinging nettle" + *-ia*]; wheal formation on the skin; commonly referred to as hives.

animals have their largest numbers of mast cells in the dermis. Mast cells are the facilitators of many allergic reactions. When presented with a recognizable allergen, a mast cell releases its histamine-containing granules. A cascade of events unfolds, resulting ultimately in inflammation. (If you would like to review the IgE-histamine hypersensitivity reaction, refer to Chapter 5.) Because the majority of mast cells in domestic animals are found predominantly throughout the dermis, hypersensitivity[11] reactions usually result in dermatitis. (Remember, other tissues of domestic animals that have relatively high numbers of mast cells are in the digestive tract and the pulmonary airways.) So, allergic dermatitis frequently results from all sorts of allergens, including contact, inhalant, and food allergens. Remember, allergic reactions cannot occur with the first exposure to an allergen. The first exposure sensitizes the animal. Once sensitized (hypersensitized with excessive amounts of IgE), these animals will overreact to subsequent (challenge) exposures to the allergen. Okay, so they'll be pruritic and scratch a lot. Big deal? Oh, these animals can scratch, bite, and rub their skin absolutely raw. Not only are they and their owners driven crazy by the pruritus, but many physiologic changes result from the dermatitis. Hyperkeratosis may be one of the resultant changes. The character of the sebum may be dramatically altered, causing seborrhea. The altered sebaceous secretions could become so thickened that some glands, including the anal glands, may become obstructed and impacted. The altered sebaceous secretions may no longer prevent colonization of commensal bacteria. The secondary bacterial overgrowth may cause pododermatitis (especially interdigitally), otitis externa, or even generalized pyoderma. These animals can be walking, breathing, oozing, encrusted messes when brought in for veterinary care. These patients can actually become septicemic. Wow, allergies can do all that? Yes, they can. That's why it's important to identify which allergens are causing the problem.

To isolate specific environmental allergens, intradermal skin testing is often performed. A series of intradermal injections is administered to the patient. Each injection contains a specified volume and concentration of an individual allergen. A positive control site is injected with histamine and a negative control site is injected with sterile saline. After the allergens have been administered, the injection sites are observed for 15 to 20 minutes for wheal[12] formation. Wheals formed in response to allergens are measured and compared with the positive and negative control sites. Any wheals less than or equal to the size of the negative control are considered negative. All others are graded on a scale of 1 to 4, with 4 being equal to or greater than the size of the positive control. (Some dermatologists carry the scale up to +6, to account for those reactions greater than the positive control.) Determination of specific allergens helps the owner remove the insulting allergens from the pet's environment. For those allergens that cannot be eliminated, the pet may be engaged in desensitization therapy. Desensitization therapy is a slow, progressive process. Allergens are injected subcutaneously, usually weekly or biweekly. Over time, the concentration of the

---

[11]Hypersensitive (hi″per-sen′sĭ-tiv); *hyper-,* above normal + *sensitive;* an exaggerated response to something, in this context an allergen.

[12]Wheal (wĕl); a smooth, raised, circumscribed, erythematous skin lesion.

allergens is increased. The goal of desensitization therapy is to administer doses of allergens that are low enough so that a hypersensitivity reaction is not stimulated, yet high enough to stimulate a different, more appropriate immune response (IgG rather than IgE) by the body. Ultimately, the animal no longer reacts adversely to challenge situations with those allergens. The therapy must be continued for the lifetime of the animal.

Flea allergy dermatitis is the most common isolate from intradermal skin testing. Dogs and cats with flea allergy dermatitis are allergic to the flea's saliva (most commonly the cat flea). It takes only one flea bite in an allergic animal to send him or her into intense dermatitis. The dermatitis from that single flea bite may last for 90 days! That is why it is so important for owners to follow through with and maintain an adequate flea control protocol. With the number of flea products on the market today that attack the flea's lifecycle from numerous angles, there is no reason for an animal to suffer from flea allergy dermatitis. Owners should consult with their veterinary professionals to determine the right combination of flea products for their pet and situation.

Food allergens are best isolated through a feeding-elimination trial. During this trial, the animal must be fed a novel food. The food must contain protein and carbohydrate sources that the animal has never eaten before. Nothing else must pass their lips. A typical feeding trial may last for 8 to 12 weeks. Why so long? It may take anywhere from 8 to 10 weeks for reactions from the previously eaten food allergens to go away. By the end of this period, the animal may become symptom free. Then, hopefully, a hypoallergenic commercial diet can be found for the animal, containing the novel protein and carbohydrate. If the owners want to determine other specific allergens, the trial can be extended and individual foods added to the diet, while observing for adverse reactions. If no reaction is observed within a week, that food can be determined hypoallergenic. That addition will be stopped and another added. If the animal reacts to a given food addition, it must be considered allergenic and removed from the diet permanently. Another food item cannot be added to the trial until the reaction to the prior food subsides. Is it necessary to know the specific food allergens involved? No. But as the owner of two food-allergic animals, that knowledge can be very useful when they have "dietary indiscretions." (That's a fancy way of saying that they ate something they shouldn't have.) Preemptive therapy may commence immediately, knowing that the allergic reaction is inevitable. This lessens the trauma for the animal as well as the owner (trust me—been there, done that).

Laminitis

Laminitis (or founder, as many horse owners call it) is a very serious condition of hoofstock. Yes, laminitis occurs more frequently in horses, but other hoofstock should not be excluded from its traumatic grips. Still, this discussion will focus on the horse. What may cause laminitis in the horse? The list is almost endless. It could be a digestive disturbance, like diarrhea. It could be an abrupt change in diet. It could be pain from colic. It could be many, many things. Whatever the inciting cause, the end result is an alteration in blood flow to the foot. That dynamic vascular event leads to laminitis. Laminitis most frequently affects the front feet (i.e., the feet that bear at least 60% of the horse's body weight at rest). Usually, both feet are involved. This condition is extremely painful and completely incapacitating for the horse.

So, what exactly is laminitis? It's an inflammation of the sensitive lamina and dermis within the hoof. Look again at Figure 16-6. Notice a few things: (1) the limited space within the hoof, (2) the position and attachment of the distal phalanx with the dorsal lamina and dermis, and (3) the attachment of the deep digital flexor tendon on the caudal aspect of the distal phalanx. Now, let's consider inflammation of the vibrant tissues (sensitive lamina and dermis) within this confining, rigid hoof wall. Isn't edema a classic symptom of inflammation? Where does the tissue have to expand? It doesn't have any space. Painful pressures will increase within the confines of the hoof wall. The connections between the sensitive and insensitive lamina will begin to break down. The tension naturally placed on the distal phalanx by the deep digital flexor tendon will, in the presence of laminar breakdown, begin to rotate the phalanx. The sole is somewhat flexible. So, rotation is permitted. In fact, the phalanx may rotate until the very point of it causes pressure necrosis and penetrates the sole. The laminar attachments can completely break down so that the hoof wall falls completely off. Often, when the condition has progressed to this level, the most humane thing to do is euthanasia.

Can this devastating disease be prevented? Perhaps. Certainly, abrupt dietary changes can be avoided. However, there are times when laminitis cannot be prevented. In those cases, early recognition of painful feet, warm hooves, and bounding digital pulses may permit us to take action to prevent some of the irreversible changes in the foot. We may be able to restore better blood flow through the foot, minimize or prevent edema, and prevent rotation of the distal phalanx. If we can do that, the horse will recover. If we cannot, nothing short of a miracle may permit the horse to walk again.

SELF-TEST

Using the previous information in this chapter, complete the following crossword puzzle using the most appropriate medical term(s). Do not use abbreviations or common names unless requested.

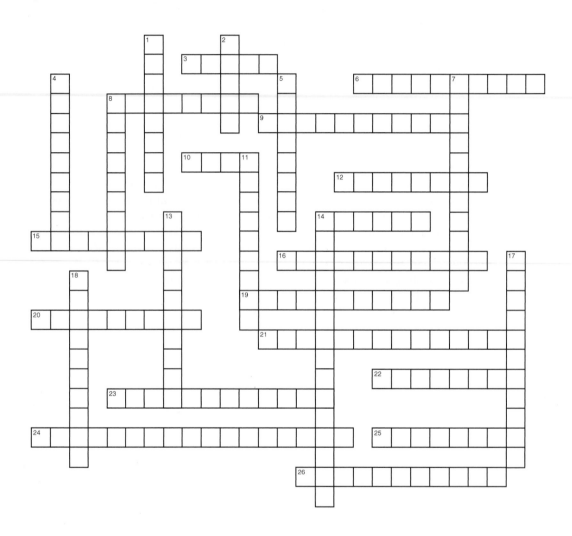

ACROSS

3	A smooth, raised, erythematous lesion resulting from intradermal skin testing
6	The black pigmented cell of the epidermis
8	The sensation of itching
9	Having extra toes
10	The palmar/plantar surface of the hoof
12	An allergy producer
14	The vascular layer of the skin, containing glands and nerves

15   Founder
16   Dehorning
19   Pertaining to within the skin
20   A malignant tumor originating from epithelial cells
21   Inflammation of foot skin
22   A WBC that secretes growth factors while debriding a wound
23   The first stage of wound healing
24   Repair of the epidermis during wound healing
25   Skin pus
26   Repair of the dermis during wound healing

DOWN
1   A ——————— (pus-containing) exudate
2   The fatty secretion of sebaceous glands
4   Hives
5   Abnormal hair loss
7   To declaw
8   A scent marker
11   The superficial layer of the skin made up of stratified epithelium
13   Pheromone-producing glands around the mouth of a cat
14   Ringworm, a skin condition caused by fungus
17   A method of medication administration across/through the skin
18   Inflammation of the skin

CHAPTER 17

Pharmacology

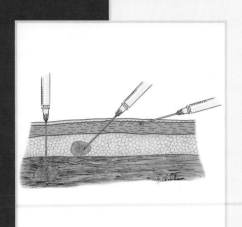

GOALS AND OBJECTIVES

By the conclusion of this chapter, the student will be able to:

1. Recognize common root words, prefixes, and suffixes related to pharmacology.
2. Divide simple and compound words into their respective parts.
3. Recognize, correctly pronounce, and appropriately use common medical terms related to pharmacology.
4. Demonstrate an understanding of the metric system with regard to weights, volumes, and conversions to apothecary and household measures.
5. Demonstrate an understanding of medication administration with regard to the five rights.
6. Demonstrate an understanding of medication administration with regard to relative rates of drug uptake per the different routes.
7. Demonstrate a basic understanding of pharmacokinetics and pharmacodynamics.
8. Demonstrate an understanding of prescription writing and transcription.

Note: The purpose of this chapter is to familiarize the student with common terminology and abbreviations used in pharmacology. Dosage calculations, drug classifications, and specific pharmacokinetics are not covered because these topics stray from the original intent of this text. It is the author's hope that the tables and descriptions of weights and volumes will provide a valuable resource for students elsewhere in their studies. It is highly recommended that this chapter be attempted only after Chapters 1 through 16 have been successfully completed. Understanding that pharmacology may fall early in some curricula, some redundancies of various terms will be contained within this chapter. These terms will serve to merely familiarize you with the various word parts, if you have not completed the other chapters. Your full understanding of their implications within a given body system will only be gained following completion of their associated chapters.

INTRODUCTION TO RELATED TERMS

Divide each of the following terms into its respective parts ("R," root; "P," prefix; "S," suffix; "CV," combining vowel).

1. **Pharmacology** (n.)   (R) _____ (CV) _____ (S) _____
   pharmacology (fahr"mah-kol'o-je; the study of medicine; clinically refers to the study of drug activity on the body)

2. **Pharmacokinetics** (n.)   (R) _____ (CV) _____ (R) _____ (S) _____
   pharmacokinetics (fahr"mah-ko-kĭ-net'iks; pertaining to drug motion [Gr. *kinesis*, movement])

3. **Pharmacodynamic** (adj.)   (R) _____ (CV) _____ (R) _____ (S) _____
   pharmacodynamic (fahr"mah-ko-di-nam'ik; pertaining to drug power [*dynamo(o)-*, power]; n. pharmacodynamics)

4. **Biotransformation** (n.)   (R) _____ (R) _____ (CV) _____ (S) _____
   biotransformation (bi"o-trans"for-ma'shun; a process of life-altering/life-changing)

5. **Hydrophilic** (adj.)   (R) _____ (CV) _____ (R) _____ (S) _____
   hydrophilic (hi"dro-fil'ik; pertaining to water loving [Gr. *philos*, loving])

6. **Lipophilic** (adj.)   (R) _____ (CV) _____ (R) _____ (S) _____
   lipophilic (lip"o-fil'ik; pertaining to fat loving)

7. **Cytotoxic** (adj.)   (R) _____ (CV) _____ (R) _____ (S) _____
   cytotoxic (si'to-tok"sik; pertaining to cell poison)

8. **Hepatotoxin** (n.)   (R) _____ (CV) _____ (R) _____ (S) _____
   hepatotoxin (hep'ă-to-tok"sin; a liver poison)

9. **Nephrotoxicity** (n.)   (R) _____ (CV) _____ (R) _____
   (S) _____
   nephrotoxicity (nef"ro-tok-sis'ĭ-te; a state/quality of kidney poisoning; *toxic(o)-* [Gr. *toxikon,* poison])

10. **Iatrogenic**   (R) _____ (CV) _____ (R) _____ (S) _____
    iatrogenic (i"at-ro-jen'ik; pertaining to physician produced; clinically refers to any disorder in a patient that results from the actions of medical personnel)

11. **Enteric** (adj.)   (R) _____ (S) _____
    enteric (en-ter'ik; pertaining to intestines [Gr. *enteron*, intestine])

12. **Parenteral**   (P) _____ (R) _____ (S) _____
    parenteral (pah-ren'ter-al; pertaining to around the intestines; clinically refers to various routes of medication administration that do not use the digestive tract)

13. **Intradermal** (adj.)   (P) _____ (R) _____ (S) _____
    intradermal (in"trah-dur'mal; pertaining to within the skin)

14. **Transdermal** (adj.)   (P) _____ (R) _____ (S) _____
    transdermal (trans-dur'mal; pertaining to across/through the skin)

15. **Subcutaneous** (adj.)   (P) _____ (R) _____ (CV) _____
                                     (S) _____
   subcutaneous (sub"ku-ta'neus; pertaining to beneath the skin "band" [L. *cutis,* skin + L. *taenia,* band]; cf. hypodermic)

16. **Intramuscular** (adj.)   (P) _____ (R) _____ (S) _____
   intramuscular (in"trah-mus'ku-lar; pertaining to within muscle)

17. **Intravenous**   (P) _____ (R) _____ (S) _____
   intravenous (in"trah-ve'nus; pertaining to within a vein)

18. **Intranasal**   (P) _____ (R) _____ (S) _____
   intranasal (in"trah-na'zal; pertaining to within the nose)

19. **Intratracheal**   (P) _____ (R) _____ (S) _____
   intratracheal (in"trah-tra'ke-al; pertaining to within the trachea)

20. **Intracardiac**   (P) _____ (R) _____ (S) _____
   intracardiac (in"trah-kahr'de-ak; pertaining to within the heart)

21. **Intraperitoneal**   (P) _____ (R) _____ (S) _____
   intraperitoneal (in"trah-per"ĭ-to-ne'al; pertaining to within the peritoneal [abdominal] cavity)

22. **Intraosseous**   (P) _____ (R) _____ (S) _____
   intraosseous (in"trah-os'e-us; pertaining to within a bone; cf. intramedullary)

23. **Kilogram**   (P) _____ (R) _____
   kilogram (kil'o-gram; one thousand grams)

24. **Deciliter**   (P) _____ (R) _____
   deciliter (des'ĭ-le"ter; ten volumes; a unit of volume in the metric system that is one tenth of a liter)

25. **Centimeter**   (P) _____ (R) _____
   centimeter (sen'tĭ-me'ter; a hundred measures; a unit of length in the metric system that is one hundredth of a meter)

26. **Milliliter**   (P) _____ (R) _____
   milliliter (mil'ĭ-le"ter; a thousand volumes; a unit of volume in the metric system that is one thousandth of a liter)

27. **Microgram**   (P) _____ (R) _____
   microgram (mi'kro-gram; a small weight; a unit of weight in the metric system that is one millionth of a gram or one thousandth of a milligram)

28. **Percent**   (P) _____ (R) _____
   percent (per-sent'; for each one hundred)

29. **Analgesic** (adj.)   (P) _____ (R) _____ (S) _____
   analgesic (an"al-je'zik; pertaining to no pain; i.e., an agent that relieves pain [Gr. *algesis,* pain]; n. analgesia)

30. **Anesthesia** (n.)   (P) _____ (R) _____ (S) _____
    anesthesia (an″es-the′zhah; a state without sensation [Gr. *aisthesis,* sensation]; adj.
    anesthetic)

31. **Agonist** (n.)   (R) _____ (S) _____
    agonist (ag′ah-nist; one that competes; i.e., a drug that activates receptors normally
    stimulated by naturally occurring substances, thereby "competing")

32. **Antagonist** (n.)   (P) _____ (R) _____ (S) _____
    antagonist (an-tag′ah-nist; one that is against competition [Gr. *antagonistes,* an
    opponent]; i.e., a drug that opposes and nullifies the action of another; a reversal agent)

33. **Antiemetic** (adj.)   (P) _____ (R) _____ (S) _____
    antiemetic (an″te-ĕ-met′ik; pertaining to against vomiting [Gr. *emetikos,* to vomit]; ant.
    emetic)

34. **Antitussive** (adj.)   (P) _____ (R) _____ (S) _____
    antitussive (an″te-tus′iv, an″ti-tus′iv; pertaining to against coughing [L. *tussis,* to cough])

35. **Anthelmintic**   (P) _____ (R) _____ (S) _____
    anthelmintic (ant″hel-min′tik; pertaining to against worms; anthelmintics are commonly
    referred to as deworming agents)

36. **Antipyretic**   (P) _____ (R) _____ (CV) _____ (S) _____
    antipyretic (an″tĭ-pi-ret′ik; pertaining to against fever; an antipyretic agent is a drug that is
    used for fever reduction)

37. **Antibiotic**   (P) _____ (R) _____ (S) _____
    antibiotic (an″tĭ-bi-ot′ik; pertaining to against life; clinically, antibiotics are drugs that are
    used to either kill or inhibit growth of bacteria)

38. **Antimycotic** (adj.)   (P) _____ (R) _____ (CV) _____ (S) _____
    antimycotic (an″ti-mi-kot′ik; pertaining to against fungus [Gr. *mykes,* fungus])

39. **Bactericidal** (adj.)   (R) _____ (R) _____ (S) _____
    bactericidal (bak-ter″ĭ-si′dal; pertaining to bacteria killing [L. *caedere,* to kill])

40. **Bacteriostatic** (adj.)   (R) _____ (CV) _____ (R) _____ (S) _____
    bacteriostatic (bak-tēr″e-o-stat′ik; pertaining to bacteria inhibition [Gr. *stasis,* a standing
    still])

41. **Antiseptic** (adj.)   (P) _____ (R) _____ (S) _____
    antiseptic (an″tĭ-sep′tik; pertaining to without/against "decay" [Gr. *sepsis,* decay], i.e.,
    infection; note: decay/decomposition of organic matter is caused by bacteria and other
    microorganisms)

42. **Virucidal** (adj.)   (R) _____ (R) _____ (S) _____
    virucidal (vi″rŭ-si′dal; pertaining to virus killing)

43. **Asepsis**   (P) _____ (R) _____ (S) _____
    asepsis (a-sep′sis; a state without "decay" (i.e., infection); cf. sterile)

44. **Indication** (n.)   (R) _____ (S) _____
    indication (in-dĕ-ka'shun; the act of indicating [L. *indicatus,* to proclaim]; i.e., declaring "advisable")

45. **Contraindication**   (P) _____ (R) _____ (S) _____
    contraindication (kon"trah-in"dĭ-ka'shun; a state opposed to the indicated; i.e., to make "inadvisable")

METRIC SYSTEM

The metric system is an unavoidable part of pharmacology. Most drug dosages are based in metric measure. Actually, compared with household measures, the metric system is quite simple. Its system is based on multiples or fractions of 10. There are three basic units of measure within the system. The meter is used for measurement of length. The liter is used for measurement of volume. Finally, the gram is used for measurement of weight. Standard prefixes are attached to each of the base units of measure to clearly indicate the multiple or fraction of 10 as appropriate (Table 17-1; note that those prefixes most commonly used in veterinary medicine are highlighted). Most of our pharmacologic discussions in this chapter will focus on weights and volumes. However, we cannot totally discount length. Metric measure is the most widely used means of noting the size of various tumors and other lesions in or on the body. Certainly, micrometers and microns are used for noting the size of microscopic organisms and cells.

Weight

Grams are a common unit of measure for weight in pharmaceuticals.[1] Dosages are frequently given as milligrams of drug per kilogram of body weight. Grams and milligrams are the most commonly used weights of pharmaceuticals. Micrograms are used less frequently. Table 17-2 shows the conversion equivalents for these commonly used weights. Beyond pharmacology, the picogram is frequently used to note various hematologic values.

Volume

Liters are a common unit of measure for volume in pharmaceuticals. Liquid drugs are frequently administered in milliliters. This is especially true when dealing with injections. Because a cubic centimeter is the equivalent volume of a milliliter, they may be used interchangeably. Table 17-3 shows the conversion equivalents for these commonly used volumes. Again, stepping outside the pharmaceutical realm, hematologic values are frequently noted in deciliters and femtoliters.

---

[1]Pharmaceutical (fahr"mah-su'tĭ-kal); pertaining to a drug or pharmacy.

TABLE 17-1 Metric Prefixes

Prefix	Phonetics	Abbreviation	Decimal Value	Scientific Notation	Meaning
tera	ter'ah	T	1,000,000,000,000	10^{12}	trillion
giga	ji'gah	G	1,000,000,000	10^{9}	billion
mega	meg'ah	M	1,000,000	10^{6}	million
kilo	**kil'o**	**k**	**1,000**	10^{3}	**thousand**
hecto	hek'to	h	100	10^{2}	hundred
deka	dek'ah	dk	10	10^{1}	ten
deci	**des'ĭ**	**d**	**0.1**	10^{-1}	**one tenth**
centi	**sen'tĭ**	**c**	**0.01**	10^{-2}	**one hundredth**
milli	**mil'ĭ**	**m**	**0.001**	10^{-3}	**one thousandth**
micro	**mi'kro**	**μ or mc**	**0.000 001**	10^{-6}	**one millionth**
nano	nan'o	n	0.000 000 001	10^{-9}	one billionth
pico	**pi'co**	**p**	**0.000 000 000 001**	10^{-12}	**one trillionth**
femto	**fem'to**	**f**	**0.000 000 000 000 001**	10^{-15}	**one quadrillionth**
atto	at'to	a	0.000 000 000 000 000 001	10^{-18}	one quintillionth

Concentration of liquid medications is expressed a number of ways. Many agents state a specific weight of the drug per volume (e.g., 10 mg/mL). Others express the concentration in percent. Because the strict definition of the term "percent" is "per one hundred," percent solutions are interpreted as weight in grams per 100 mL. For instance, a 5% solution of Lasix (furosemide) contains 5 g of drug in every 100 mL of solution. To transition from these larger weights and volumes to a clinically useful mg/mL, convert everything to the same prefix (i.e., milli-). Let's see, a milligram is much smaller than a gram, right? It's a thousandth smaller to be exact. If you find thinking in terms of thousandths difficult, then try this: there are 1000 milligrams in every gram. (That's comparable with saying that there are 100 pennies in every dollar. Do whatever it takes to keep it simple in making these relationships real and functional.) If there are 1000 mg/g, then for our 5% solution example that will give us 5000 mg per 100 mL. Now we simply need to cross out zeros to figure out that a 5% solution actually contains 50 mg/mL of the drug. How easy was that?! Some manufacturers will express concentration in ratios (e.g., 1:1000). In such a ratio, the number preceding the colon represents the drug weight in grams and the number following the colon represents the volume of fluid in milliliters. So, let's figure this out. A concentration of 1:1000 solution is interpreted as containing 1 g of drug in every 1000 mL of fluid. Shall we try to reduce this to a simple fraction as we did before? Again, convert everything to the same prefix, giving us 1000 mg of drug in 1000 mL of fluid. Simplifying this to milligrams per milliliter is now so easy you could do it blindfolded without a calculator. It's all about using a common language to compare apples with apples and oranges with oranges. Once you have a good

TABLE 17-2   Metric Weights

Weight	Symbol	Equivalency
1 kilogram	1 kg	1000 grams
1 gram	1 g	1000 mg; (1/1000 kg)
1 milligram	1 mg	0.001 gram; 1/1000 gram; (1000 mcg)
1 microgram	1 mcg	0.000001 gram; 1/1,000,000 gram; (1/1000 mg)

TABLE 17-3   Metric Volumes

Volume	Symbol	Equivalency
1 liter	1 L	1000 mL
1 milliliter	1 mL	0.001 liter; 1/1000 liter
1 cubic centimeter	1 cc	0.001 liter; 1/1000 liter

handle on the relationship between each of the commonly used prefixes, your dosage calculations will be a walk in the park.

Conversion to Apothecary and Household Systems

The metric system is understood throughout the world. Metrics are universal in medicine. Ah, but the average client may not be as familiar with metric weights and volumes. For their sake, we may need to make conversions between metrics and apothecary[2] or household units of measure. This is particularly true in the United States. Think about it. How many people know the weight of themselves or their animals in kilograms? I would venture to guess, very few, if any. Why? Most U.S. scales provide weight in pounds not kilograms. Unfortunately, many medications are dosed as milligrams per kilogram. So, we'll have to convert the patient's body weight in pounds to kilograms before any dosage calculation may be completed. Even if our final dosage calculation gives us a volume to be administered in milliliters, many of our clients may have no means to measure such volumes. What do they have in the kitchen? Teaspoons, tablespoons, cups, and so forth. Sure, we could simply send home a syringe or two with them. In some cases, we may have noncompliant pet owners if we do. Some elderly clients may have arthritic hands, making it difficult for them to move the plunger of the syringe. They may have visual deficits, making it very difficult to read the tiny markings on the barrel of the syringe. Frankly, they may be more compliant with administration of the medication if they can simply use a very familiar means of measuring it. Remember, the medication will do our patients no good if they don't receive it because of

---

[2]Apothecary (ah-poth'ĕ-ka"re); from [Gr. *apotheke,* storehouse]; refers to a pharmacy or pharmacist.

TABLE 17-4 Metric, Apothecary, and Household Equivalencies

Metric	Apothecary	Household
Weight		
1 kg	2.2 lb	2.2 lb
453.6 g	16 oz	1 lb
~ 30 g (31.1 g)	1 oz	
1 g	~ 15 gr (15.4 gr)	
~ 65 mg	1 gr	
~ 16 mg	$\frac{1}{4}$ gr	
~ 0.5 mg	$\frac{1}{120}$ gr	
Volume		
3.8 L	128 fl oz	1 gal (4 qt)
946.3 mL	32 fl oz	1 qt (2 pt)
473.2 mL	16 fl oz	1 pt
~ 240 mL (236.6 mL)	8 fl oz	1 c
~ 30 mL	1 fl oz	2 tbsp
~ 15 mL	0.5 fl oz (4 fl dr)	1 tbsp (~3 tsp)
~ 5 mL	1 fl dr	1 tsp

Note that approximate (~) weights and volumes in the table above are commonly used for calculation purposes. Actual equivalencies follow some approximations in parentheses.

noncompliance or if they receive the wrong volume. Bottom line: be prepared to convert to and from metric, apothecary, and household units of measure. Table 17-4 has been provided for this purpose.

MEDICATION ADMINISTRATION

Five Rights of Medication Administration

Within the veterinary health care team, everyone on the team must ensure that no harm comes to the patient. The patient and its welfare must come first. To that end, we must think, cross-check, and double-check every step leading up to the administration of any medication. It's when we become rushed and/or complacent that tragic iatrogenic complications result. Yes, sadly those iatrogenic complications are at times fatal. Most such complications can be avoided if each of us simply follows the "five rights" of medication administration. The five rights provide a simple checklist to ensure correct administration of medications. All one has to do is ask himself or herself the following questions: "Do I have the right patient? The right drug? The right dosage?" "Am I giving it via the right route?" and "Is this the right time?"

Right Patient?

Remember, it's all about the patient. The patient comes first. Can our patients speak for themselves or question what we're doing? No. We must be our patients' advocates, always being mindful of their needs and condition.

Veterinary patients who are hospitalized should be identified with labels on the cage or stall, as well as on the animal itself. Many small animal hospitals prefer to remove personal collars and harnesses to prevent injury. Without distinctive physical characteristics or other mechanisms for identifying patients, mistakes are more likely to occur. Think of the consequences in the case of an antibiotic to be administered to one of two black Labradors who look identical. Suppose that the antibiotic is contraindicated for use in one of those two dogs because the dog is severely allergic to it. If we give the drug to the wrong dog, that dog may die. Adequate identification of each Labrador would help prevent a fatal error in this situation. Veterinary practices may purchase any of a number of commercial patient identification devices that are safe and cost-effective. Regardless of how patients are marked for identification, anyone administering medications should make every effort to ensure that the right patient is receiving the drug. Imagine a situation in which two patients named "Buffy" are hospitalized because of unexplained fever. A drug order has been given for one Buffy to receive an antipyretic. Buffy the dog can safely receive most of the common antipyretic agents, like aspirin or Tylenol (acetaminophen). Buffy the cat, however, cannot. Tylenol, even in small doses, is highly toxic and can be lethal in cats. Even aspirin can have toxic effects in cats. Taking just a moment to clarify the drug order for a correct patient can avert an iatrogenic crisis.

Right Drug?

Several things must be checked to ensure that one has the right drug. Verify the veterinarian's drug order. Compare the drug order with the drug label. Evaluate the label for the drug name, concentration, and expiration date. Evaluate the contents of the container for spoilage or contamination. Check to see that the drug is in the correct form. Table 17-5 provides common prescription abbreviations for the various forms of medications. Are you unfamiliar with this particular drug? Then look it up! This is particularly important for veterinary technicians. Although technicians may not prescribe the pharmaceuticals, they must be familiar with the agents they administer. Again, we are all a part of a health care team. Each of us must do our utmost to ensure quality health care for our patients. What if the veterinarian writing the order misspelled the drug name? What if the veterinarian, in trying to juggle a number of critical patients, wrote down the wrong drug because he or she was thinking about another patient at the time? What if the veterinarian is unaware of a change in the physical condition of the patient and that condition makes administration of this particular drug contraindicated? Whose responsibility is it to ensure that the right drug is administered to any of these patients? The veterinary technician charged with administering the drug is responsible. Take your mind off of yourself and place your patient first. You are your patient's advocate. By addressing the error with the prescribing veterinarian, you may save the life of your patient. The other value in looking up unfamiliar drugs is that you will be aware of appropriate versus inappropriate reactions to the medication, after it's given. In fact, that knowledge may permit us to be preemptive by having an antagonist readily available, in anticipation of adverse reactions.

TABLE 17-5 **Medication Form Abbreviations**	
R$_x$ Abbreviation	**Meaning**
aq	Water [L. *aqua*]
cap	Capsule
elix	Elixir
emuls	Emulsion
ext	Extract
mixt	Mixture
supp	Suppository
susp	Suspension
syr	Syrup
tab	Tablet
tinct	Tincture [L. *tinctura*]
ung	Ointment [L. *unguentum*]

Right Dosage?

This may sound like a broken record, but verify the veterinarian's drug order. Is the order dosed per pounds body weight or per kilograms body weight? Whenever calculating drug dosages, always be certain to carry through with the appropriate units in the mathematical equation. Label the final answer of the calculation in the units that are to be administered. Be clear in what you record. There is a very big difference between giving 1 mL of a 2-mg/mL solution of acepromazine versus 1 mL of a 1% solution. When you draw the drug up into the syringe, look at it to ensure that the volume drawn up is the volume calculated. Plus, look at it and ask yourself, "Does this make sense?" Think about it. Many of the preanesthetic agents that we administer to dogs and cats are usually in very small volumes, often given using a tuberculin (1 mL) syringe. Now, as you stand there ready to give one of those same drugs to a 5-pound kitten with a 5-mL syringe full, red flags should go up. Stop, look, and if it doesn't seem right don't give it. Better to err on the side of caution than to kill a patient with haste or carelessness. What if it's an oral medication, using enteric-coated tablets? You can't split or crush enteric-coated tablets because you'll alter the absorption of the drug or it may cause gastritis. Capsules absolutely cannot be split. So, what if the calculated dosage in milligrams doesn't work out evenly to a whole tablet or capsule? Consult with the ordering veterinarian. He or she may alter the dosage, to accommodate the available sizes of the tablets or capsules. All it takes is a simple question to ensure that the right dosage is administered to the patient for an optimal, harmless result. Table 17-6 gives common units by which drugs are administered.

Right Route?

Remember—verify the veterinarian's drug order. How or where is the medication to be administered? Is the form of drug and the in-hand volume appropriate for the ordered route? If the in-hand volume seems to exceed that which may be reasonably given by the ordered route, double-check the calculations. If the calculations are found to be correct, perhaps the veterinarian who gave the order should be consulted. The veterinarian may deem the calculated volume within acceptable

TABLE 17-6	Medication Unit Abbreviations				
Abbreviation	**Meaning**	**Abbreviation**	**Meaning**	**Abbreviation**	**Meaning**
kg	kilogram	gal	gallon	gt	drop [L. *gutta*]
g, gm	gram	qt	quart	gtt	drops [L. *guttae*]
mg	milligram	pt	pint	U	unit
mcg, μg	microgram	fl oz	fluid ounce	lb, #	pound
cc	cubic centimeter	fl dr	fluid dram	oz	ounce
L	liter	TBL, tbsp	tablespoon	gr	grain
ml, mL	milliliter	tsp	teaspoon	dr	dram
mEq	milliequivalent				

limits of the selected route, or he or she may choose an alternate route or an alternate drug. Did you misinterpret the order? Could not clearly read to know for certain whether the order is for intramuscular (IM) or intravenous (IV) administration? If it is ordered for intravenous administration, it should be a transparent solution that you're giving. (There are only rare exceptions to "never giving an opaque fluid intravenously." Those exceptions include drugs like propofol and nutritive suspensions like total parenteral nutrition.) Even though the prescription simply states "IV," the technician administering the agent may need to determine an appropriate vein to use for the administration. Highly caustic or hypertonic solutions often require rapid dilution with a large blood volume. That means we need to select a larger vein. It may even mean that we have to place a central line to avoid iatrogenic phlebitis. Plus, is this a one-time dose or will there be repeated dosages? Is an IV catheter in order or not? What's going to be best for the comfort of our patient? Perhaps an IV route using an indwelling catheter will be tolerated better by our patient than multiple IM injections. Never assume anything. Always consult with the attending clinician to ensure that the appropriate action is taken. Remember, the only stupid question is the one that is never asked. Don't live with the regret of harming your patient because you gave something by the wrong route. Table 17-7 contains prescription abbreviations and their meanings for commonly used routes of medication administration.

Right Time?

Hello! Verify the veterinarian's drug order. How frequently is the medication to be administered? Should the medication be given before a meal for optimal absorption? Should the medication be given after meals to avoid gastric upset? The timing of medication administration is very important. Giving a drug too frequently could result in toxic side effects. Giving a drug beyond the prescribed period (i.e., late) could result in low blood levels of the agent, consequently making it ineffective and jeopardizing the health of the patient. Most medication administration periods are based on the half-life of the drug. The time schedule for administration of medications should be strictly adhered to, *as written in the prescription.* If the order states b.i.d., then twice daily is what should be written on the dispensing label to go home with the patient. If the clinician wants the medication given every 12 hours, then q12h should be written in the prescription.

TABLE 17-7   Route of Medication Administration Abbreviations

R$_x$ Abbreviation	Meaning
AD	Right ear [L. *auris dextra*]
AS	Left ear [L. *auris sinistra*]
AU	Both ears [L. *auris uterque*]
IC	Intracardiac
ID	Intradermal
IM	Intramuscular
IO	Intraosseous
IP	Intraperitoneal
IT	Intratracheal
IV	Intravenous
OD	Right eye [L. *oculus dexter*]
OS	Left eye [L. *oculus sinister*]
OU	Both eyes [L. *oculus uterque*]
PO	By mouth [L. *per os*]
PR	By rectum [L. *per rectum*]
SQ, SC	Subcutaneous

Your dispensing label should follow suit with a very specific "every 12 hours" written on the label. Again, never assume anything. For legal reasons, never alter the drug order based on common knowledge or assumptions. ("Hmm, he wrote q6h but I'm sure he meant 4 times daily." No!) If you want to be certain that the frequency at which you are giving a drug or that you are instructing an owner for giving a drug is correct, ask the clinician. Table 17-8 contains prescription abbreviations and their meanings for common times of medication administration.

Routes of Medication Administration

Per Os
Per os (PO) administration is one of the most widely used routes of medication administration. Many would advocate, "if the gut works, use it." When the length of time for uptake of a drug is not critical, per os administration is useful. The per os route provides one of the slower routes for uptake of drugs. Giving per os medications to animals does present challenges at times, particularly if the agent is not palatable. Anthelmintics are probably one of the most frequently used per os medications. Most of the paste and liquid anthelmintics are manufactured to be palatable, to facilitate easier administration. Antibiotics are also frequently administered per os. As mentioned earlier, if you are unfamiliar with a drug, look it up. If you discover that stomach upset is a common side effect, you may be prompted to ask the clinician if he or she wants the drug given with food. Perhaps you'll discover that a drug like the tetracyclines should not be given with dairy products, but you know that this cat's owner always gives it a small bowl of milk every day. Knowing that, you'll be able to appropriately counsel the owner about not feeding milk while the cat is receiving this medication.

TABLE 17-8   Time of Medication Administration Abbreviations

R$_x$ Abbreviation	Meaning
a.c., ac	Before meals [L. *ante cibum*]
ad lib.	As desired [L. *ad libitum*]
b.i.d., BID	Twice daily [L. *bis in die*]
c̄	With
h	Hour [L. *hora*]
hs	At bedtime [L. *hora somni*]
noct.	At night [L. *nocte*]
NPO	Nothing by mouth [L. *nil per os*]
p.c., pc	After meals [L. *post cibum*]
per	By
PRN	As needed [L. *pro re nata*]
q	Every [L. *quaqua*]
qAM	Every morning
qd	Every day [L. *quaqua die*], cf. s.i.d.
qh	Every hour [L. *quaqua hora*]
q2h	Every 2 hours
q4h, qqh	Every 4 hours [L. *quaqua quarta hora*]
q6h	Every 6 hours
q8h	Every 8 hours
q12h	Every 12 hours
q.i.d., QID	Four times daily [L. *quarta in die*]
q.o.d., QOD	Every other day
s.i.d., SID	Once daily [L. *semel in die*], cf. qd
s̄	Without
Sig., SIG:	Give [L. *signa*]
STAT	Immediately [L. *statim*]
t.i.d., TID	Three times daily [L. *ter in die*]

Some antibiotics, as well as other drugs, have the tendency to cause gastritis. For such agents, manufacturers have produced enteric-coated tablets. The enteric coating protects the stomach from the drug because the coating is only fully removed from the tablet once it is in the intestinal tract, hence the name, "enteric coated." The enteric coating controls the rate of absorption of the drug. To break or crush an enteric-coated tablet may dramatically alter the absorption of the drug. It could even result in acute overdose. Be certain that your clients understand this, if enteric-coated tablets are dispensed.

With regard to volumes of medication that can be administered per os, the only limiting features are the patient's stomach size and the correct dosage of the specific drug to be given. Realistically, the patient's stomach size is probably not going to be a limiting feature for most medication administration. In general, most per os medications are administered in manageable, diminutive doses. Per os administration is one of the easiest routes to use, particularly for most pet owners. Even if an owner cannot master "pilling" his or her pet, tablets and capsules can be easily hidden in tasty treats for the pets, provided that the food is not contraindicated. If food is contraindicated or if you have one of those

patients who manages to chew around the pill and spit it out every time, you'll need to poke it down. A rule of thumb that I've always advocated is: poke it down until you gag and it will probably be far enough to ensure your success.

Parenteral

Parenteral routes of medication administration include any of the injectable modalities. Each of the methods of injection is briefly discussed in the following sections. Which parenteral route is chosen depends on the patient, the drug, how rapidly the drug's activity is desired, and perhaps the veterinarian's personal preference. The dosage may vary, depending on the prescribed parenteral route. Even the speed of delivery may need to be controlled. The manufacturer will specify by which routes the medication may be given, as well as specifying any additional instructions (e.g., "give IV *slowly*"). Figure 17-1 shows the needle placement and angle for some of the more common parenteral routes of medication administration.

Subcutaneous

Subcutaneous injections can be administered nearly anywhere that enough loose skin can be found on the animal. This route is frequently used for administration of immunizations, antibiotics, and (in small animals) subcutaneous fluids. The uptake of drug from subcutaneous sites is slower than from intramuscular and intravenous sites because of the lesser blood supply in the subcutis. Depending on the drug given, the subcutaneous route does provide a faster uptake than that of per os. Most subcutaneous injections are less than 5 to 10 cc in volume. If subcutaneous fluids are to be administered to a dog or a cat, the size and conformation of the animal must be considered. In general, 20 to 50 mL is an acceptable range per site for subcutaneous fluids in dogs and cats. Large volumes of fluids are rarely, if ever, administered to large animals subcutaneously (SQ).

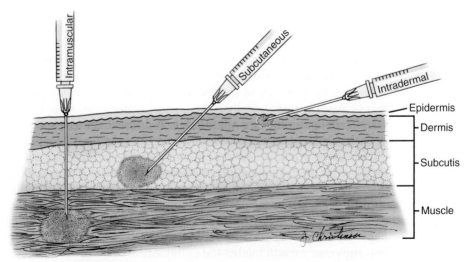

FIGURE 17-1 Common parenteral routes of administration.

Intramuscular

Intramuscular injections are administered into large muscle masses. Specific intramuscular injection sites are discussed in Chapter 6. The uptake of drug from intramuscular injection sites is far more rapid than from either the per os or subcutaneous routes. The excellent blood supply to skeletal muscle facilitates the rapid redistribution of the drug. There are greater volumetric limitations to intramuscular injections than in most of the other routes. Obviously, species, breed, size, and muscular condition of the animal play major roles in determining reasonable volumes that may be administered intramuscularly. Generally accepted per-site volume ranges for intramuscular injections are 3 to 6 mL in dogs and cats, and 10 to 20 mL in cattle and horses.

Intravenous

Intravenous administration of medications provides the fastest onset of any of the routes. Specific phlebotomy/intravenous injection sites are discussed in Chapter 7. For any agents for which a very rapid onset is indicated, or that will be potentially caustic to perivascular tissues, or that require large fluid volumes to be given concurrently, the intravenous route is the administration method of choice. Usually, only transparent, sterile solutions are acceptable for intravenous administration. As mentioned earlier, there are few exceptions to this rule. With the exceptions of total parenteral nutrition and propofol (an anesthetic agent), unless the solution is transparent (i.e., no suspended particles), intravenous administration is contraindicated. The intravenous route is the modality of choice for fluid therapy. Volumes of fluids for both deficit replacement and hydration maintenance are based on the body weight of the individual patient. Any parenteral injection requires adherence to aseptic protocols, but because of the direct entry into the bloodstream, asepsis is very critical for intravenous injections.

Intraosseous

Intraosseous fluid administration is being used more and more frequently in emergency and critical care medicine. Certainly for hypovolemic patients in whom we cannot successfully enter a vein for fluid administration, the intraosseous route gives us a viable option to improve the circulating blood volume. Most often the intramedullary cavity of a long bone, like the femur or humerus, is chosen for delivery of the fluids. It is more painful than an IV catheter placement? Yes. Does that really matter when it becomes a life or death decision to use an intraosseous site? No. What's a little discomfort compared with death?

Intratracheal

While we're on the subject of emergency medicine, we have to point out the value of the intratracheal (IT) route for emergency drugs. We're not talking about large volumes being administered via this route. Ah, but we are talking about very rapid absorption from this route that is comparable with giving an IV injection. Let's say that a dog goes into cardiac arrest and we don't have an IV catheter in yet. How can we administer the epinephrine to the dog to give us rapid absorption and not traumatize the dog? The IT route. We will likely need to increase

the small volume of the drug with sterile water or saline, to carry it down to the lower airways. For a patient in cardiac arrest we want rapid delivery of drug to the heart, right? Well, the intratracheal route gives us rapid absorption from the lungs with one short "hop" to the heart. (You'll want to read Chapters 7 and 8, to fully appreciate the anatomy and physiology behind this emergency route.) The only way to get it to the heart faster is to inject it directly into the heart.

Intracardiac
While we're discussing cardiac arrest, we might as well talk about giving emergency drugs directly into the heart. Yes, it can be and is done. It is typically left to a last resort. For emergency drugs, our first choice is usually IV. If we don't have an IV catheter, our second choice is often IT. If the intratracheal administration does not give life-saving results, then we may give it by the intracardiac (IC) route. Why is it the last resort? Think about it. How risky do you suppose it is to be poking needles into the heart? How "angry" do you suppose the heart muscle is going to be from being poked? That, in and of itself, could cause abnormal heart rhythms. That's why we save IC injections for last.

Intradermal
Intradermal (ID) injections are used predominantly in veterinary medicine for allergy skin testing and tuberculosis testing. The latter is routinely performed in cattle and primates. The ID site most commonly used for tuberculosis testing in cattle is the tail fold. In primates, the eyelid is used. Because of the minute tissue thickness of the dermis, volumes that may be injected are significantly restricted. In general, volumes less than 0.3 mL are acceptable for ID injection sites. Obviously, given the limited blood supply found in the dermis, uptake of agents injected intradermally is negligible. Most activity remains localized at the injection site. So, any reaction to the antigen or allergen injected there will remain localized to the injection site.

Transdermal
Transdermal administration is limited in veterinary medicine, compared with human medicine. One of the limiting characteristics of domestic animals is their fur. Does that prohibit the transdermal route in animals? Absolutely not. All we need to do is carefully clip the fur from the area intended for the application. Notice that I said we need to *carefully* clip the fur. If we scratch, scrape, or abrade the skin while clipping, those traumatic marks will likely increase the rate of absorption of the drug. Probably the most frequently used transdermal medications are narcotic analgesic patches, like fentanyl. Fentanyl is an extremely potent narcotic that we don't want rapidly absorbed in large doses. That's why fentanyl transdermal patches should *never* be cut (e.g., cutting a 25-mcg patch in half, thinking that you'll create a 12.5-mcg patch. The rapid absorption from the cut edge could kill an animal.). The absorption needs to occur at a reasonable, safe rate. In fact, in most dogs it may take 12 hours before therapeutic levels of analgesia are achieved. Once there, the prolonged absorption from the transdermal patch will provide the animal with analgesia for approximately 3 days. Obviously, there is a wide range of differences in transdermal absorption from animal to animal. Plus, there is really

no control over the absorption. That's why transdermal analgesics are usually supplemented with other analgesics in other forms and via other routes.

Intraperitoneal

Intraperitoneal injections are used most frequently in small laboratory animals, such as mice. Uptake of medications by this route is comparable with that of intramuscular injections. Occasionally, intraperitoneal fluids are administered to large animals, such as sheep and goats. In dogs and cats, intraperitoneal dialysis may be performed in patients with renal failure. Finally, when trying to carefully warm a severely hypothermic patient, intraperitoneal lavage may be used. Intraperitoneal lavage warms the core organs first to maintain adequate blood flow to them. If severely hypothermic patients are warmed too rapidly from the periphery, peripheral vessels may dilate, causing a critical loss of blood pressure.

Intranasal

The most common use of the intranasal route of administration is for certain vaccines. The active components of these vaccines are most often infectious respiratory organisms. These vaccines may be killed or modified-live (attenuated).

Topical

Anything that is applied to the surface of the skin, eyes, or ears is considered a topical agent. Most ophthalmic and otic preparations are sterile. Therefore, care must be taken to avoid contamination of the applicator tip when the drug is administered. Ophthalmic and otic solutions are generally prescribed to be given by the drop. Ophthalmic solutions should always be applied before ophthalmic ointments. Dermatologic agents come in a variety of forms. For those that cannot or should not be applied directly from the original container, gloves or another suitable device should be used to apply the drug. This protects the patient's wounds from contamination by human skin; it also protects the person applying the medication from absorbing the agent. The issue of personnel safety is very important when topical pesticides[3] are being applied to patients.

PHARMACOKINETICS

What is it? Well, pharmacokinetics looks at how drugs move into, through, and out of the body. We've already addressed part of that story by looking at various routes of administration. How slowly or quickly a drug is absorbed into the system is important. What influences the rate of absorption? Well, blood flow to the area is one thing. That alone does not completely dictate the rate of absorption. Take a drug that's administered subcutaneously. If the drug given SQ is hydrophilic, it will probably diffuse fairly rapidly through the extracellular fluid. Why? Extracellular fluids are aqueous. A lipophilic drug injected SQ may take longer to simply reach the capillaries, because oil and water don't mix. In contrast, think about a

---

[3]Pesticide (pes'tǐ-sīd); to kill pests; any of a number of chemical poisons used to destroy various pests, including insects, arachnids, and fungi.

lipophilic drug being administered PO. Once the medication has dissolved in the digestive tract, it will fairly readily diffuse across cellular membranes. Why? Most cellular membranes have a phospholipid structure, making passive diffusion of a lipophilic drug relatively easy. A hydrophilic drug in the digestive tract will probably need an active transport mechanism to get through those cellular barriers.

Okay, so we want to get medications (regardless of the route of administration) into the bloodstream for distribution. Can the circulation from the site of administration impact the distribution of the drug? You bet it can. Now, many drugs undergo biotransformation in the liver (e.g., metabolized by the liver). Let's say that we have a drug that is rapidly biotransformed by the liver. Would it make sense to give that drug PO? No. Circulation from the digestive tract goes immediately to the liver. If the liver is very efficient, we may never achieve therapeutic concentrations of the drug. Perhaps a parenteral route will provide distribution of the drug to the needed tissues, by temporarily taking the liver out of the loop. Of course, once it is freely circulating in the bloodstream, the drug will eventually reach the liver and systemic concentrations will be reduced. Most medications, once in circulation, will be distributed to well-perfused tissues and organs (including the liver and kidneys). The liver and kidneys are excellent points for the drugs and their metabolites to exit the system through excretion. Unfortunately, being a "clearinghouse" for drugs also makes the liver and kidneys targets for toxicity. It's one thing to have a localized cytotoxic reaction to an injected medication. It's quite another to be hepatotoxic or nephrotoxic. That's why you'll commonly find contraindications for certain medications in patients with liver or kidney disease. If the drug has a high probability of damaging those organs (like some antimycotic agents), giving it to patients with existing pathology of the liver or kidneys will only make the pathology worse.

PHARMACODYNAMICS

Pharmacodynamics is just a very big word for looking at the actions of drugs on the body (i.e., the "power" that they exert over the body). How a drug exerts its power over specific tissues or organs depends on the drug's compatibility with cellular receptors. You might think of these receptors as on and off switches that control very specific functions. Specific pharmacodynamic effects result from the drug flipping particular switches. The pharmaceutical industry has done a fabulous job of researching and finding very specific receptors that control very specific activities within the body. Then they have formulated drugs to fit those specific receptors to achieve a desired effect. It's sort of like Cinderella[4] and the glass slipper. It has to be a perfect fit or it won't work.

Let's look at opioid[5] analgesics for a moment, to demonstrate this receptor idea. Of course, the whole purpose behind narcotic agonists is to relieve pain. They do this by binding at specific cellular receptors in the central nervous

---

[4]Cinderella: a popular fairy tale written by French author, Charles Perrault, in 1697.
[5]Opioid (o'pe-oid); synthetic narcotics that have similar actions to that of opium but are not derived from opium.

system along pain pathways. That's fantastic, and as expected, when an analgesic is given we expect the patient to experience relief of pain. Unfortunately, when these powerful agonists are given systemically, they may be so powerful in their effects that they critically depress vital functions, like cardiac and respiratory functions. (Think about it, the analgesics are depressing neuronal activity in the brain. Depress brain function and those things that it controls will also be depressed.) The beauty of narcotic agonists is, when adverse actions become significant, a narcotic antagonist may be administered. How does that work? It's sort of like a competitive game show. Let's envision a game show in which two participants must compete to sit in a single chair. Let's look at our competitors. Competitor number one (our agonist) is about 5 feet tall, very fit, but weighs only about a 100 pounds dripping wet. Competitor number two (our antagonist) is about 6 feet tall, muscular, and weighs about 200 pounds. They both fit in the chair. As they race to the chair, the antagonist will likely beat the agonist there because of his stride and muscular strength. Even if the agonist is quick and sits down first, the antagonist could easily push him off the chair and sit down. Once our antagonist is sitting there, he's not going to budge and our agonist can't do a thing about it. Okay, that's a silly game show. What about the body? Well, a narcotic antagonist will sit on those receptors and not allow the agonist to exert its effects. This will for all practical purposes reverse the effects of the agonist (remember the cardiopulmonary depression we were talking about?). With regard to the adverse effects that the agonist was creating, that's a very good thing. Ah, but I'll bet you're concerned about the analgesia that we're no longer providing. Well, there are many other narcotic and nonnarcotic analgesics available. Perhaps another analgesic or combination of analgesics will provide the necessary pain relief, without compromising the patient's vital functions. Perhaps we can use an agonist-antagonist that will provide reversal of the original agent while providing its own analgesic effects. Perhaps we can provide analgesia through a different route, like epidural[6] analgesia, avoiding the systemic complications altogether. Never fear. One way or another, we will be able to provide the needed analgesia.

While we're on the subject, let's look at the pharmacodynamics of local anesthetic agents like lidocaine. If you have ever experienced the intradermal and subcutaneous infusion of a local anesthetic agent, you know how quickly they desensitize the area. Did you ever wonder how they do it? If you remember from Chapter 9, neurotransmission depends in part on sodium and potassium diffusion. Lidocaine binds at receptors that block the sodium channels. No sodium can diffuse. Therefore, no neurotransmission can occur for any painful sensations to be transmitted. Of course, based on what we know about pharmacokinetics, blood flow to the infused skin will rapidly remove the lidocaine from the area. So, for lidocaine alone to be used for local anesthesia, it had better be a very quick procedure (perhaps 20 minutes or less). Gee, if it's the blood flow

---

[6]Epidural (ep″ĭ-doo′ral); pertaining to upon the dura mater; epidural analgesia is achieved by injecting the agent into the vertebral canal and infusing it over the dura mater. This effectively blocks pain impulses from reaching the brain.

to the area that's removing the lidocaine too quickly, can't we do something to alter the blood flow locally? We sure can. That's why lidocaine with epinephrine is used so often for local anesthesia. The epinephrine targets alpha-adrenergic receptors on the vessels in the area causing vasoconstriction. This limits the blood flow to the area, prolonging the desired effects of the lidocaine. How cool is that? (Refer to Chapters 9 and 15 to learn more about epinephrine.)

Understanding pharmacodynamics is important to know the intended effects of the drug. As veterinary professionals, our understanding must go beyond the indications or purpose of various drugs. To simply know that an antitussive will relieve a cough or that an antiemetic will stop the vomiting episodes is not enough. We need to understand how the drugs create those effects. Why? Take anthelmintics and pesticides, for instance. You wouldn't believe the amount of research behind those agents, to pinpoint very specific receptors. Many of these agents target neurologic receptors to kill the worms or other pests via paralysis. Who cares how the parasites die, as long as they die, right? Not so fast. You see, animals and people may have similar neurologic receptors. Under the right conditions, perhaps in high enough doses, those agents could create the same effects in the animal being treated or in the people administering them (depending on the route). So, it is of value to understand the pharmacodynamics of a drug, to know the kinds of adverse reactions that might occur. Bottom line—always look up drugs that you are unfamiliar with, before administering them. Acting on that knowledge may save a patient's life.

ANTIMICROBIALS

Wow. This area of pharmacology is HUGE. Do you realize that the pharmaceutical industry has developed most of the antimicrobials used today since World War II? Before that time, microbes and the diseases that they caused were poorly understood. Certainly, controlling diseases caused by these microscopic creatures was symptomatic at best, because there was no means to eradicate the organisms. Through years of research the pharmaceutical industry developed numerous antibiotics, antimycotics, and even some antiviral drugs. Today, we have a better understanding of the importance of asepsis (particularly in surgery). We understand the importance of using antiseptics to directly treat open wounds or to prepare the skin before surgery. Even the disinfectants[7] that we use throughout our facilities to prevent nosocomial[8] transmission to our patients have been developed through the labors of the pharmaceutical industry. Do we need to know how they work? Of course we do! Plus, we need to know something about the pathogens themselves. Why? Well, let's see, if a virus has a

---

[7]Disinfectant (dis″in-fekt′tant); an agent used to disinfect (make free of pathogenic organisms) inanimate objects. Both disinfectants and antiseptics are antimicrobials, but antiseptics are used on living tissue.

[8]Nosocomial (nos″o-ko′me-al); pertaining to disease caretaking; nosocomial diseases are those that originate from the medical facility, usually from pathogens contaminating the facility [Gr. *nosos*, disease + Gr. *komeion*, to take care of].

lipid envelope, do we want to use a hydrophilic disinfectant or a lipophilic disinfectant to clean the contaminated cage? Which agent is more likely to give us the virucidal effects that we desire? Well, the lipophilic agent of course. By the way, please read and follow the manufacturer's instructions for mixing antiseptics and disinfectants. Remember, years of research have gone into developing these chemicals and determining which concentrations will be most effective against certain pathogens. More is not necessarily better. Some agents, like iodophors,[9] have virtually no antimicrobial activity until they are appropriately diluted. That's because iodophor solutions have stabilizing agents bound to the iodine to extend the life of the product in storage. It's free iodine that provides the antimicrobial activity. So, iodophors must be diluted. The other factor to be considered, when diluting antiseptics like iodophors, is where will this be used? Stronger concentrations can safely and effectively be used on intact skin, for surgical preparation for instance. Those same concentrations used in an open wound will likely be cytotoxic and prolong the healing of that wound. Which concentration is going to provide bacteriostatic effects versus antimycotic effects? Is there a concentration that will give very good broad-spectrum antimicrobial activity? We won't know unless we read the label. Another thing to pay close attention to is contact time. Great that you've mixed the perfect concentration of the agent, but if you don't leave it in contact long enough you won't do anything except "slap the microbes' little wrists." Can you say "superbug"? That's precisely how we've created so many antibiotic-resistant bacteria. Often, people do not follow through with the full duration of antibiotic therapy. Once they or their pet begin to feel better, they stop the antibiotic therapy. What have they done? If this was a bactericidal drug, they have successfully killed off the weaker bacteria. Those that are stronger are left to survive. Not only have they survived, but they have gained valuable insight into how that antibiotic worked. Now they may adapt to protect themselves if they are exposed to the same antibiotic in the future. The next time those bacteria may simply "thumb their noses and laugh" at the antibiotic. That's how resistant bacteria develop, either they are treated with same antibiotic over and over again (allowing for familiarity for adaptation), or they are treated with insufficient concentrations of the antibiotic, or they are simply not treated long enough. Strains of bacteria that are resistant to multiple drugs are very dangerous. The dangers of these microbes reach far beyond veterinary patients. They may affect animals and people globally. As veterinary professionals, we not only care for animals but also must protect public health. We need to take care, regardless of the type of antimicrobial being used, that it is used appropriately as the manufacturer designed it to work. Failure to do our part here may not only jeopardize our patients, but humanity as well. That's a big responsibility that should not be taken lightly.

---

[9]Iodophor (i-o'-do-for); antiseptic and disinfectant compounds of iodine with various carriers.

PRESCRIPTION WRITING AND TRANSCRIBING

Until now, we have been talking about various pharmaceuticals, how they can be given and how they work. What we haven't discussed is the specialized language of pharmacology with regard to prescriptions. For our medical records and communication with pharmacists, we need a very succinct and precise language. That's why we have all of those mind-boggling abbreviations. It's sort of like shorthand for pharmacology. Once you have absorbed the prescription abbreviations contained in this chapter's tables, transcription to and from layman's terms should be easy. We'll talk about transcription a little later. Let's look at those "foreign" prescriptions first. Prescriptions are written in a fairly standardized format. Each written prescription begins with the superscription or heading symbol "R_x." What follows this "recipe" symbol is information regarding the specific drug to be given. This information should include the name of the drug, its concentration, its form, its quantity, and any relevant compounding instructions. The signature (represented by the symbol "S." or "Sig.," meaning "mark" or "give") contains specific instructions for patient dosing that should be included on the container for the owner or that should be followed by the personnel administering the drug to a hospitalized patient. Of course, it goes without saying that pertinent patient information, the date, and veterinarian's name and signature should also be included on the written prescription. If the veterinarian issued the prescription verbally or by telephone, the notation "VO" (verbal order) or "TO" (telephone order) should accompany the order in the patient's medical record. The date, time, and initials of the person entering this prescription in the patient's medical record should also accompany the entry. If the person entering the information is not the veterinarian, then "per Dr. ..." should also be written with the entry. Figure 17-2 provides an example of a written prescription.

Think of how overwhelmed you probably feel right now, learning all of these pharmaceutical abbreviations. There is no way that we could possibly expect a pet owner to read and understand the abbreviated instructions of a prescription. Like any foreign language, it needs to be translated for those who do not speak the language. So, the prescription information must be transcribed into a form understood by the average person. All of the information found in the written prescription must be included on the dispensing label. In addition, the initials of the person filling the prescription, as well as the drug's expiration date, should be included on the dispensing label. Figure 17-3 is representative of the label that should be placed on the bottle to be sold to the owner of the preceding patient. Finally, to ensure owner compliance, when dispensing a medication we need to be sure to verbally explain the label instructions to avoid any misinterpretations. For some medications, we may actually have to physically show the owner how to administer the medication. (Explain, demonstrate, and, if necessary, have the owner explain and show you that he or she can do it.) This is very true for things like ophthalmic medications. If multiple medications are being dispensed, we also need to be clear about any order or time delays between their administrations. For instance, with ophthalmic medications, if a solution and an ointment have been dispensed for b.i.d. application, it should be explained that the solution is to be applied first. (Oil and water don't mix. Ointments typically have a petroleum base. So, any solution applied after an ointment will simply run off and never reach the eye.) It is usually recommended that there be a 5-minute delay between applications of multiple ophthalmic agents. This is to permit optimal contact and absorption of each agent. Adequate communication, both written and verbal, is often the key to owner compliance. Never assume anything, particularly that an owner will ask if he or she doesn't understand. Think about yourself as a student. Do you always ask every question that comes to mind in the classroom? Probably not. Why not? Most of the time it's probably because you think your question will make you look stupid, right? Remember that when dealing with clients, they're human too. Always remember too, it's all about the patient—the patient comes first. You need to do whatever it takes to ensure that the patient receives the optimal care, whether in the hospital or at home.

Veterinary Medical Center, P.C.
3000 S. Fork Road
Anytown, MI 01234
(012) 345-6789
J. A. Smith, DVM

Patient: *"Sadie" Christenson*   I.D. # *642351*

R$_x$: *Prednisolone, 5 mg tabs, #30*

Sig: *1 tab PO bid pc × 5d, then 1 tab PO qd pc × 5d, then 1 tab PO qod pc until gone*

0   Refills

Dr. *J.A. Smith*   Date: *7-25-08*

FIGURE 17-2   Prescription example.

Veterinary Medical Center
3000 S. Fork Rd., Anytown, MI 01234
(012) 345-6789
Dr. J. A. Smith   Date: 07-25-08
Patient: Sadie Christenson #642351
R$_x$: Give 1 tablet orally twice daily after meals for 5 days, then give 1 tablet orally once daily after a meal for 5 days, then give 1 tablet orally every other day after a meal until gone.
30 Prednisolone 5 mg tablets   0 Refills
Expiration date: 7-25-08   dec

FIGURE 17-3   Prescription label.

SELF-TEST

Using the previous information in this chapter, complete the following crossword puzzle using the most appropriate medical term(s). Do not use abbreviations unless requested.

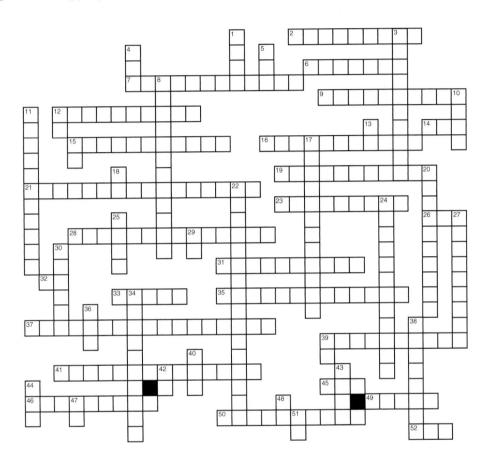

ACROSS

2	An agent that kills viruses
6	For each hundred
7	The study of drugs
9	A disease that results from the actions of a medical professional
12	An agent used to suppress vomiting
14	Pharmaceutical abbreviation for "twice daily"
15	An injection into the skin
16	An agent used to destroy fungus
19	An agent, like an NSAID, used to reduce fever
21	The movement of drugs into, through, and out of the body
23	An agent used to relieve pain
26	Pharmaceutical abbreviation for "three times daily"

28	An agent that inhibits bacterial growth
31	Any route of medication administration that does not use the digestive tract
32	Pharmaceutical abbreviation for "intraperitoneal"
33	Prefix meaning "within"
35	An injection into muscle
37	Metabolism of a drug
39	One thousandth of a liter
41	A state of liver poisoning
45	Pharmaceutical abbreviation for "ointment"
46	Pertaining to cellular poison
49	Prefix meaning "small" or "one millionth"
50	A state without sensation
52	Pharmaceutical abbreviation for "milliequivalent"

DOWN

1	Combining form for "fat"
3	A reversal agent
4	Pharmaceutical abbreviation for "teaspoon"
5	Pharmaceutical abbreviation for "nothing by mouth"
8	A "dewormer"
10	Combining form meaning "to kill"
11	A type of agent that easily diffuses into aqueous fluids
12	Pharmaceutical abbreviation for "left ear"
13	Pharmaceutical abbreviation for "by mouth"
15	Pharmaceutical abbreviation for "intravenous"
17	A route of administration using the medullary cavity of a bone
18	Pharmaceutical abbreviation for "after meals"
20	One hundredth of a meter
22	A reason making it inadvisable to give a medication
24	An injection into the heart
25	Pharmaceutical abbreviation for "immediately"
27	One tenth of a liter
29	Pharmaceutical abbreviation for "subcutaneous"
30	Combining form for "kidney"
34	A disease contracted from a medical facility
36	Pharmaceutical abbreviation for "as needed"
38	One thousand grams
39	Pharmaceutical abbreviation for "milligram"
40	Pharmaceutical abbreviation for "four times daily"
42	Pharmaceutical abbreviation for "both eyes"
43	Prefix meaning "against"
44	Pharmaceutical abbreviation for "microgram"
47	Pharmaceutical abbreviation for "right eye"
48	Pharmaceutical abbreviation for "intratracheal"
51	Pharmaceutical abbreviation meaning "at bedtime"

Chemical Symbol–Element Cross Reference

Atomic No.	Symbol	Name	Atomic No.	Symbol	Name	Atomic No.	Symbol	Name
1	H	hydrogen	38	Sr	strontium	75	Re	rhenium
2	He	helium	39	Y	yttrium	76	Os	osmium
3	Li	lithium	40	Zr	zirconium	77	Ir	iridium
4	Be	beryllium	41	Nb	niobium	78	Pt	platinum
5	B	boron	42	Mo	molybdenum	79	Au	gold
6	C	carbon	43	Tc	technetium	80	Hg	mercury
7	N	nitrogen	44	Ru	ruthenium	81	Tl	thallium
8	O	oxygen	45	Rh	rhodium	82	Pb	lead
9	F	fluorine	46	Pd	palladium	83	Bi	bismuth
10	Ne	neon	47	Ag	silver	84	Po	polonium
11	Na	sodium	48	Cd	cadmium	85	At	astatine
12	Mg	magnesium	49	In	indium	86	Rn	radon
13	Al	aluminum	50	Sn	tin	87	Fr	francium
14	Si	silicon	51	Sb	antimony	88	Ra	radium
15	P	phosphorus	52	Te	tellurium	89	Ac	actinium
16	S	sulfur	53	I	iodine	90	Th	thorium
17	Cl	chlorine	54	Xe	xenon	91	Pa	protactinium
18	Ar	argon	55	Cs	cesium	92	U	uranium
19	K	potassium	56	Ba	barium	93	Np	neptunium
20	Ca	calcium	57	La	lanthanum	94	Pu	plutonium
21	Sc	scandium	58	Ce	cerium	95	Am	americium
22	Ti	titanium	59	Pr	praseodymium	96	Cm	curium
23	V	vanadium	60	Nd	neodymium	97	Bk	berkelium
24	Cr	chromium	61	Pm	promethium	98	Cf	californium
25	Mn	manganese	62	Sm	samarium	99	Es	einsteinium
26	Fe	iron	63	Eu	europium	100	Fm	fermium
27	Co	cobalt	64	Gd	gadolinium	101	Md	mendelevium
28	Ni	nickel	65	Tb	terbium	102	No	nobelium
29	Cu	copper	66	Dy	dysprosium	103	Lr	lawrencium
30	Zn	zinc	67	Ho	holmium	104	Rf	rutherfordium
31	Ga	gallium	68	Er	erbium	105	Ha	hahnium
32	Ge	germanium	69	Tm	thulium	106	Sg	seaborgium
33	As	arsenic	70	Yb	ytterbium	107	Bh	bohrium
34	Se	selenium	71	Lu	lutetium	108	Hs	hassium
35	Br	bromine	72	Hf	hafnium	109	Mt	meitnerium
36	Kr	krypton	73	Ta	tantalum			
37	Rb	rubidium	74	W	tungsten			

Common Veterinary Medical Abbreviations

Abbreviation	Meaning
ac	before meals
ACE	angiotensin-converting enzyme
ACTH	adrenocorticotropic hormone
AD	right ear
ad lib	as desired
ADH	antidiuretic hormone
AI	artificial insemination
ALT	alanine transaminase
ANS	autonomic nervous system
AP	anteroposterior
APTT	activated partial thromboplastin time
AS	left ear
AST	aspartate transaminase
ATP	adenosine triphosphate
AU	both ears
AV	atrioventricular
BAL	bronchoalveolar lavage
BAR	bright alert and responsive
BCS	body condition score
BCV	bovine coronavirus
BHV	bovine herpes virus
BID	twice daily
BMR	basal metabolic rate
BRSV	bovine respiratory syncytial virus
BSE	bovine spongiform encephalopathy
BUN	blood urea nitrogen
BVD	bovine viral diarrhea
cap	capsule
CAT	computed axial tomography
CAV-1	canine adenovirus type 1 (hepatitis virus)
CAV-2	canine adenovirus type 2
CBC	complete blood count
cc	cubic centimeter
CCV	canine coronavirus
CdCr	caudocranial
CHF	congestive heart failure
cm	centimeter
CMT	California mastitis test
CNS	central nervous system
CO	carbon monoxide

Abbreviation	Meaning
COPD	chronic obstructive pulmonary disease
COX	cyclooxygenase
CP	conscious proprioception
CPR	cardiopulmonary resuscitation
CPV	canine parvovirus
CrCd	craniocaudal
CRT	capillary refill time
CSF	cerebrospinal fluid
CT	computed tomography
CVP	central venous pressure
CWD	chronic wasting disease
DA	displaced abomasum
DIC	disseminated intravascular coagulopathy
DJD	degenerative joint disease
DLH	domestic long hair
DNA	deoxyribonucleic acid
dr	dram
DSH	domestic short hair
DTM	dermatophyte test medium
DV	dorsoventral
ECG	electrocardiogram
EDTA	ethylenediaminetetraacetic acid
EEE	eastern equine encephalomyelitis
EEG	electroencephalogram
EHV	equine herpes virus
EIA	equine infectious anemia
ELISA	enzyme-linked immunosorbent assay
EMG	electromyogram
EPI	exocrine pancreatic insufficiency
EPM	equine protozoal encephalomyelitis
ERG	electroretinogram
EVA	equine viral arteritis
FAD	flea allergy dermatitis
FCV	feline calicivirus
FeLV	feline leukemia virus
FIP	feline infectious peritonitis
FIV	feline immunodeficiency virus
fL	femtoliter
FLUTD	feline lower urinary tract disease
FSH	follicle-stimulating hormone

Abbreviation	Meaning
FVR	feline viral rhinotracheitis
g	gram
GABA	gamma-aminobutyric acid
gal	gallon
GDV	gastric dilatation volvulus
GGT	gamma-glutamyltransferase
GH	growth hormone
GI	gastrointestinal
GOT	glutamic-oxaloacetic transaminase
GPT	glutamic-pyruvic transaminase
gr	grain
gtt	drops
HGE	hemorrhagic gastroenteritis
HBC	hit by car
HCl	hydrochloric acid
HCM	hypertrophic cardiomyopathy
hs	at bedtime
IBS	irritable bowel syndrome
IBR	infectious bovine rhinotracheitis
IC	intracardiac
ID	intradermal
IFA	immunofluorescence assay
IGR	insect growth regulator
IM	intramuscular
IO	intraosseous
IOP	intraocular pressure
IP	intraperitoneal
IT	intratracheal
IU	international unit
IV	intravenous
IVDD	intervertebral disc disease
IVP	intravenous pyelogram
KCS	keratoconjunctivitis sicca
kg	kilogram
kV	kilovolt
kVp	kilovolts peak
L	liter
LAR-PAR	laryngeal paralysis
LDA	left displaced abomasum
LH	luteinizing hormone
LM	lateromedial
LMO	lateromedial oblique
LUTD	lower urinary tract disease
mA	milliampere
MAC	mean alveolar concentration
MAO	monoamine oxidase
mAs	milliampere seconds
mcg	microgram
mEq	milliequivalent
mg	milligram
ML	mediolateral
mL	milliliter
MLO	mediolateral oblique
mm	millimeter
MRI	magnetic resonance imaging
MRSA	methicillin-resistant *Staphylococcus aureus*
MSDS	material safety data sheet
NG	nasogastric
NPO	nothing by mouth
NRBC	nucleated red blood cell
OCD	osteochondritis dissecans
OD	right eye
OG	orogastric
OHE	ovariohysterectomy

Abbreviation	Meaning
OS	left eye
OU	both eyes
oz	ounce
PA	posteroanterior
pc	after meals
pCO_2	partial pressure carbon dioxide
PCR	polymerase chain reaction
PCV	packed cell volume
PDA	patent ductus arteriosis
pg	picogram
PHF	Potomac horse fever
PI-3	parainfluenza virus type 3
PLR	pupillary light reflex
PNS	peripheral nervous system
PO	by mouth
pO_2	partial pressure oxygen
PRN	as needed
pt	pint
PTH	parathyroid hormone
PTT	partial thromboplastin time
PU/PD	polyuria/polydipsia
q12h	every 12 hours
q4h	every 4 hours
q6h	every 6 hours
q8h	every 8 hours
qd	once daily
qh	every hour
QID	four times daily
QOD	every other day
qt	quart
RBC	red blood cell
RDA	right displaced abomasum
RNA	ribonucleic acid
SID	once daily
SIV	swine influenza virus
SOAP	subjective, objective, assessment, plan
STAT	immediately
syr	syrup
T3	triiodothyronine
T4	thyroxine
tab	tablet
tbsp	tablespoon
TGE	transmissible gastroenteritis
TID	three times daily
TP	total protein
TPR	temperature, pulse, respiration
TS	total solids
TSH	thyroid stimulating hormone
tsp	teaspoon
U	unit
UA	urinalysis
ung	ointment
URI	upper respiratory infection
UTI	urinary tract infection
VD	ventrodorsal
VEE	Venezuelan equine encephalomyelitis
VPC	ventricular premature complex
VSD	ventricular septal defect
vWF	von Willebrand factor
WBC	white blood cell
WEE	western equine encephalomyelitis
WNV	West Nile virus

Index

Page numbers followed by *f* indicate figures; *t,* tables; *b,* boxes.